BSAVA Manual of Advanced Veterinary Nursing

D1586816

Editor:

Alasdair Hotston Moore MA VetMB CertSAC CertVR MRCVS

Lecturer in Small Animal Soft Tissue Surgery,
Division of Companion Animals,
Department of Clinical Veterinary Science,
University of Bristol, Langford House,
Langford, Bristol BS40 5DU

Series Editor for BSAVA Manuals of Veterinary Nursing

Gill Simpson BVM&S MRCVS

Rose Cottage, Edgehead,
Midlothian EH37 5RL

Published by:
British Small Animal Veterinary Association
Woodrow House, 1 Telford Way, Waterwells Business Park,
Quedgeley, Gloucester GL2 4AB, United Kingdom

A company limited by guarantee in England.
Registered company no. 2837793.
Registered as a charity.

A catalogue recorded for this book is available from the British Library.

ISBN 0 905412 51 X

The publishers and contributors cannot take responsibility for information
provided on dosages and methods of application of drugs mentioned in
this publication. Details of this kind must be verified by individual users
from the appropriate literature.

It must be remembered that the veterinary nurse must at all times work
within the guidelines of the Veterinary Surgeons Act.

Typeset by: Fusion Design, Fordingbridge, Hampshire.

Printed by: Lookers, Upton, Poole, Dorset.

Other titles in the BSAVA Manuals of Veterinary Nursing series:

Manual of Veterinary Care
Edited by Sue Dallas

Manual of Veterinary Nursing
Edited by Margaret Moore

Other BSAVA manuals:

Manual of Canine and Feline Emergency and Critical Care
Manual of Canine and Feline Gastroenterology
Manual of Canine and Feline Nephrology and Urology
Manual of Canine and Feline Wound Management and Reconstruction
Manual of Companion Animal Nutrition and Feeding
Manual of Canine Behaviour
Manual of Exotic Pets
Manual of Feline Behaviour
Manual of Ornamental Fish
Manual of Psittacine Birds
Manual of Raptors, Pigeons and Waterfowl
Manual of Reptiles
Manual of Small Animal Anaesthesia and Analgesia
Manual of Small Animal Arthrology
Manual of Small Animal Clinical Pathology
Manual of Small Animal Dentistry, 2nd edition
Manual of Small Animal Dermatology
Manual of Small Animal Diagnostic Imaging
Manual of Small Animal Endocrinology, 2nd edition
Manual of Small Animal Fracture Repair and Management
Manual of Small Animal Neurology, 2nd edition
Manual of Small Animal Oncology
Manual of Small Animal Ophthalmology
Manual of Small Animal Reproduction and Neonatology

Contents

Contributors

Wendy Adams BVSc MRCVS
University of Liverpool Small Animal Hospital, Crown Street, Liverpool L7 7EX

David J. Argyle BVMS PhD
Department of Veterinary Clinical Studies, University of Glasgow Veterinary School, Bearsden Road, Bearsden, Glasgow G61 1QH

Carole J. Clarke MA VetMB MRCVS
Mill House Veterinary Surgery, 20 Tennyson Avenue, King's Lynn, Norfolk PE30 2QG

Cathy Garden VN DipAVN(Surgical)
Novartis Animal Health UK Ltd, Whittlesford, Cambridge CB2 4XW

Tim Greet BVMS MVM CertEO DESTS MRCVS
Beaufort Cottage Stables, High Street, Newmarket, Suffolk CB8 8JS

Alasdair Hotston Moore MA VetMB CertSAC CertVR MRCVS
Division of Companion Animals, Department of Clinical Veterinary Science, University of Bristol, Langford House, Langford, Bristol BS40 5DU

Clare M. Knottenbelt BVSc MSc DSAM MRCVS
Flat 2F4, 7 Albert Street, Leith, Edinburgh EH7 5HL

Anna Meredith MA VetMB Cert LAS Cert Zoo Med MRCVS
Department of Veterinary Clinical Studies, RDSVS, Hospital for Small Animals, Easter Bush Veterinary Centre, Roslin, Midlothian EH25 9RG

Jacqueline Niles BVetMed MRCVS
The Ohio State University Veterinary Hospital, 601 Vernon L Tharp Street, Columbus, OH 43210-1089, USA

Kostas Papasouliotis DVM PhD
Department of Clinical Veterinary Science, University of Bristol, Langford House, Langford, Bristol BS40 5DU

Sharon Redrobe BSc BVetMed CertLAS MRCVS
Zoo Veterinary Officer, Bristol Zoo Gardens, Clifton, Bristol BS8 3HA

James W. Simpson BVM&S SDA MPhil MRCVS RCVS Specialist Inernal Medicine
Department of Veterinary Clinical Studies, RDSVS, Hospital for Small Animals, Easter Bush Veterinary Centre, Roslin, Midlothian EH25 9RG

Deborah J. Smith BVSc DVR CertSAS MRCVS
PDSA, 1 Shamrock St, Glasgow G4 9JZ

Garry Stanway BVSc CertVA MRCVS
Hird & Partners, 10 Blackwell, Halifax HX1 2BE

Foreword

This trilogy of veterinary nursing manuals marks another significant landmark in the history of BSAVA Publications. The rise in status of the veterinary nurse within companion animal practice together with the new syllabus under the S/NVQ training scheme has meant that, after three editions spanning 15 years, *Practical Veterinary Nursing* has reached the end of its useful life. However, it was felt that there still was a need for a publication to complement the established textbook *Veterinary Nursing* (formerly Jones's Animal Nursing) published by Butterworth Heinemann on behalf of the BSAVA.

Based on the extremely successful BSAVA Manual formula of a logical, user-friendly approach, this exciting new series of three manuals caters for all levels of staff working with animals, whether it be in veterinary practice or other areas of animal care.

The editors of each of the manuals, Sue Dallas, Margaret Moore and Alasdair Hotston Moore, together with the series editor Gill Simpson, are to be congratulated on bringing together a wide range of talented contributors, both veterinary surgeons and veterinary nurses, to write individual chapters in an impressively easy-to-read format. They have succeeded in the difficult task of maintaining a continuity of style throughout. Each chapter opens with a summary of the information contained therein. The liberal use of tables and illustrations adds to the appeal of the layout, making the information accessible and highly practical in nature.

The *Manual of Veterinary Care* is a perfect introduction to those wishing to pursue a career working with animals. The *Manual of Veterinary Nursing* is written for student veterinary nurses studying for the new vocational qualification. The *Manual of Advanced Veterinary Nursing* has been designed for qualified veterinary nurses who are already working in practice and who either wish to take the Diploma in Advanced Veterinary Nursing (Surgical) or (Medical) or who just wish to expand their knowledge and further their education. There is, at present, no textbook that deals with the advanced course. This book provides both the necessary theoretical background and practical information, all in an easy-to-read style.

This three-volume series is certain to become an essential addition to the libraries of veterinary practices, training colleges and a wide range of animal care establishments.

P. Harvey Locke BVSc MRCVS
BSAVA President 1999–2000

Series preface

The veterinary profession has developed rapidly in recent years and the role of the ancillary staff in the small animal veterinary practice has increased in importance and diversity. Small animal practice in the new millennium will focus on the team approach to total animal care. Within this team should be adequately and appropriately trained personnel.

The aim of the BSAVA Manuals of Veterinary Nursing is to assist in the training and education of staff who are responsible for the care of animals, either within the veterinary practice or in other establishments which have responsibility for the welfare of animals. The series has been produced for the use of animal care personnel through to veterinary nurses studying for Advanced Diploma but the books fundamentally address the requirements for good nursing care.

The first book, the *Manual of Veterinary Care*, acts as an introduction to the care of small animals kept as pets, exploring the opportunities available for employment with animals, then progressing to describe basic animal care techniques. The second volume, the *Manual of Veterinary Nursing*, aims to assist those student veterinary nurses who are training for a formal qualification. It has been compiled with the needs of the Vocational Qualification in Veterinary Nursing in mind. With the development of veterinary nursing as a profession in its own right the remit of the qualified veterinary nurse is expanding. The objective of the *Manual of Advanced Veterinary Nursing* is to aid qualified veterinary nurses in developing their knowledge and skills. The inclusion of more advanced techniques should assist these nurses in fulfilling their essential role in the modern veterinary practice.

Multiple authors, both veterinary surgeons and veterinary nurses, have been involved in writing these books. Indeed, many sections have been co-written by veterinary surgeons and veterinary nurses working together to give a comprehensive approach to subject areas. Where appropriate, authors have contributed to more than one book, which gives continuity of content and style.

Having been associated with the education and training of veterinary nurses for some years, I am delighted to have been involved with these publications. I am grateful to all the authors who have contributed. Many thanks to Marion Jowett from BSAVA for directing the project and to the volume editors who have worked extremely hard to ensure these manuals are succinct and well presented. In particular I should like to thank BSAVA, who have supported the concept and publication of these manuals with the aim not only to improve the education of veterinary nurses but to improve animal care at all levels.

Gill Simpson
August 1999

 It must be remembered that the veterinary nurse must at all times work within the guidelines of the Veterinary Surgeons Act.

Preface

This volume of the Manuals of Veterinary Nursing is aimed at veterinary nurses, who up until now have only had textbooks available intended for use prior to qualification and often of limited use after that time. Their only source of information at a level beyond that has been material intended for veterinary surgeons or veterinary undergraduates, whose perspectives are often quite different.

The authors and editors of this volume have attempted to do two things: introduce techniques carried out in veterinary practice of which many veterinary nurses may be aware but have no personal experience; and review techniques that nurses themselves may wish to use now or in the future as the legislative framework develops. The Manual has been written to provide information not only on what veterinary nurses need to know, but also on what they want to know.

This book is not intended as a course textbook; additional material may be found in the companion volumes, other BSAVA manuals and through the indicated Further Reading. Given the large and expanding field of nursing, it is not posssible to include all in one book. The syllabuses of the Diplomas in Advanced Veterinary Nursing are wide ranging and cannot be addressed in their entirety within this volume, but this book should provide a lead into these areas.

What has been produced includes material on a wide range of areas from a set of authors who have great enthusiasm for their fields and the work of veterinary nurses. Although fewer nurses are included in the authorship than in the companion volumes, nationally and internationally recognized authorities have contributed.

The coverage of internal medicine introduces the concept of the problem-based approach which is not seen in other nursing texts. The surgery chapter includes techniques for nursing patients with major surgical problems. Laboratory medicine includes advanced techniques and their interpretation. Equine nursing is a developing field and is covered in a nursing text for probably the first time. Critical care nursing and anaesthesia are areas of great interest and, again, material has been included that is not generally available. The imaging chapter includes both advanced radiography techniques and the other imaging modalities, seldom described in other general nursing texts. Practice management and the nursing of exotic species are also covered in a depth not found in the traditional texts.

I enjoyed reading all the chapters here tremendously and I thank the authors for their hard work. I hope our readership similarly enjoy, use and are inspired by their work.

Alasdair Hotston Moore
August 1999

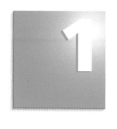

Clinical medicine: a problem-based approach

James W. Simpson and David J. Argyle

This chapter is designed to give information on:

- The investigative approach to common presenting syndromes in small animal medicine
- Interpretation of findings associated with the physical examination of the patient
- A description of the various diagnostic techniques used in small animal medicine
- A brief introduction to small animal therapeutics

Introduction

Internal medicine is a very large subject, requiring a sound knowledge of diseases affecting all internal body systems. The depth of knowledge on these diseases continues to increase, making it increasingly difficult for the clinician to remember all the aspects of every disease. Consequently the approach to internal medicine has changed from learning all the clinical features, diagnostic tests and treatment of each disease, to a problem-solving approach.

Whole textbooks have been written on the subject of internal medicine and clearly provision of this level of information is not possible within the confines of this chapter. The aim of the chapter is to introduce the veterinary nurse to the more advanced aspects of investigative medicine. The chapter has been divided into four sections covering: common syndromes in small animal medicine; interpretation of physical findings; investigative techniques; and therapy.

It must be remembered that veterinary nurses are not legally allowed to make a diagnosis but they are frequently involved in the investigations and diagnostic procedures required to allow the veterinary surgeon to reach a diagnosis.

Clinical syndromes

As our depth of knowledge regarding the different diseases that can affect the dog and cat continues to increase, so does the complexity of the investigations required to reach a definitive diagnosis. Many dogs and cats present with atypical clinical symptoms, making a diagnosis even more difficult to establish. For these reasons, a problem-solving approach to clinical cases is now the method used by most clinicians.

This section considers the investigative problem-solving approach to some of the most common presenting complaints in dogs and cats. The importance of the clinical examination (history and physical examination) is discussed, together with the differential diagnoses and diagnostic procedures that can be used to reach a definitive diagnosis.

Dysphagia

Dysphagia may be defined as difficulty or inability in eating or drinking. This is usually associated with a mechanical or functional disorder of the swallowing process. It must be differentiated from anorexia, which is defined as a loss of desire to eat. Dysphagia may be further differentiated into oral, pharyngeal or oesophageal in origin.

History

The owner may report that the animal is 'vomiting' when in fact it is retching or regurgitating. The latter symptoms are common in dysphagic patients and careful questioning is required to differentiate these patients from those that are actually vomiting.

Although the history should include questions about all body systems, where dysphagia is suspected the following questions should be asked:

- Has there been any recent trauma to the animal?
- How long have the symptoms been present?
- Does the animal salivate?
- Is the animal losing weight?
- Can the animal drink fluids without difficulty?
- Is the animal still willing to eat?
- Can it pick up food from its dish?
- Does it choke, cough, gag or retch when trying to swallow?
- Does the animal appear to swallow normally but shortly afterwards arch its neck and regurgitate the food just eaten?
- Does the animal actually vomit? This is an active process with a prodromal phase of anxiety followed by marked abdominal contractions, prior to food being forced out of the stomach and out through the mouth.

Physical examination

A full detailed examination of all body systems should be carried out in case there is a systemic disease causing the dysphagia:

- Presence of facial asymmetry?
- Does the tongue hang out of the mouth?
- Is the patient salivating?
- Are there any food or fluids coming down the nose?
- Is the patient able to hold its mouth closed?
- Are there any signs of trauma, foreign body or tumour within the mouth?
- Is the mandible intact?
- Is there a gag reflex present?
- Does palpation of the pharynx detect any mass or discomfort?
- Is the patient's breathing disturbed?
- Is the patient pyrexic?

Observation of eating behaviour

At this point there is considerable value in observing the patient eating. Place the animal in a stress-free environment and provide some of its favourite food in a suitable bowl. Stand back and observe the eating behaviour.

- *Oral dysphagia:* The patient will try to eat, indicating it is hungry. Food may be picked up but immediately dropped out of the mouth. There may be evidence of persistent chewing without swallowing. Food may be held in the mouth or cheeks
- *Pharyngeal dysphagia:* After picking up food from the bowl the animal will gag, choke, retch and cough when attempting to swallow. This is associated with food entering the airways and may result in food or fluid coming down the nose

- *Oesophageal dysphagia:* The animal is able to pick up food from the bowl and swallow it without obvious difficulty. However, after a variable period of time the neck will be arched and a 'sausage' of food regurgitated. There is no evidence of abdominal contraction with this process.

Differential diagnosis

Following the clinical examination and observation of eating behaviour, it should be possible to differentiate between animals with oral, pharyngeal and oesophageal dysphagia. Use of appropriate radiographic techniques and endoscopy may assist in obtaining a definitive diagnosis (Figure 1.1) . Neurological examination may be employed in cases where there is believed to be a neurological component.

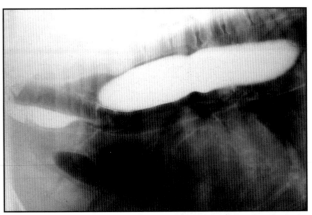

1.2   *Megaoesophagus. Lateral radiograph of the thorax showing a dilated oesophagus filled with barium sulphate. The entire oesophagus is dilated.*

1.1   Differential diagnosis and diagnostic procedures for dysphagia

Condition	Neurological examination	Radiography	Endoscopy
Oral dysphagia			
Cranial nerve defect	Valuable	No	No
Fractured mandible	No	Plain radiographs	No
Cleft palate	No	No	No
Foreign body	No	Plain radiographs	No
Tumour	No	Plain radiographs	Valuable
Pharyngeal dysphagia			
Cranial nerve defect	Valuable	No	No
Tumour	No	Plain radiographs	Valuable
Foreign body	No	Plain radiographs	Valuable
Lymphadenopathy	No	Plain radiographs	No
Tonsillitis	No	No	No
Oesophageal dysphagia			
Megaoesophagus	No	Plain and contrast studies (Figure 1.2)	No
Vascular ring anomaly	No	Plain and contrast studies (Figure 1.3)	
Oesophagitis	No	No	Valuable (Figure 1.4)
Foreign body	No	Plain radiographs (Figure 1.5)	Valuable
Tumour	No	Plain radiographs	Valuable
Stricture	No	Plain and contrast studies	Valuable (Figure 1.6)

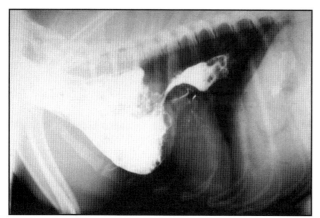

1.3 *Vascular ring anomaly. Lateral radiograph of the thorax showing a dilated oesophagus, filled with barium sulphate, cranial to the heart base. This is a typical view in young dogs with vascular ring anomaly.*

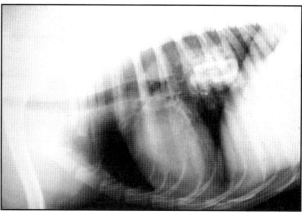

1.5 *Foreign body. Lateral radiograph of the thorax showing a radiodense foreign body lying in the oesophagus between the base of the heart and the diaphragm.*

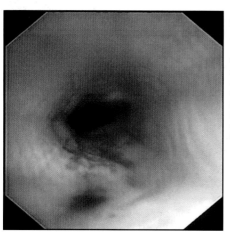

1.4 *Oesophagitis. This endoscopic view of the distal oesophagus shows blood and ulceration associated with oesophagitis. The cardia can be seen in the distance.*

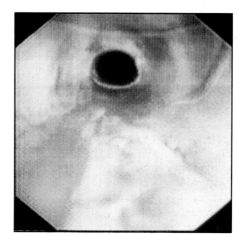

1.6 *Stricture. This endoscopic view of the canine oesophagus shows annular narrowing of the lumen due to a fibrous tissue structure.*

Polyphagia

Polyphagia describes the state of increased hunger. The animal is not satisfied by its normal diet and seeks additional sources of food. It may steal food and may even have a 'depraved' appetite, eating abnormal items such as soil or stones, or licking concrete. The polyphagia may be associated with weight gain or with weight loss.

History
Polyphagia should be related to the animal's body weight. Is the animal eating excessively in the face of weight gain or loss? The answer to this question will assist in reaching a diagnosis. In addition to all the usual questions regarding all body systems, the following questions may be of particular value:

- What is the animal's normal diet?
- Is the animal being fed an adequate amount of food?
- Is the animal gaining weight or losing weight while polyphagic?
- Is there any evidence of vomiting or diarrhoea?
- Is the animal polyuric or polydipsic?
- Is there any change in abdominal size?
- Is there any evidence of alopecia?
- Is there a history of exercise intolerance?
- Is the animal receiving any medication?

Physical examination
Polyphagia falls into two major types:

- Where the animal has lost the ability to assimilate food, such as in exocrine pancreatic insufficiency (EPI), inflammatory bowel disease (IBD) or liver disease
- Associated with systemic disease, especially endocrine diseases.

The physical examination should supplement the history and aim to determine to which group the patient belongs. In particular, the following should be addressed:

- Is the animal adequately hydrated? Especially important if polyuric
- Is there evidence of weight loss and particularly loss of muscle mass?
- If alopecia is present, where has this occurred and to what extent?
- Is there a change in the animal's abdominal size?
- Is there a 'sweet' or foul smell on the animal's breath?
- Is there any evidence of lymphadenopathy or other masses on palpation?

Differential diagnosis
The clinical examination will indicate the degree of polyphagia present and whether the patient is gaining or losing weight. From this information a differential diagnosis can be determined and the diagnostic tests required to reach a definitive diagnosis selected (Figure 1.7).

Differential diagnosis and diagnostic procedures for polyphagia

Condition	History	Blood tests	Radiography	Other tests
Polyphagia plus weight gain				
Drug use	Valuable	No	No	No
Dietary	Valuable	No	No	No
Insulinoma	No	Blood glucose and insulin	No	Ultrasonography of pancreas and liver
Acromegaly	Valuable	IGF-1	No	No
Polyphagia plus weight loss				
Dietary (poor quality)	Valuable	No	No	No
Dietary (increased demand)	Valuable	No	No	No
Hyperadrenocorticism	Valuable	SAP; white cell count; cholesterol	Plain radiography of the abdomen	ACTH stimulation test Dexamethasone tests
Diabetes mellitus	Valuable	Blood glucose, ketones	No	Urinalysis
Neoplasia	Valuable	Hype rcalcaemia	Plain radiographs	Ultrasonography
Parasitism	Valuable	No	No	Faecal worm egg count
Hyperthyroidism	Valuable	T4 levels	No	Ultrasound
Exocrine pancreatic insufficiency	Valuable	TLI test	No	Faecal for undigested food
Inflammatory bowel disease	No	Serum folate and cobalamin	No	Endoscopy and biopsy
Pyrexia of unknown origin	No	Haematology Biochemistry	Plain radiographs	Urinalysis Blood culture Immune tests

ACTH = adrenocorticotropic hormone; IGF-1 = insulin-like growth factor 1; SAP = serum alkaline phosphatase; T4 = thyroid hormone; TLI = trypsinogen-like immunoreactivity

Vomiting

Vomiting is defined as the active forceful ejection of stomach contents up the oesophagus and out through the mouth. It involves the fixation of the diaphragm, cessation of respiration, and forceful contraction of abdominal muscles.

History

It is important to differentiate vomiting from regurgitation, which is a more passive process associated with oesophageal disease. More importantly, it is essential to remember that vomiting may not be associated with gastric disease but may be secondary to some systemic disorder, toxaemia, drug interaction or vestibular disease. When collecting a history it is therefore important to ask questions regarding all body systems and also drugs that the animal may be taking. In particular, questions should include:

- Is the animal fully vaccinated?
- What is the normal diet and does the animal scavenge?
- Has the animal been wormed regularly?
- Is there any history of ingesting poisons?
- What is the duration and frequency of vomiting?
- What does the vomitus contain?
- Has the animal's vomition been associated with travelling?
- Are there any signs of incoordination or ataxia?
- Is there a history of polyuria and polydipsia?

- Is the animal on any drug regimes?
- If the patient is female, is she spayed?
- When was her last season? And is there any vaginal discharge?
- Is there any associated diarrhoea or constipation?
- Is there evidence of abdominal enlargement?
- Is there evidence of weight loss?
- Is the patient still eating or anorexic?

Physical examination

The physical examination should supplement the information obtained from the history. In particular, look for signs of systemic disease and note the following:

- Is the animal dehydrated? If so to what degree?
- What is the general demeanour of the animal?
- Is the breath uraemic or ketoacidotic?
- Are there ulcers in the mouth?
- Is there a vaginal discharge?
- Is there pain on palpation of the abdomen? If so, involving which organs?
- Is the abdomen tympanic?
- Is there a mass detectable in the abdomen?
- Is there fluid within the intestinal loops?

Differential diagnosis

The information gathered above should allow a decision to be made as to whether a gastric (primary) or systemic disease (secondary) is present. A differential diagnosis list can then be compiled and more specific diagnostic tests performed (Figure 1.8).

Differential diagnosis and diagnostic procedures for vomiting

Condition	Radiography	Endoscopy	Blood analysis	Other tests
Primary				
Acute gastritis	No	No	No	No
Chronic gastritis	Plain radiographs	Valuable	No	No
Gastric ulcer	Plain and contrast studies	Valuable (Figure 1.9)	No	No
Gastric neoplasia	Plain and contrast studies (Figure 1.10)	Valuable	No	Ultrasonography
Pyloric stenosis	Plain and contrast studies (Figure 1.11)	No	No	No
Gastric torsion	Plain radiographs	No	No	Stomach tube
Secondary				
Intestinal obstruction	Plain and contrast studies (Figure 1.12)	No	No	Exploratory surgery
Colitis	No	Valuable	No	No
Pancreatitis	Plain radiographs	No	Amylase, lipase, TLI	Ultrasonography
Hepatitis	Plain radiographs	No	SALT, SAP, Bile acids	Ultrasonography and biopsy
Renal failure	No	No	Blood urea, creatinine	Urinalysis
Diabetes mellitus	No	No	Blood sugar, ketones	Urinalysis
Chemotherapy	No	No	No	History
Pyometra	Plain radiographs	No	White cell count	Exploratory surgery

TLI = trypsinogen-like immunoreactivity; SALT = serum alanine aminotransferase; SAP = serum alkaline phosphatase

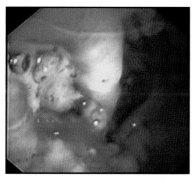

1.9

Gastric ulcer. Endoscopic view of the canine stomach showing (right) the opening into the pyloric antrum and (left) a large gastric ulcer.

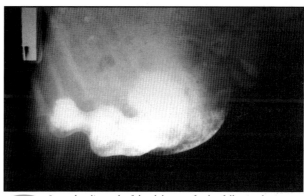

1.11 *Lateral radiograph of the abdomen of a dog following barium administration. No barium has left the stomach after 2 hours, suggesting a pyloric stenosis.*

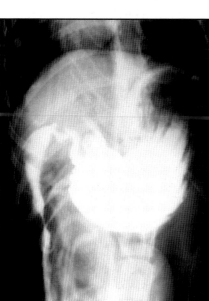

1.10

Dorsoventral radiograph of a barium study, showing a filing defect near the pylorus which was observed over a series of radiographs. This is suggestive of a gastric neoplasm. Endoscopic examination of the stomach could be used to confirm the diagnosis.

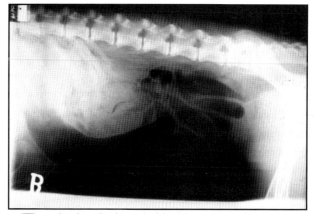

1.12 *Plain lateral radiograph of the abdomen of a dog showing gas-filled loops of intestine bunched together. This is the typical appearance of an intussusception.*

Diarrhoea

Diarrhoea may be defined as the passage of faeces with an increased water and/or nutrient content, resulting in an alteration in consistency.

History

It is important to note that diarrhoea may be caused by a primary intestinal disorder or may be associated with a systemic disease. Diarrhoea is very common in dogs, usually associated with some form of dietary indiscretion, but less common in cats, where vomiting is the predominant symptom of intestinal disease.

It is important to take a detailed history regarding all body systems. In particular, the following questions may provide valuable information:

- Is the animal fully vaccinated?
- Has it been regularly wormed?
- What is the animal's normal diet and how much is fed each day?
- Is the animal still eating?
- Is the animal fed titbits or other foods?
- Is there any knowledge of scavenging behaviour?
- What is the colour, consistency and frequency of defecation?
- Is there any mucus or blood present in the faeces?
- Is the animal straining to pass faeces (rectal tenesmus)?
- Is the diarrhoea associated with weight loss?

Physical examination

The information collected here should help to substantiate the historical findings and determine the severity of the animal's clinical condition. All body systems should be thoroughly examined and, in particular, the following should be assessed:

- Is the animal clinically dehydrated?
- What is its general demeanour?
- Is there evidence of weight loss?
- Does palpation of the abdomen detect pain, a mass, fluid-filled intestines or organ enlargement?
- Is there evidence of systemic disease?

Differential diagnosis

From the clinical examination it should be possible to determine whether the patient has a systemic disease or a primary intestinal disorder. If the latter is suspected, an attempt should be made to determine whether there is a small or large intestinal problem (Figure 1.13) . Once the location of the problem has been identified, the underlying disorder can be determined using the diagnostic procedures shown in Figure 1.14.

Enlarged abdomen

History

An increase in the size of the abdomen may occur in many disease states. When the contents of the abdomen are considered, it is clear that many different causes may result in abdominal enlargement. Rather than considering all the conditions which may enlarge the abdomen, it is better to consider what may actually cause the abdominal size to increase. As a guide to remembering the possible differential diagnosis for an enlarged abdomen, a simple phrase can be used: Consider the five Fs – fat, faeces, fluid, fetus, flatus.

When collecting a history from an animal with an enlarged abdomen it is important to ask questions regarding all body systems but in particular to consider:

- How quickly did the abdomen become enlarged?
- How long has the abdomen remained enlarged?
- Does the animal appear to be in distress?
- Is there any evidence of vomiting or diarrhoea?
- Is the animal constipated?
- How is the animal's appetite?
- Is the animal a female? If so is she spayed?
- If intact could she have been mated?
- Is there any evidence of limb swelling?
- Is there a history of breathing difficulty or coughing?
- Is there a history of weight loss?

Physical examination

The physical examination is particularly important, especially as any sudden onset of abdominal enlargement in the dog always suggests the possibility of gastric torsion, which is a life-threatening condition and a true emergency. As always the whole animal should be examined but in particular the following may be helpful:

- Is the animal in distress?
- Does percussion of the abdomen suggest tympany?
- Does palpation of the abdomen cause pain?
- Is there evidence of organomegaly on abdominal palpation?
- Is there any evidence of breathing difficulty?
- Does percussion of the chest suggest hydrothorax?
- Is there evidence of subcutaneous oedema?
- Is there a vaginal discharge?
- Does a rectal examination suggest constipation?
- Has the animal lost muscle mass?

Differential diagnosis

From the clinical examination it may be possible to determine a cause for the enlargement of the abdomen; for example, a

1.13 Small versus large intestine problems

Parameter	Small intestine	Large intestine
Weight loss	Present	Absent
Steatorrhoea	Present	Absent
Faecal tenesmus	Absent	Present
Faecal mucus	Absent	Present
Faecal blood	Absent	Present
Faecal frequency	Three times daily	Six times daily

Differential diagnosis and diagnostic procedures for diarrhoea

Condition	Faecal analysis	Blood tests	Endoscopy	Other tests
Small intestine				
Dietary	No	No	No	History
Exocrine pancreatic insufficiency	Undigested food	TLI test	No	History
Inflammatory bowel disease	Worm egg count and bacteriology	Serum folate and cobalamin	Valuable	Intestinal biopsy
Parasitism	Worm egg count	No	No	No
Small intestinal bacterial overgrowth	No	Serum folate and cobalamin	Duodenal aspirate culture	No
Bacterial infection	Bacteriology	No	No	No
Viral infection	ELISA tests	No	No	Viral isolation
Neoplasia	No	No	Valuable	Radiography
Large intestine				
Colitis	Worm egg count and bacteriology	No	Valuable, plus biopsy	Radiography
Parasitism	Worm egg count	No	Valuable	No
Bacterial infection	Bacteriology	No	No	No
Neoplasia	No	No	Valuable, plus biopsy	Radiography
Systemic				
Hyperthyroidism	No	T4 levels	No	Thyroid scan
Hypoadrenocorticism	No	Sodium, potassium	No	ACTH test, ECG
Renal failure	No	Blood urea, creatinine	No	Urinalysis
Hepatitis	No	SALT, SAP, bile acids	No	Ultrasonography, biopsy

ACTH = adrenocorticotropic hormone; SALT = serum alanine aminotransferase; SAP = serum alkaline phosphatase; T4 = thyroid hormone; TLI = trypsinogen-like immunoreactivity

large mass may be felt in the abdomen, or the colon may appear to be distended with faeces. However, in a significant number of cases palpation of the abdomen will not permit such a definitive conclusion to be made. In most cases further investigation is warranted. The causes and types of diagnostic procedure that might be used in such an investigation are shown in Figure 1.15.

Abnormal free abdominal contents
True transudate:

- Usually associated with hypoproteinaemia
- There may also be fluid accumulations in the thorax and under the skin
- Causes of hypoproteinaemia include malnutrition, burns, hepatic failure, renal failure and protein-losing enteropathy.

Modified transudates:

- Usually pink but may vary from clear to yellow, so care must be taken with visual interpretation
- Associated with local hypertension due to conditions such as portal hypertension or with tumours obstructing venous flow. May also be associated with cardiac disease.

Exudates:

- Usually red; may be turbid; occasionally yellow. Always have high cell and protein contents
- Always associated with infections within the peritoneal cavity. Good examples include nocardiosis and feline infectious peritonitis (FIP).

Chyle:

- Rarely difficult to recognize due to its characteristic white colour
- Presence in the abdomen implies lymphatic vessel rupture
- May be due to trauma, neoplasia or inflammation; occasionally associated with cardiac disease.

Gut contents:

- Always associated with perforation of the alimentary tract
- Trauma is the most common reason
- Pressure necrosis from a longstanding foreign body, ulceration and neoplasia may be implicated.

Condition	Clinical examination	Radiography	Blood tests	Other tests
Fat				
Sublumbar and omental fat	Valuable	Plain	No	No
Obesity	Valuable	Plain	No	No
Hyperadrenocorticism	Valuable	Plain	SAP, haematology	ACTH test
Organomegaly	Valuable	Plain	No	Ultrasonography
Hepatic lipidosis	Valuable	No	SALT, SAP, GGT	Ultrasonography, biopsy
Faeces				
Constipation	Valuable	Plain (Figure 1.16)	No	No
Megacolon	Valuable	Plain (Figure 1.16)	No	No
Intestinal obstruction	Valuable	Plain and contrast studies	No	Exploratory surgery
Overeating	Valuable	Plain	No	No
Fluid (see Figure 1.17)				
Atonic bladder	Valuable	Plain	Blood urea, creatinine	Catheterization
Intestinal perforation	Valuable	Plain	No	Paracentesis
Free urine	Valuable	Plain	Blood urea, creatinine	Paracentesis
Bile duct rupture	Valuable	Plain	No	Paracentesis
True transudate	Valuable	Plain	No	Paracentesis
Modified transudate	Valuable	Plain	No	Paracentesis
Exudate	Valuable	Plain	White cell count	Paracentesis and culture
Chyle	Valuable	Plain	No	Paracentesis
Fetus		Plain		
Pregnancy	Valuable	Plain	No	Ultrasonography
Pseudopregnancy	Valuable	Plain	No	Ultrasonography
Pyometra	Valuable	Plain	White cell count	Ultrasonography
Flatus				
Gastric torsion	Valuable	Plain	No	Stomach tubing
Free gas	No	Plain	No	Ultrasonography, exploratory surgery
Intestinal tympany	Valuable	Plain	No	Exploratory surgery

ACTH = adrenocorticotropic hormone; GGT = γ-glutamyl transferase; SAP = serum alkaline phosphatase; SALT = serum alanine aminotransferase

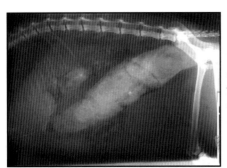

1.16 *Lateral radiograph of the abdomen of a cat, showing gross accumulation of faeces in the descending colon associated with constipation and megacolon.*

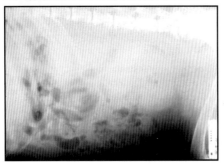

1.17 *Lateral radiograph of the abdomen of a dog, showing loss of detail and contrast in the image associated with fluid accumulation (ascites).*

Urine:

- When paracentesis yields urine, ensure cystocentesis has not occurred by accident. Check the location of needle insertion is not too far caudal and check a plain radiograph to see if the urinary bladder is intact or enlarged
- Free urine in the abdomen is associated with bladder rupture which may be due to trauma, obstruction to urine flow or neoplasia
- Occasionally free urine is associated with rupture of the renal pelvis or ureter.

Bile:

- Free bile in the abdomen is always associated with gall bladder rupture
- Most common cause is a road traffic accident
- Rarely, gall bladder rupture is associated with choleliths or tumours causing obstruction and perforation of the bile duct
- Careless placement of a biopsy needle within the liver may also cause bile leakage into the abdomen.

Laboratory analysis of abdominal fluids

Fluid	Specific gravity	Protein content	Cell content	Bacteria	Colour
True transudate	<1.018	<25 g/l	$<1 \times 10^9$/l	None	Clear
Modified transudate	1.018 to 1.025	25–35 g/l	$<5 \times 10^9$/l	None	Pink
Exudate	>1.025	>25 g/l	$>5 \times 10^9$/l	Likely	Red
Chyle	1.018	25–35 g/l	$1–2 \times 10^9$/l	None	White
Gut content	Variable	Variable	High	Many	Brown
Urine	>1.015	20–30 g/l	1×10^9/l	Variable	Yellow
Bile	>1.015	>30 g/l	$>2 \times 10^9$/l	Variable	Green
Blood	>1.015	>30 g/l	High	None	Red

Blood:

- Free whole blood in the abdominal cavity is associated with haemorrhage
- May be due to trauma, such as a ruptured spleen
- May also occur with neoplastic disease, especially haemangiosarcoma
- Clotting disorders, such as warfarin poisoning, may lead to haemorrhage
- Look for other sites of bleeding.

The types of fluid that may accumulate can be differentiated by laboratory tests (Figure 1.18).

Urinary incontinence

The inappropriate voiding of urine. The passage of urine from the urinary bladder without conscious control.

Control of bladder function is very complex, involving input through sympathetic and parasympathetic nerves and conscious control through the CNS. Voluntary control of bladder emptying requires coordination between detrusor muscle contraction and relaxation of the internal and external urethral sphincters.

History
Collection of a detailed history is extremely important where the owner suspects urinary incontinence has developed. Although it is important to collect information regarding all body systems, there are specific questions which can assist in reaching a diagnosis:

- Is the animal neutered?
- How old is the animal?
- Is the animal drinking excessively?
- Is the animal able to pass urine normally as well as being incontinent?
- Is there any evidence of urinary tenesmus?
- Is there any evidence of faecal incontinence, hindlimb weakness or inability to use the tail?
- Does the urine produced appear to be normal?
- When does the animal appear to be incontinent?
- Is the animal aware of voiding urine?

Physical examination
A careful examination of the patient will assist in confirming the history and hopefully provide further useful information. A complete physical examination should be carried out in all cases, as apparent urinary incontinence can be a feature of systemic disease. Parts of the examination which should receive special attention include:

- Palpation of the abdomen to assess bladder size and position
- Palpation of the kidneys to assess size and evidence of pain
- Examination of the prepuce or vagina for abnormalities
- Assessing the state of hydration
- Checking for evidence of a uraemic or ketotic breath
- A complete neurological examination with special attention to hindlimb function, ability to use the tail and anal tone
- In male dogs, rectal examination to check the size and position of the prostate gland.

Differential diagnosis
Based on data collected from the clinical examination it may be possible to reach a tentative diagnosis. For example, if the animal is only 8 months old, voids urine normally but also dribbles urine continuously, this is likely to be an ectopic ureter. However, if the animal is 10 years old, incontinent and has haematuria, the diagnosis is more likely to involve bladder neoplasia. Further diagnostic tests are required to reach a definitive diagnosis (Figure 1.19).

Urinary tenesmus

Urinary tenesmus refers to an animal's straining to pass urine. It should not be confused with dysuria, which is difficulty in passing urine, although both may be present at the same time.

History
Urinary tenesmus associated with obstruction is much more common in the male than the female, due to the shorter and wider urethra in the latter. However, because of this anatomy, females are more likely to develop cystitis. A detailed history should always be collected and, in particular, questions regarding the function of the urinary system should be included:

- How long has the animal been straining to pass urine?
- What sex is the animal?
- Does the animal void urine normally and then strain?
- Is the animal unable to pass urine at all and but continues to try?
- What is the appearance of the urine which is voided?
- Is the animal showing any signs of incontinence?

1.19 Differential diagnosis and diagnostic procedures for urinary incontinence

Condition	Radiography	Ultrasonography	Urinalysis	Other tests
Congenital				
Ectopic ureter	Intravenous urethrography (Figure 1.20)	Valuable	No	Surgical exploration
Hypoplastic bladder	Plain, pneumocystogram	Valuable	No	No
Intrapelvic bladder	Plain, pneumocystogram	No	No	No
Bladder neck abnormality	Plain and contrast studies	Valuable	No	No
Patent urachus	Plain and contrast studies	Valuable	No	Surgical exploration
Adult female				
Sphincter mechanism incompetence	Urethrography	No	Valuable	Clinical examination
Uterine stump abnormality	Plain	Valuable	No	Surgical exploration
Other				
Prostatic disease	Plain (Figure 1.21)	Valuable	Valuable	Rectal examination, prostatic wash cytology, ultrasonography
Neoplasia	Plain and contrast studies	Valuable (Figure 1.22)	Valuable	Cytology
Uroliths	Plain and contrast studies (Figure 1.23)	Valuable	Valuable	Ultrasonography
Spinal lesions	Spinal	No	No	Neurological examination
Fear, stress	No	No	No	Clinical examination
Cystitis	No	No	Valuable	Culture
Polyuria/polydipsia	No	No	Valuable	Blood tests

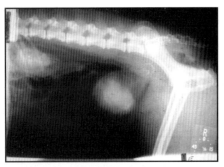

1.20 *Lateral view of the abdomen of a dog during intravenous urography, showing contrast medium in the ureter opening beyond the bladder into the vagina – an ectopic ureter.*

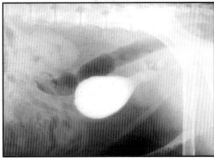

1.21 *Lateral radiograph of the abdomen of a male dog showing the bladder full of contrast medium. The space between the neck of the bladder and the pelvis contains a large prostate gland.*

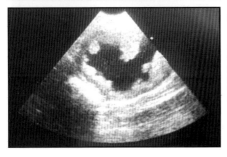

1.22 *Ultrasound image of the urinary bladder showing a thickened and irregular bladder wall associated with neoplasia.*

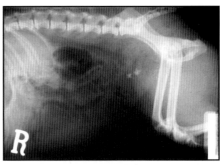

1.23 *Lateral radiograph of the abdomen of a dog showing radiodense calculi lying in the urinary bladder.*

Physical examination

A careful examination of the entire animal is required but particular attention should be centred around the urinary tract. In particular, the following are important:

- Abdominal palpation for position and size of the bladder
- Is the patient adequately hydrated?
- Carry out a rectal examination to examine the prostate and pelvic canal
- Examine the urethra by extruding the penis in males and examining the vagina in females
- Pass a catheter along the urethra to assess patency.

Differential diagnosis

The clinical examination should allow a detailed assessment of the process of micturition to be obtained. It is rarely possible to make a definitive diagnosis at this stage; further diagnostic tests are required (Figure 1.24). One of the first and most important tests involves urethral catheterization in order to determine if there is obstruction to the flow of urine.

1.24 Differential diagnosis and diagnostic procedures for urinary tenesmus

Condition	Radiography	Urinalysis	Ultrasonography	Other tests
Cystitis	No	Valuable	No	Urine culture and sensitivity
Urethritis	No	Valuable	No	Urine culture and sensitivity
Prostatic disease	Plain	Valuable	Valuable	Prostatic wash
Uroliths	Plain and contrast	Valuable	Valuable	Urine mineral assay
Neoplasia	Plain and contrast	Valuable	Valuable	Cytology
Reflex dyssynergia	No	No	No	Neurological examination
Penile trauma	No	No	No	Catheterization and examination
Retroflexed bladder	Plain	No	Valuable	Catheterization

Polyuria and polydipsia

- Polyuria(PU): Increased daily urine production – >50 ml/kg/day
- Polydipsia (PD): Increased daily fluid intake – >100 ml/kg/day.

Water consumption and urine production are carefully controlled by the interactions of the kidney, hypothalamus and pituitary gland. Increases in plasma ion concentration stimulate osmoreceptors in the hypothalamus and lead to the feeling of thirst. To conserve water, antidiuretic hormone (ADH) is secreted by the pituitary gland and acts on the kidney collecting ducts.

History
As PUPD can be associated with many systemic conditions a detailed history should always be collected. In particular the following questions should be addressed:

- What is the age and breed of the patient?
- If female, is she entire?
- When was her last season?
- Vaccination status?
- Speed of onset and duration of PUPD?
- Actual daily water intake?
- Frequency of urination?
- Is nocturia present?
- Are there any other systemic symptoms, such as vomiting, diarrhoea, anorexia, weight loss?
- Has the patient been prescribed any medications?
- Is the patient frequently left alone for long periods?

Physical examination
A thorough physical examination should always be carried out in order to support the history and determine the likely cause of the PUPD. In particular, attention should be paid to the following:

- Presence of abnormal breath: uraemic or ketotic
- State of hydration
- Presence of any vaginal discharge
- Enlargement of the abdomen
- Activity level of the patient
- Presence of alopecia
- Size of the peripheral lymph nodes
- Bodily condition.

Differential diagnosis
The information gained may help to suggest the likely cause of the PUPD but in all cases further investigative tests are needed in order to obtain a definitive diagnosis (Figure 1.25).

1.25 Differential diagnosis and diagnostic procedures for polyuria/polydipsia

Condition	Urinalysis	Blood tests	Hormone assays	Other tests
Diabetes mellitus	Valuable	Blood sugar, ketones	No	No
Diabetes insipidus	Valuable	No	ADH test	Water deprivation test
Hyperthyroidism	No	No	T4	Thyroid imaging
Hyperadrenocorticism	Valuable	Haematology, biochemistry	ACTH stimulation test, LDDT, HDDT	Ultrasonography of adrenal glands
Hypoadrenocorticism	Valuable	Haematology, biochemistry	ACTH stimulation test	ECG, sodium, potassium
Renal failure	Valuable	Blood urea, creatinine	PTH	Calcium, phosphorus
Hypercalcaemia	No	Blood calcium	PTH	Radiography, cytology
Pyometra	No	Haematology	No	Radiography, ultrasonography
Hepatic disease	Valuable	Haematology, biochemistry	No	Ultrasonography, biopsy
Psychogenic polydipsia	Valuable	No	ADH	Water deprivation test
Drug-induced	No	No	No	History

ACTH = adrenocorticotropic hormone; ADH = antidiuretic hormone; LDDT = low-dose dexamethasone test; HDDT = high-dose dexamethasone test; PTH = parathyroid hormone; T4 = thyroid hormone

Alopecia

Alopecia is the absence of hair from areas of the skin where it is normally present. It may be partial or complete and reversible or irreversible, depending on cause.

Alopecia may be due to a primary disease of the hair follicles or may be secondary to other diseases or influences on the skin.

History
A detailed history should be collected including information on:

- Age, sex and breed of the patient
- When did the alopecia start?
- Which part of the patient was first affected?
- Is there evidence of pruritus?
- What is the patient's diet and has it been changed recently?
- Are there any other symptoms such as PUPD, weight loss, vomiting or diarrhoea?.

Physical examination
A thorough physical examination is carried out, paying special attention to the skin and checking for signs of systemic disease:

- Is there evidence of skin inflammation?
- Is there evidence of skin pigmentation or thickening?
- Is there evidence of self-trauma?
- Are there any obvious parasites?
- Is there any evidence of pyoderma?

Differential diagnosis
Alopecia carries a large and varied differential diagnosis. Carefully carrying out the clinical examination will ensure the detection of primary or systemic disease. Figure 1.26 shows the differential diagnosis and diagnostic procedures which will enable a definitive diagnosis to be made.

Pruritus

Pruritus is the sensation that elicits the desire to scratch the skin and is one of the most common presentations in small animal practice.

History
Collect a detailed history including:

- What is the age, sex and breed of the patient?
- How long has the patient been pruritic?
- How extensive and severe is the pruritus?
- Have there been any new carpets, cleaning agents or bedding introduced?
- Has the diet been changed recently?
- Are there any other pets with pruritus?
- Is the owner pruritic?
- Is there a history of recent kennelling?
- Is there evidence of hair loss?
- Are there any systemic symptoms?
- Is there any vomiting or diarrhoea?
- In what season of the year did pruritus start?

1.26 Differential diagnosis and diagnostic procedures for alopecia

Condition	Diagnostic procedures
Primary alopecia	
Hereditory/congenital agenesis of hair follicles Follicular dysplasia Inflammation of the hair follicle	Clinical examination; skin biopsy and histopathology
Endocrine disorders	
Hypothyroidism Hyperadrenocorticism (Figure 1.27) Sertoli cell tumours Sex hormone alopecia	Haematology and biochemistry; ACTH stimulation test; TSH test; sex hormone assay
Nutritional disease	
Vitamin A deficiency Malnutrition Deficiency in essential fatty acids	Dietary history
Parasites	Examination of the skin – skin scrapings, coat brushings; skin biopsy
Infections	Culture of discharge and biopsies with sensitivity testing
Drug-induced	History

ACTH = adrenocorticotropic hormone;
TSH = thyroid stimulating hormone

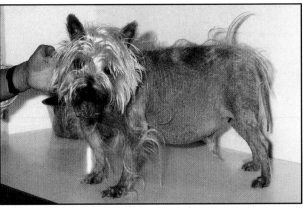

1.27 Alopecia. This dog demonstrates the degree of alopecia that can occur in hyperadrenocorticism. Note that there is no evidence of inflammation or self-trauma. The alopecia is hormonally induced.

Physical examination

- Carefully examine the skin of affected and apparently normal regions
- Is there any sign of parasitism?
- Is the skin inflamed, if so which regions?
- Is there evidence of alopecia?

Differential diagnosis
From the information gathered above some indication as to the cause of the pruritus should be possible. Further diagnostic tests can be carried out in order to confirm the diagnosis (Figure 1.28).

1.28 Differential diagnosis and diagnostic procedures for pruritus

Condition	Diagnostic procedures
Allergic	
Flea allergy Atopy Food allergy Contact allergy	Clinical examination; intradermal skin testing; patch testing; dietary trials
Pyoderma	Culture skin sample or discharge; biopsy and histopathology
Parasitic	
Sarcoptes *Demodex* *Cheyletiella* *Trombicula* Lice *Otodectes*	Skin examination; scrapings, adhesive tape samples; microscopic examination
Fungal	
Malassezia	Culture, cytology
Miscellaneous	
Drug reactions Hepatocutaneous syndrome Seborrhoea	History; serum biochemistry; skin examination and biopsy

Coughing

Coughing is an expiratory effort producing an expulsion of air from the lungs, usually to clear the lungs of foreign material. This expiratory effort is accomplished against a closed glottis.

Coughing is a feature of respiratory disease but is not an indicator of it. Nocturnal coughing is classically associated with cardiac disease and tracheal collapse. Cardiac coughing becomes more noticeable during the day as the condition progresses. Coughing due to pneumonia and other infections, tumours and allergies is usually worse during the day.

It is important to remember that tuberculosis is on the increase and that coughing can be associated with this important zoonosis.

History

Coughing may be divided into those described as 'dry' and 'soft' coughs. Obtaining the owner's perception on this assists in the differential diagnosis. The following information should be obtained:

- What is the age, breed and sex of the patient?
- What is its vaccination status?
- Is there a recent history of kennelling?
- What is the speed of onset and duration of the cough?
- Is coughing more common at night or during the day?
- Is coughing associated with exercise?
- Does the patient appear to be in respiratory distress?
- Is the cough productive? If so what is produced?

Physical examination

The clinician should also be able to assess the type of cough present while carrying out the physical examination.

- Is the patient pyrexic?
- What is the respiratory rate and character of breathing?
- Are there changes on auscultation of the lungs?
- Are there changes on auscultation of the heart?
- Are there changes in the pulses?
- What is the mucous membrane colour?
- What is the capillary refill time?
- Are there changes on examination of the oral and pharyngeal cavity?
- Check the peripheral lymph nodes.

Differential diagnosis

The information collected above should assist the clinician is determining the cause of coughing. Figure 1.29 shows the differential diagnosis and diagnostic procedures that may be used in the coughing patient.

1.29 Differential diagnosis and diagnostic procedures for coughing

Condition	Diagnostic procedures
Tracheobronchitis	History, vaccination status, clinical signs
Chronic bronchitis	Radiography, bronchoscopy, BAL
Pneumonia	Radiography, bronchoscopy, BAL
Tumours	Radiography; BAL; search for primary tumour if pattern is metastatic
Cardiac disease	Radiography, ECG, ultrasonography
Asthma	Clinical examination, radiography, bronchoscopy, BAL
Foreign body inhalation (usually right lung)	Radiography, bronchoscopy
Parasitic (e.g. *Oslerus osleri*)	Radiography, bronchoscopy, BAL; faecal examination
Tracheal collapse	Radiography, fluoroscopy, bronchoscopy

BAL = bronchoalveolar lavage

Dyspnoea and tachypnoea

- Dyspnoea is an inappropriate degree of respiratory effort in the context of respiratory rate, rhythm and character. The term is used interchangeably with respiratory distress.
- Tachypnoea is an increased rate of breathing, not necessarily an indicator of distress. While tachypnoea can arise from dyspnoea, it can also arise through physiological reasons such as exercise, anxiety and panting in hot weather.

Dyspnoea and tachypnoea may be features of respiratory tract disease or may be associated with systemic disease, including central nervous system disorders, cardiac disease and disorders of the red blood cells.

Primary respiratory disorders can be divided into obstructive and restrictive disorders. Obstructive disorders arise through obstruction of any site in the respiratory system and are usually divided into upper (above the thoracic inlet) and lower (below the thoracic inlet) airway diseases:

- Upper airway disease is clinically manifest by increased *inspiratory* effort
- Lower airway disease is clinically manifest by increased *expiratory* effort.

History
Collection of a detailed history is essential to determine whether a systemic or primary respiratory disease is present. Careful questioning of the owner may help in this differentiation.

- What is the age, sex and breed of the patient?
- What is its vaccination status?
- Is there any history of trauma?
- Has there been any known access to poisons?
- Are there any other symptoms present?

Physical examination
Although a thorough physical examination should be carried out, particular attention should be paid to the following:

- What is the colour of the mucous membranes?
- Is the patient pyrexic?
- What is the capillary refill time?
- Observation of the patient's breathing pattern
- Careful examination of the oral cavity and pharynx
- Auscultation of the thorax for both lung and cardiac function
- Checking the femoral pulses
- Looking for signs of other body system involvement.

Differential diagnosis
Information derived from the clinical examination and further diagnostic procedures should be used to work through the differential diagnosis as shown in Figure 1.30.

Nasal discharge
Nasal discharge is a common presenting feature of primary diseases affecting the nasal passages and sinuses. In some circumstances a nasal discharge may also result from systemic disease such as distemper and cat 'flu in which case the discharge is usually acute in nature. A nasal discharge is considered chronic if it has been present for more than 3 weeks.

- Acute nasal discharge in the dog and cat is most commonly the result of systemic disease or localized respiratory infection
- Chronic nasal discharge may arise from prolongation of acute disease, especially where secondary infection becomes established following viral infection.

History
A detailed history should be collected to help determine whether systemic disease is present. In particular the following information may be of value:

- What is the age, breed and sex of the patient?
- What is its vaccination status?
- Is there a recent history of kennelling?
- Are other pets in the household affected?
- What is the nature of the discharge: blood, serous, mucoid, mucopurulent?
- Is it a unilateral or bilateral discharge?
- Is the patient able to breath through its nose?
- Is there any coughing, sneezing or dysphagia?
- Has there been any history of facial trauma?

Physical examination
The physical examination should support the findings of the history and help the clinician determine whether the problem appears to be primarily respiratory or a systemic disease. The following should be carefully assessed:

1.30 Differential diagnosis and diagnostic procedures for dyspnoea and tachypnoea

Condition	Diagnostic procedures
Obstructive disorders	
Laryngeal paralysis Tracheal collapse Asthma Pneumonia Pharyngeal/laryngeal tumours Neoplasia Bronchitis Paraquat poisoning	History; physical examination; endoscopy of the pharynx, larynx and lower airways; bronchoalveolar lavage; radiography; fluoroscopy
Restrictive disorders	
Pneumonia (with failure to expand lungs) Pneumothorax Pleural effusions Trauma/haemothorax Diaphragmatic rupture Mediastinal tumours	Radiography; thoracocentesis; fine needle aspiration of masses; ultrasonography
Red blood cell disorders	
Anaemia Methaemoglobinaemia	Routine haematology; reticulocyte count; history of access to poisons
Cardiac disease	Radiography; ECG; ultrasonography
Central nervous system disorders	Look for signs of pain; look for evidence of head trauma; radiography; neurological examination

- Is there any evidence of pyrexia?
- Is there any asymmetry of the face?
- Is there any facial swelling?
- Is there any facial pain?
- Can the patient breathe through each nostril?
- What is the character of the nasal discharge?
- If blood, is there evidence of bleeding elsewhere?
- Are the submandibular lymph nodes enlarged?
- Are there any associated oral lesions?

Differential diagnosis

From the information collected above the clinician should be able to make a short list of differential diagnoses and carry out the necessary tests in order to reach a definitive diagnosis (Figure 1.31).

1.31 **Differential diagnosis and diagnostic procedures for a nasal discharge**

Condition	Diagnostic procedures
Viral rhinitis	Viral isolation; clinical examination
Secondary bacterial rhinitis	Culture and sensitivity testing
Nasal tumours	Radiography; endoscopy and biopsy
Aspergillosis	Radiography; endoscopy and biopsy for culture; serology
Chronic rhinitis	Endoscopy and biopsy for histopathology
Foreign body	Radiographs; endoscopy

Weight loss

History

Animals lose weight as a consequence of many different clinical conditions. The degree of weight loss present and the speed at which the loss has occurred can provide a very useful indicator of the severity of disease. Thus, an animal that has lost 30% of its body weight in 2 weeks is much more seriously ill than one which has been unwell for 2 months but has lost only 10% of its body weight.

It is also useful to view weight loss in association with the animal's eating behaviour (see Polyphagia). Where the animal is polyphagic but losing weight this may suggest a problem associated with the utilization of nutrients, neoplasia or some systemic endocrine disease.

Physical examination

Where an animal has lost a considerable amount of weight, its serum protein levels may also be reduced, i.e. the animal becomes hypoproteinaemic. The physical examination does not always reveal evidence of hypoproteinaemia, though it may be manifest as ascites, hydrothorax and/or subcutaneous oedema. If weight loss and consequent hypoproteinaemia occur slowly, compensatory mechanisms may prevent these symptoms from developing. In all cases where there is marked weight loss, serum protein levels should be checked.

Differential diagnosis

So large is the list of differential diagnoses associated with weight loss that it is rarely listed when investigating clinical cases. If the animal is hypoproteinaemic, the differential diagnosis can be reduced. Rather than looking at weight loss as

a differential diagnosis, therefore, it should be used as a marker of severity of disease.

Weight gain may be used as a monitor of success in the treatment of many conditions. Where the animal gains weight following instigation of a treatment regime, this should be viewed as a good prognostic sign.

The bleeding patient

Haemorrhage may be acute or chronic and may have a number of causes, including abnormalities of the blood clotting process. Haemostasis is a complex physiological process involving the interaction of the blood vessels, the platelets, the coagulation cascade and the fibrinolytic mechanism.

- The vascular response and the platelet response constitute *primary haemostasis*
- The coagulation cascade is *secondary haemostasis*
- The fibrinolytic pathway constitutes *tertiary haemostasis*.

Primary haemostasis begins when the vascular endothelium is damaged. The blood vessel wall constricts, reducing the size of the damage. Exposed subendothelial structures attract platelets and induce their loose aggregation. These mechanisms in turn initiate the generation of thrombin and eventually fibrin, which aggregates platelets irreversibly and causes the formation of a clot. This is secondary haemostasis (Figure 1.32). Simultaneously, limiting processes are activated that confine haemostasis to the site of injury. Finally, lysis of the platelet fibrin network occurs when vascular endothelium has regenerated.

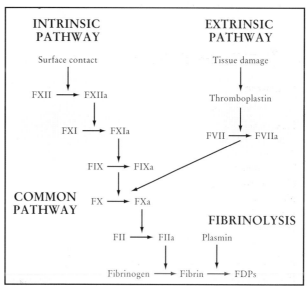

1.32 *The coagulation cascade, showing secondary and tertiary haemostasis.*

History

The complicated process of haemostasis can often be daunting to the clinician faced with a bleeding patient. It is therefore particularly important to collect a detailed history of events including:

- At what age was bleeding was first noticed?
- What is the frequency of bleeding?
- Is bleeding associated with major or minor trauma?

- Is there a family history of bleeding?
- Has there been any access to poisons, such as warfarin?
- Is there any evidence of bleeding into urine, faeces or body cavities?
- How is the bleeding manifest?
- Is there any evidence of coughing, haematemesis or melaena?
- Is the patient receiving drugs such as oestrogens, sulphonamides, chloramphenicol, aspirin or other non-steroidal anti-inflammatory agents?
- Has the animal had surgery?

Physical examination

Figures 1.33 and 1.34 illustrate possible clinical presentations of bleeding. A thorough physical examination should be carried out, with particular attention being paid to the type of bleeding observed in the patient.

- Are there petechial haemorrhages on the mucous membranes or sclera?
- Is there evidence of oral bleeding or epistaxis?
- Is there evidence of prolonged bleeding after venepuncture?
- Is there evidence of bleeding occurring into a body cavity?
- Are there any subcutaneous haematomas?
- Is haematuria, haematemesis, melaena or haematochezia present?
- Look for an underlying systemic condition.

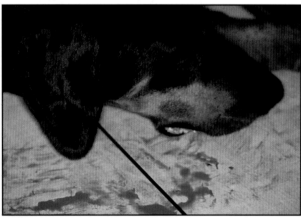

1.33 *Dog with persistent bleeding associated with von Willebrand factor disease.*

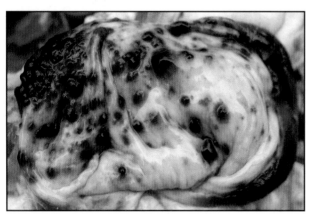

1.34 *Gastric mucosa from a dog with severe immune-mediated thrombocytopenia. Multiple petechial (pinpoint) and ecchymotic (paint brush) haemorrhages can be seen.*

Differential diagnosis

Figure 1.35 shows the differential diagnostic procedures used in acute and chronic haemorrhage. From the information collected above it should be possible to determine whether the bleeding is associated with a primary or secondary haemostatic disorder. Primary defects manifest as prolonged bleeding following venepuncture and petechial haemorrhages. Secondary disorders are manifest as epistaxis, haematuria and haematoma formation. Within each of these main categories there exists a number of differential diagnoses (Figure 1.35). The relationship between the clotting cascade and coagulation tests is shown in Figure 1.36.

1.35 Differential diagnoses and diagnostic procedures for haemorrhage

Condition	Diagnostic procedures
Acute	
Trauma	Routine haematology,
Surgical	thrombocyte count, examination
Ruptured viscera	for external bleeding, examination
Coagulopathies	of body cavities, check clotting
Thrombocytopenia	factors, radiography
Chronic	
Gastrointestinal ulceration	Examination of faeces for fresh blood or melaena, worm egg
Internal neoplasms	count in faeces, drug history,
Hookworm infection	radiography, ultrasonography

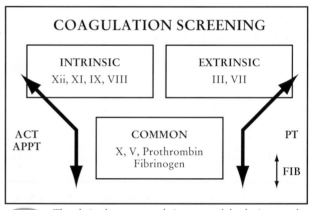

1.36 *The relation between coagulation tests and the clotting cascade. Prothrombin time (PT) is a measure of the integrity of the extrinsic pathway. The activated clotting time (ACT) and activated partial thromboplastin time (APPT) are measures of the integrity of the intrinsic pathway. Fibrinogen (FIB) measurement evaluates the common pathway.*

It is important not to rely on automated platelet (thrombocyte) counts as they are unreliable. Some animals produce large platelets which are then counted as red blood cells, thus giving an artificially low platelet count. Where a low platelet count is found but there is no evidence of bleeding, carry out a manual platelet count to determine the count more accurately.

The normal platelet count should be in the range of 200 to 500 x 10^9/l. Thrombocytopenia is considered present when the count falls below 40 x 10^9/l. Spontaneous bleeding occurs when the platelet count falls below 20 x 10^9/l. A low platelet count may be the result of:

- Reduced production of platelets from the bone marrow
- Increased consumption of platelets
- Immune-mediated disease with destruction of platelets.

All the clotting factors involved in the secondary haemostatic mechanism are produced in the liver. When there is severe disease of the liver, clotting factors may become deficient and bleeding may occur.

Disseminated intravascular coagulation (DIC) is a common acquired coagulopathy seen in a number of disease states including trauma, neoplasia and certain haemolytic disorders. It occurs when there is diffuse activation of haemostatic mechanisms *in vivo*. For activation to occur there must be either a release of tissue factors into the circulation or endothelial damage with exposure of components of the blood vessel wall. It may also occur when there has been vascular stasis with acidosis and electrolyte imbalances.

Episodic weakness

In clinical terms, weakness can be considered to include fatigue (lack of energy), asthenia (generalized muscle weakness) and syncope (fainting).

Episodic weakness and syncope are common reasons for presentation to the veterinary surgeon. With syncope the patient actually loses consciousness for a variable period of time. The difference between fatigue and asthenia is subjective and there is no clear demarcation between the two states.

History
There is a very large differential diagnosis list for these conditions, so it is particularly important to collect a detailed history, which should include the following questions:

- What is the age, breed and sex of the patient?
- Did the clinical signs develop suddenly?
- How long has the patient exhibited weakness?
- Is there any change in the patient's demeanour?
- Is there any change in appetite?
- Is there any change in thirst?
- Is the patient able to exercise?
- Does exercise bring on an episode of weakness?
- Is there any coughing or respiratory distress?
- Is there any weight loss?
- Is there any evidence of alopecia?

Physical examination
The information collected above should be substantiated and supplemented by carrying out a full physical examination. In particular the following should be noted:

- Heart rate and rhythm, presence of heart murmurs, pulse deficits or dysfunction
- Colour of the mucous membranes and the capillary refill time
- Respiratory rate and rhythm – by auscultation, percussion and compression of the thorax
- Thorough neurological examination.

In many cases where there is episodic weakness or collapse, it is rarely observed in the clinic. The patient may appear completely normal between episodes. In some cases it may be useful to keep the patient in the clinic for observation or to simulate the circumstance under which weakness occurs. This latter procedure must be carried out with great care.

Differential diagnosis
The differential diagnosis of weakness or collapse is diverse, as are the types of diagnostic procedures required in order to reach a definitive diagnosis (Figure 1.37).

Seizures

A seizure is an episode that results from disturbance of the electrical activity of the brain.

Seizures are one of the most common causes of collapse in the dog. The seizure starts within the brain at a focus which consists of a group of neurons that demonstrate a reduced threshold of excitability and lack sufficient control from inhibitory neurons. Status epilepticus is a term used to describe successive or prolonged seizure activity without recovery of consciousness.

History
Although in the young adult dog, seizures may be idiopathic – often termed idiopathic epilepsy – there are many other causes

1.37 **Differential diagnosis and diagnostic procedures for episodic weakness**

Condition	Blood tests	Urinalysis	Cardiac assessment	Other tests
Anaemia	Haematology	No	No	Bone marrow biopsy
Hypoglycaemia	Glucose, insulin	No	No	Ultrasonography
Cardiac disease	No	No	Valuable	Radiography, ultrasonography
Pulmonary disease	Haematology, biochemistry	No	No	Bronchoalveolar lavage, bronchoscopy, radiography
Hypoadrenocorticism	Haematology, biochemistry	Valuable	No	ACTH stimulation test
Hyperadrenocorticism	Haematology, biochemistry	Valuable	No	ACTH stimulation test
Diabetes mellitus	Biochemistry	Valuable	No	Urinalysis
Hypothyroidism	Haematology, biochemistry	No	No	TSH test
Myasthenia gravis	ACh receptor test	No	No	Edrophonium test
Renal failure	Haematology, biochemistry	Valuable	No	Ultrasonography, urinalysis
Hepatic failure	Haematology, biochemistry	Valuable	No	Ultrasonography, biopsy
Generalized myopathy	Haematology, biochemistry	No	No	Electromyogram, muscle biopsy
Hypocalcaemia	Biochemistry	No	No	History

ACh = acetylcholine; ACTH = adrenocorticotropic hormone; TSH = thyroid stimulating hormone

of seizures that should be considered. It is important to remember that it is very rare to observe a seizure occurring and most patients appear clinically normal on physical examination. Collection of a detailed history is therefore of particular importance in this condition. The following questions may be of value in determining the cause of seizure activity:

- What is the age, sex and breed of the patient?
- What is the vaccination status?
- Is there a previous history of distemper?
- How is the patient's appetite?
- Is there any evidence of PUPD?
- Is the patient losing weight?
- How many seizures has the patient had?
- How long do the seizures last?
- What is the patient doing just prior to having a seizure?
- Describe in detail what happens during a seizure.
- How does the patient behave just after a seizure?
- What is the general responsiveness of the patient?
- Is there any history of access to poisons?

Physical examination

Even though the patient may be apparently 'normal' at the time of presentation, it is important to carry out a detailed physical examination, as seizures may be a feature of systemic disease. In particular pay attention to the following:

- Is the patient pyrexic?
- What is the demeanour of the patient?
- Is the patient responsive?
- Is there any evidence of halitosis – ketotic or uraemic?
- Is cardiac function normal?
- Is there any evidence of head trauma?

Differential diagnosis

Based on the information gathered from the clinical examination it may be possible to determine whether the seizures are occurring as a consequence of an intracranial or extracranial disorder. Within these categories there is a number of differential diagnoses. In order to determine the exact cause of the seizure, further diagnostic procedures are required (Figure 1.38).

Ataxia, paresis and paralysis

Ataxia, paresis and paralysis are gait alterations associated with abnormalities of the central or peripheral nervous systems.

Ataxia

Ataxia is a failure of muscle coordination which may follow loss of sensory perception or dysfunction of the vestibular system or cerebellum.

History

A detailed history is essential when considering a patient with ataxia. In particular, the following questions may be of value:

- How old is the patient?
- What is the vaccination status of the patient and its mother?
- Is there any history of trauma?
- Is the patient aware of its surroundings and is it responsive?
- Does the patient turn continuously in circles to the right or left?
- Is there a head tilt present?
- Does the patient fall over?
- Does the patient's eye flick from side to side?
- Does the patient bump into objects, suggesting blindness?

Physical examination

- Is there evidence of trauma?
- Is there evidence of strabismus or nystagmus?
- Is there a head tilt?
- Are there any other cranial nerve defects?
- Does the patient circle?

1.38 Differential diagnosis and diagnostic procedures for seizures

Condition	Blood tests	Urinalysis	Imaging	Other tests
Intracranial				
Meningitis	No	No	No	CSF tap
Neoplasia	No	No	MRI, CT	CSF tap
Infections	Haematology	No	No	CSF tap and culture
Epilepsy	No	No	No	History
Toxicity (lead)	Haematology, biochemistry	No	No	History
Trauma	No	No	Valuable	Neurological examination
Extracranial				
Hypoglycaemia	Blood sugar, insulin	No	No	Exploratory surgery
Hepatoencephalopathy	SALT, SAP, bile acids, ammonia	Biurate crystals	Plain radiography, ultrasonography	Biopsy
Uraemia	Blood urea, creatinine	Valuable	Ultrasonography	
Hypocalcaemia	Serum calcium	No	Plain radiography of bones	History? Lactation?
Ketoacidosis	Blood sugar	Valuable	No	No

CSF = cerebrospinal fluid; CT = computed tomography; MRI = magnetic resonance imaging; SALT = serum alanine aminotransferase; SAP = serum alkaline phosphatase

- Is the patient responsive?
- Is there evidence of ear infection?
- If the patient is a cat, is there a history of feline enteritis infection in the household?

Differential diagnosis
The information provided from the clinical examination will assist in reaching a diagnosis. Figure 1.39 lists the possible differential diagnoses.

1.39 Differential diagnosis of ataxia

Condition	Features
Peripheral vestibular disease	Head tilt, ataxia, strabismus, nystagmus Usually responsive to therapy within one week May be associated with ear infection or Horner's syndrome
Central vestibular disease	As for above but also includes generalized loss of postural and proprioceptive function Multiple cranial nerve deficits
Cerebellar ataxia	Usually neonatal kitten or puppy. Queen may have had feline enteritis while pregnant Ataxia, intention tremor and dysmetria affecting all limbs

Paresis and paralysis

- Paresis is a partial loss of voluntary motor function in a body part.
- Paralysis is the complete loss of voluntary motor function of a body part
  - *Quadriplegia* describes the loss of motor function in all four limbs
  - *Paraplegia* describes the loss of motor function in the hindlimbs. It implies a spinal lesion between T3 and S1
  - *Hemiplegia* describes the loss of motor function on a fore and hindlimb involving one side of the patient.

The key to the successful management of these cases relies on determining the precise location of the lesion in the nervous system by a careful and logical neurological examination (see below).

- Paresis or paralysis of both fore and hindlimbs suggests disease affecting the cervical spinal cord or brain. It may also occur when there is a diffuse peripheral nerve disorder
- Paresis or paralysis predominantly affecting the forelimbs suggests disease affecting the cervical spinal cord
- Paresis or paralysis affecting predominantly the hindlimbs suggests disease affecting the thoracic or lumbar spinal cord
- Paresis or paralysis of a single limb suggests damage to a peripheral nerve supplying that limb.

To understand the clinical outcomes of diseases affecting the spinal cord, the peripheral nerves are considered to be either lower motor neurons (LMNs) or upper motor neurons (UMNs) (Figure 1.40). The former carry impulses from the spinal cord to the muscle; the latter carry impulses to and from the brain within the spinal cord.

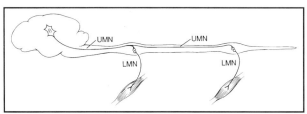

1.40 *Diagrammatic representation of upper (UMNs) and lower motor neurons (LMNs) supplying the limbs. The UMNs are shown as a single pathway and interneurons are not shown. Reproduced from* BSAVA Manual of Small Animal Neurology.

- Signs of LMN disease can result in paresis or flaccid paralysis with loss of normal reflexes
- Signs of UMN disease can also lead to paresis or paralysis where muscle tone is retained. However, this muscle tone may be altered in character.

History
Always carry out a detailed history but in particular include the following questions:

- How old was the animal when symptoms were first noted?
- What is the vaccination status of the patient?
- Is there a history of trauma?
- How quickly did the clinical signs develop?
- How long have the clinical signs been present?
- Is the patient responsive and aware?
- Are there any other clinical symptoms present?

Physical examination
A thorough physical examination is required and in this case must include a detailed neurological examination in order to determine the location of the lesion:

- Observe the patient's ability to move and assess which limbs are affected
- Carry out a detailed neurological examination
  - Cranial nerve function
  - Sensory perception
  - Muscle tone
  - Reflexes (see Figure 1.41)
  - Conscious proprioception
  - Pain response
  - Bladder function
  - Anal tone
  - Tail function
- Look for signs of trauma even if owner suggests this has not occurred.

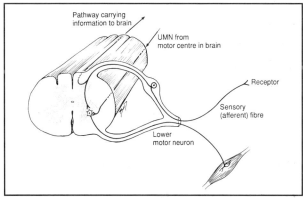

1.41 *Diagrammatic representation of a simple reflex arc that can be clinically tested. Damage to lower motor neurons and/or the sensory fibre will interrupt the reflex. Damage to the upper motor neurons or spinal cord will not affect the reflex. Reproduced from* BSAVA Manual of Small Animal Neurology.

Differential diagnosis and diagnostic procedures for paresis and paralysis

Condition	Diagnostic procedures
Spinal cord disease	
Traumatic spinal injury Intervertebral disc protrusion Congenital spinal lesions Cervical spondylopathy (Wobblers syndrome) Spinal tumours Discospondylitis Chronic degenerative radiculomyopathy	Clinical examination; neurological examination; radiography; myelography; cerebrospinal fluid analysis
Peripheral nerve disorders	
Traumatic nerve damage Polyreticuloneuritis	Neurological examination; nerve biopsy; electromyography; nerve conduction velocity
Myopathies	
Myasthenia gravis Hyperadrenocorticism	Acetylcholine receptor antibody test; serum biochemistry; ACTH stimulation test; dexamathasone tests; electromyography

ACTH = adrenocorticotropic hormone

Differential diagnosis

From the clinical examination of the patient it may be possible to reach a diagnosis. However, in most cases further diagnostic procedures will require to reach a definitive diagnosis (Figure 1.42).

Physical signs

The physical examination of the patient involves a careful assessment of many parameters including rectal temperature, mucous membrane colour, and evaluation of peripheral lymph nodes. In addition, abnormal findings such as nasal discharge, evidence of bleeding and neurological deficits may be detected. The purpose of this section of the chapter is to interpret the causes of changes and abnormalities.

Pyrexia

Pyrexia (fever) is a rise in body temperature above reference values as a normal physiological response to infection (acute or chronic), excitement, pain, tumours or anxiety.

The body's 'thermostat' resides in the hypothalamus of the brain and keeps body temperature within a narrow range. Pyrexia arises through the release of endogenous pyrogens which reset the hypothalamus thermostat to a higher level. Normal rectal temperatures for dogs and cats are:

- Dogs: 38.3 to 38.7°C
- Cats: 38.0 to 38.5°C.

When an elevated rectal temperature is detected in a patient, the history and physical examination are used to look for a possible cause for this alteration in homeostasis. Information which may help in determining the cause of pyrexia includes:

- The age, sex and breed of the patient
- The vaccination status
- How long has the patient has been ill?
- Was the onset sudden (acute), slow (chronic) or does the body temperature fluctuate?
- Is the patient lame?
- Is there evidence of exercise intolerance?
- Is there changes in body weight?
- Are symptoms such as vomiting, diarrhoea or PUPD present?
- Is there evidence of pain?
- Has the owner detected any masses?
- What is the patient's demeanour?
- Are there any discharges?
- Is there joint swelling or pain?
- Are there changes in the heart and lungs?
- Are there abnormalities on palpation of the abdomen?
- Is there evidence of lymphadenopathy (see below)?
- Are there any skin changes?

It is important to consider other key points at the time of the clinical examination. Car journeys to the surgery cause stress and excitement and may elevate body temperature. Pyrexia may induce shivering or thirst leading potentially to dehydration. Depression, lethargy and unresponsiveness increase as body temperature rises.

Differential diagnosis

Most cases of pyrexia encountered in small animal practice are of infectious origin. Often the history and physical examination will identify the underlying problem and the most appropriate therapy can be initiated. However, there are instances where the cause is not clear and in these cases the term pyrexia of unknown origin (PUO) is used. These cases always require an investigation in order to find the underlying cause. Ultimately PUO cases can be divided equally into infectious, immune-mediated or neoplastic causes. Figure 1.43 shows the most likely differential diagnosis and diagnostic procedures of value to the clinician.

Differential diagnosis and diagnostic procedures for pyrexia

Condition	Blood tests	Imaging	Culture	Other tests
Infectious				
Acute (distemper)	Haematology	Thoracic radiography	Discharge for secondary infection	Serology
Subacute (e.g. cat bites)	Haematology	No	Useful	Sensitivity testing
Chronic (e.g. pyelonephritis)	Haematology	Ultrasonography	Urine culture	Sensitivity testing
Non-infectious				
Immune-mediated diseases	Haematology, Coombs' test, antinuclear antibody	Joints	No	Cytology, bone marrow biopsy
Tumours	Haematology, biochemistry	Very useful	No	Fine needle biopsy, cytology

Mucous membrane colour

Examination of the mucous membranes forms an integral part of the physical examination. Many systemic diseases will manifest themselves in mucous membrane changes such as pallor, jaundice, congestion, cyanosis and petechial haemorrhages.

Pallor

The two main causes of this change are shock and, perhaps more commonly, anaemia. Pallor in shocked animals can be the result of closure of small capillary beds in the peripheral circulation in order to maintain adequate perfusion of the heart and brain. Typically, animals that are shocked are recumbent and have cool extremities and rapid pulses.

Shock is discussed in the *BSAVA Manual of Veterinary Nursing*, Chapter 3. The remainder of this section will focus on anaemia.

Anaemia

Anaemia may be defined as a reduction in the packed cell volume (PCV), red blood cell count (RBCs) and haemoglobin (Hb) concentration of the blood when compared with the accepted normal values for the appropriate species, age and sex.

Anaemia is always associated with an underlying disease. It arises (Figure 1.44) because of:

- Inadequate production of erythrocytes (RBCs) by the bone marrow
- Increased destruction of RBCs (haemolysis)
- Increased loss of RBCs from the vasculature (haemorrhage).

1.44 **Causes of anaemia**

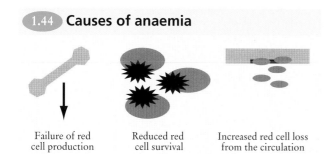

| Failure of red cell production | Reduced red cell survival | Increased red cell loss from the circulation |

The inevitable consequence of anaemia is reduced oxygen carrying capacity of the blood. The clinical features of the anaemic patient are therefore due to inadequate tissue oxygenation. In addition there will be clinical signs associated with the underlying cause.

The clinical features are also determined by the speed of development of the anaemia. In chronically anaemic patients there are certain physiological mechanisms that allow the patient to compensate for the low haemoglobin concentration in the blood. Consequently the chronically anaemic patient may show modest clinical signs compared to the patient with acute anaemia, for example from a large acute haemorrhage. The general clinical symptoms exhibited by anaemic patients include:

- Pallor of the mucous membranes
- Weakness
- Tachycardia
- Tachypnoea
- Haemic cardiac murmur
- Bounding pulse.

The key to determining the cause of anaemia is collection of a detailed history from the client and a thorough physical examination. Specific questions which may assist in determining the cause of the anaemia include:

- What is the age, breed and sex of the patient?
- What is its vaccination status?
- How quickly has the patient become ill?
- Is there any history of exercise intolerance?
- Has the patient collapsed, fainted or appeared lethargic?
- Is there any evidence of external blood loss?
- Is there any recent history of drug administration?
- Has there been access to poisons?
- What colour is the urine?
- Are there any other signs of systemic disease, e.g. PUPD?

When examining the patient, particular attention is paid to the following:

- Evidence of shock
- Capillary refill time
- Is cardiac function normal?
- Can a cardiac murmur be detected?
- Is the patient adequately hydrated?
- Is the patient pyrexic?
- Is there any peripheral lymphadenopathy?
- Is there any evidence of hydrothorax or ascites?

The first step in evaluating the anaemic patient is routine haematology of a blood sample. The packed cell volume will indicate the extent to which the patient is anaemic (Figure 1.45).

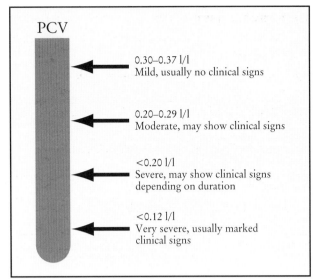

PCV

0.30–0.37 l/l
Mild, usually no clinical signs

0.20–0.29 l/l
Moderate, may show clinical signs

<0.20 l/l
Severe, may show clinical signs
depending on duration

<0.12 l/l
Very severe, usually marked
clinical signs

1.45 *Packed cell volume is a guide to the severity of anaemia. The values may be given as a percentage (0.30 l/l = 30%).*

The next step is to determine whether the anaemia is regenerative or non-regenerative (Figure 1.46). This is achieved by measuring the number of reticulocytes present in the circulating blood. If the reticulocyte count is below 1%, the anaemia is said to be non-regenerative.

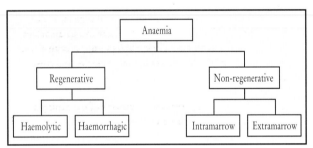

1.46 *Anaemia is either regenerative or non-regenerative. The hallmark of regenerative anaemia is the presence of reticulocytes in the circulation.*

Regenerative anaemias occur in situations where there is an increased production of red cells to compensate for the increased loss. Regenerative anaemias occur after haemorrhage (see above) or haemolysis (Figure 1.47). When red blood cells are destroyed within the blood vessels this is called intravascular haemolysis (Figure 1.48). When the red cells are removed from the circulation by mononuclear phagocytes this is called extravascular haemolysis (Figure 1.49). Extravascular haemolysis occurs more commonly than intravascular haemolysis. Figure 1.50 shows the differential diagnosis and diagnostic factors for haemolysis.

Non-regenerative anaemias are defined as where there is a reticulocyte count below 1%. There are essentially two broad classifications:

- Extra-bone marrow disease, for example where there is a lack of erythropoietin production in renal disease
- Intra-bone marrow disease, for example where there is a generalized marrow dysfunction such as in leukaemia.

Diagnostic factors for the differentiation of these are shown in Figure 1.51.

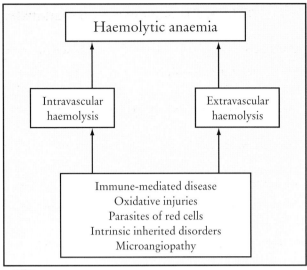

1.47 *Causes of haemolytic anaemia.*

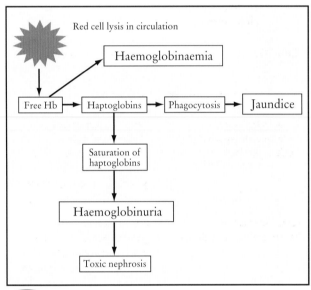

1.48 *Intravascular haemolysis.*

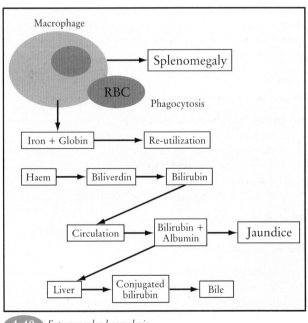

1.49 *Extravascular haemolysis.*

Differential diagnoses and diagnostic procedures for haemolysis

Condition	Diagnostic procedures and pointers
Immune-mediated anaemia	Haematology reveals spherocytes; Coombs' test usually positive; slide agglutination test positive
Methaemoglobinaemia (e.g. paracetamol poisoning)	Chocolate brown coloured blood; Heinz body formation; history of access; possible liver failure
Haemobartonella felis infection	Haematology; look for parasitaemia (cyclical) using Wright's stain on blood smear
Pyruvate kinase deficiency	Very rare; examine for specific enzyme deficiency
Microangiopathy (e.g. splenic haemangiosarcoma)	Haematology reveals mechanical shearing of red blood cells
Copper toxicity	Bedlington Terrier; associated liver disease

1.51 Non-regenerative anaemia: extra- versus intra-bone marrow disease

Condition	Diagnostic procedures
Extra-bone marrow disease	
Anaemia of chronic disease Chronic renal failure Hypothyroidism Hypoadrenocorticism FeLV infection	Examine patient for underlying disease; renal function tests; check thyroid and adrenal gland function; check cats for FeLV infection; measure serum erythropoietin levels
Intra-bone marrow disease	
Aplastic anaemia Myeloproliferative disease	Routine haematology for pancytopenia, leukaemias, cytopenias of single cell lines; bone marrow biopsy

Cyanosis

Cyanosis is a bluish colour of the mucous membranes (or skin) as a result of an increased amount of deoxygenated haemoglobin in the blood. Cyanosis can be considered to be either central or peripheral in origin.

History

As part of the history ask questions regarding the following:

- Did the cyanosis occur suddenly?
- How long has the patient been cyanotic?
- Is the patient on any medications?
- Has there been any access to poisons?
- Is the patient in pain?
- Has there been any syncopal episodes?

Physical examination

A thorough physical examination should be carried out and should assess the following:

- Is there a patent airway?
- What is the nature of the patient's respirations?
- Is there evidence of weakness, paresis or paralysis?
- Are there changes on auscultation of the thorax?
- Are there any abnormalities of the extremities?

Differential diagnosis

From the information obtained in the clinical examination it should be possible to determine whether the cyanosis is central or peripheral:

- Central cyanosis is a generalized condition that affects all mucous membranes and the skin. It arises either through lack of oxygen in the arterial blood or through increased methaemoglobin formation
- Peripheral cyanosis occurs in a localized region of the body. It is usually associated with occlusion of an artery, such as occurs with thromboembolism, hypercoagulable disease such as nephrotic syndrome, or cold agglutinin disease.

The differential diagnosis and methods of obtaining a definitive diagnosis are shown in Figure 1.52.

1.52 Differential diagnosis and diagnostic procedures for cyanosis

Condition	Diagnostic procedures
Central	
Poor oxygenation at anaesthesia	Examine patient for patent airway
Failure of muscles of ventilation	Auscultation of thorax
Pneumonia	Radiography
Airway obstruction	Radiography, endoscopy
Tracheal collapse	Bronchoscopy
Anatomical shunting of blood; venous blood in arteries	Blood gas analysis
Peripheral	
Thromboembolism	Check routine haematology
Nephrotic syndrome	Check renal function, urinalysis
Cold agglutinin disease	Check serum proteins; electrophoresis of serum proteins

Jaundice

Jaundice (icterus) is an abnormal staining of the mucous membranes and skin with bilirubin or bilirubin complexes.

Bilirubin is a waste product of the metabolism of haem when old red blood cells are broken down. The normal production of bilirubin is summarized in Figure 1.53. Increased serum levels of bilirubin arise is the following ways:

- Pre-hepatic: increased production of bilirubin following excess red cell destruction
- Hepatic: normal bilirubin production exceeds the liver's ability to eliminate the waste product
- Post-hepatic: there is obstruction to the flow of bile down the bile duct into the intestine.

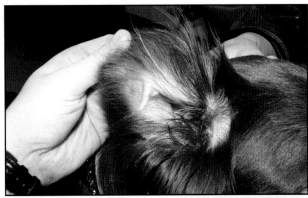
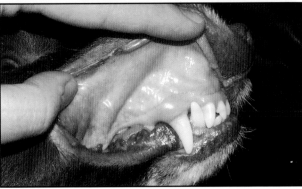

1.54 *The pinna and oral mucous membranes of a dog with severe jaundice.*

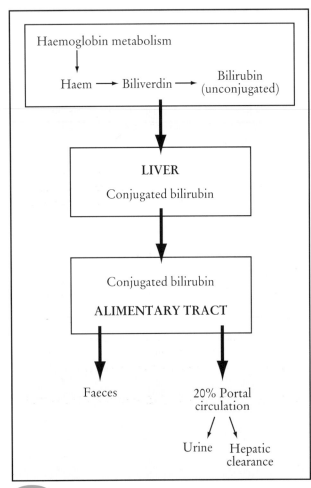

1.53 *The normal production of bilirubin.*

Bile pigments have a strong affinity for elastic tissue and thus the yellow colour can be readily seen on the sclera and mucous membranes (Figure 1.54). The serum bilirubin level gives an indication of the degree of icterus present. In the dog the level of serum bilirubin is normally less than 6 mmol/l but clinical jaundice occurs when the value exceeds 30 mmol/l.

History

The history plays an important part in determining which of the three types of jaundice described above is present. In addition to asking questions regarding all body systems the following specific questions may be of value:

- What is the age, breed and sex of the patient?
- What is its vaccination status?
- How long has the patient been jaundiced?
- Is there any other significant history, such as vomiting, diarrhoea, weight loss or PUPD?
- What colour are the faeces?
- Is there any evidence of abdominal enlargement?
- Has the patient's behaviour changed?
- Is there any exercise intolerance, weakness or collapse?

Physical examination

A thorough physical examination will assist in determining the cause of the jaundice. In particular the following should be addressed:

- Has the patient any signs of tachycardia, weak fast pulse, tachypnoea?
- Is there a haemic murmur present?
- Is there any evidence of haemoglobinuria?
- Does palpation of the abdomen reveal a change in liver size?
- Is there any hepatic pain on palpation?
- Has the patient lost weight?
- Is there any evidence of ascites?
- On rectal examination are the faeces acholic?

Differential diagnosis

From the above examination it should be possible to suspect whether the jaundice is due to severe red cell destruction, hepatic disease or biliary obstruction. There are various causes for each of these categories and different diagnostic tests are required to confirm their presence (Figure 1.55).

1.55 Differential diagnosis and diagnostic procedures for jaundice

Condition	Diagnostic procedures
Pre-hepatic	
Autoimmune haemolytic anaemia	Routine haematology; Coombs' test
Copper toxicosis	Assessment of copper levels
Haemobartonella felis	Blood smears with Wright's stain for parasitaemia
Hepatic	
Acute/chronic hepatitis Cholangiohepatitis Leptospirosis Infectious canine hepatitis Cirrhosis Hepatic lipidosis Feline infectious peritonitis	SALT, SAP, bile acids, ammonia; serum bilirubin levels; pre- and postprandial bile acids; radiography; ultrasonography; clotting factor assessment; liver biopsy
Post-hepatic	
Bile duct obstruction – cholelith – tumour Pancreatic tumour (obstructing the bile duct) Acute pancreatitis (especially cats)	Serum bilirubin; urine urobilinogen; faecal examination for fat; radiography; ultrasonography; exploratory laparotomy

SALT = serum alanine aminotransferase; SAP = serum alkaline phosphatase

Congested mucous membranes

Congested/injected mucous membranes are deep red; this may be indicative of polycythaemia, toxaemia or carbon monoxide poisoning.

History and physical examination

As congested mucous membranes are always associated with some form of systemic disease, a detailed history and physical examination are essential when looking for the underlying cause. In particular, the following should be considered:

- Is the patient dehydrated?
- Is there any history of being within a car or building where an engine is running?
- What is the sex of the patient?
- If female, is she spayed? If not, when was the last oestrus and is there any evidence of vaginal discharge?
- Check the cardiac and respiratory function carefully.

Differential diagnosis

There is a limited number of differential diagnoses for congested mucous membranes (Figure 1.56).

Lymphadenopathy

Lymphadenopathy literally means disease of the lymph nodes but the term is commonly used to describe enlarged lymph nodes. Lymphadenopathy may be solitary, regional or generalized.

History

When considering a patient with lymphadenopathy the following historical factors may be of value:

- When were the enlarged lymph nodes first observed?
- Has the patient been abroad?
- How has the patient's general health been recently?
- Has the owner noted any other symptoms?
- Are there any changes in body weight?
- Are there any cutaneous or hair coat changes?

1.56 Differential diagnosis and diagnostic procedures for congested mucous membranes

Condition	Diagnostic procedures
Polycythaemia	
Relative (dehydration)	Check PCV and total protein
Absolute (primary erythrocytosis)	Erythropoietin levels can be measured
Secondary to respiratory/cardiac disease	Assess respiratory function; radiography, bronchoscopy; alveolar lavage; assess cardiac function; ECG; ultrasonography
Toxaemia	
Bacterial infections	Blood culture
Pyometra	Radiography of abdomen; culture of discharges
Cat bite abscess	History and clinical examination; aspiration
Uraemia	Check renal function
Carbon monoxide poisoning	History

Physical examination

Figures 1.57 and 1.58 show typical clinical presentations. Where lymph node enlargement has been found, the physical examination should assess the extent of the problem:

- Are all the peripheral lymph nodes enlarged?
- Are the lymph nodes painful?
- Are the lymph nodes hard but not painful?
- Can other lymph nodes which are not normally palpable be detected?
- If a single lymph node is enlarged, are there any lesions within its drainage area?

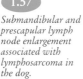
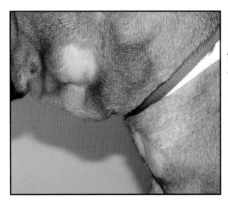

Submandibular and prescapular lymph node enlargement associated with lymphosarcoma in the dog.

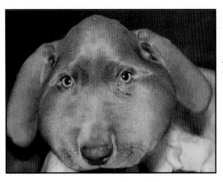

Head swelling and lymphoderitis in a puppy with 'head gland' disease.

Differential diagnosis

The commonest causes of lymph node enlargement are shown in Figure 1.59, together with the diagnostic procedures which may assist in their detection.

 Differential diagnosis and diagnostic procedures for lymphadenopathy

Condition	Diagnostic procedures
Reactive lymphadenopathy: – Immune-mediated disease – Systemic infection	Routine haematology, biochemistry; blood culture; lymph node aspiration; antinuclear antibody test
Lymphosarcoma	Aspiration or biopsy of lymph nodes
Metastatic disease	Aspiration or biopsy of lymph nodes; examine drainage region for primary tumour; radiography and ultrasonography

Diagnostic procedures

This section describes the various diagnostic procedures that have been mentioned earlier and gives some insight into how they are carried out, the nurse's role in carrying out the tests and interpretation of the results.

Sampling/biopsy techniques

Paracentesis

In this procedure the abdominal wall is aseptically prepared and a sterile 23 gauge x 1.5 inch needle is inserted attached to a sterile 20 ml syringe. The point of entry depends on the amount of fluid present but is usually behind the umbilicus on the midline.

The types of fluid that may accumulate can be differentiated by laboratory analysis as shown in Figure 1.18.

Nasal biopsy

This is indicated whenever nasal mucosal abnormalities are visualized (see Rostral rhinoscopy, below) and especially when tissue growth is present. A general anaesthetic is essential.

- 'Grab' biopsies can be performed by passing clamshell-type biopsy forceps (Figure 1.60). Care should be taken not to pass forceps beyond the medial canthus of the eye
- In some cases (especially larger dogs) a large-bore (3–5 mm) cannula attached to a 10 ml syringe can be used for nasal biopsy
  - The cannula is passed up the nostril and into the mass after premeasuring on a radiograph
  - Once the cannula is in the mass, suction is applied to aspirate the mass effectively
  - When the cannula has been removed, the core is forcefully expelled using the syringe
  - The sample is then fixed in formalin and sent for pathological examination
- In small dogs and cats, samples can also be taken using a bone curette to 'scoop' some of the mass from the nasal passages
- All of the above procedures are likely to be associated with post-biopsy haemorrhage and the animal should be monitored following the procedure.

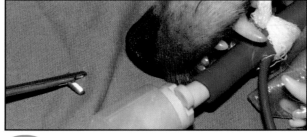

1.60 *Nasal biopsy using clamshell forceps.*

Bronchoalveolar lavage (BAL)

This is the recovery of cells or infectious agents (e.g. bacteria) from the airways for cytological examination or for the culture of organisms and the selection of the most appropriate antibiotic therapy.

Indications

- Investigation of chronic airway disease
- Suspected neoplasia
- Suspected pulmonary infiltrate with eosinophilia (PIE)
- Suspected cases of pneumonia.

Equipment

- Readily available and inexpensive
- Portex bronchoscope biopsy catheter (Figure 1.61a)
- Bitch urinary catheter
- Syringes
- Sampling solution (warm sterile saline)
- Bijou bottles
- Fixative material
- Jugular through-the-needle catheter if blind transtracheal sampling is to be performed (Figure 1.61b).

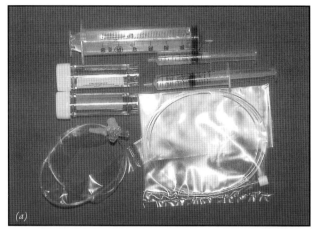

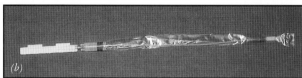

1.61 *The basic equipment required for airway sampling is readily available and inexpensive. (a) Examples of sampling equipment: Portex bronchoscope biopsy catheter, bitch urinary catheter, syringes, Bijou bottles and fixative material (Cytofix®, Shandon Ltd, UK). (b) Jugular through-the-needle catheter for transtracheal sampling.*
Reproduced from the BSAVA Manual of Small Animal Cardiorespiratory Medicine and Surgery, *edited by V. Luis Fuentes and S. Swift.*

Techniques

The bronchoscopic, blind sampling and transtracheal/translaryngeal techniques are described in Figure 1.62. Figure 1.63 shows the anatomical placement of the catheters for transtracheal/translaryngeal sampling.

Skin punch biopsy

Indications

- Suspected neoplastic condition
- Persistent ulceration of the skin
- Skin conditions not responding to conventional treatment
- Vesicular-type skin conditions.

Biopsy may be incisional or excisional (under general anaesthetic) but a punch biopsy is simple and inexpensive to perform.

Equipment
4–6 mm biopsy punch.

Technique
Taking a skin biopsy is described in Figure 1.64.

1.62 Techniques for bronchoalveolar lavage

Bronchoscopic technique

- Endoscope (with catheter in biopsy channel) is passed into bronchus serving lung area of interest
- Aliquot of saline (2 ml for cats, 2–15 ml for dogs) is injected and immediately aspirated
- Approximately 50% recovery of fluid
- Recovered fluid is divided, some for cytological examination and some for culture
- Procedure is repeated two or three times.

Blind sampling

- Where endoscope is not available
- Sampling catheter is passed as far as possible into respiratory tract
- Solution is infused and aspirated as described above, with about 20–30% recovery.

Transtracheal and translaryngeal sampling

- Site is clipped and aseptically prepared
- Patient is sedated and local anaesthetic used through to airway lumen
- With animal in sternal recumbency, 2–4 mm skin incision is made and wide-bore (12–14 G) hypodermic needle is inserted into airway lumen (between tracheal rings or through cricothyroid ligament)
- Catheter is advanced through needle (by pre-determined distance)
- Solution is instilled and aspirated as described above.

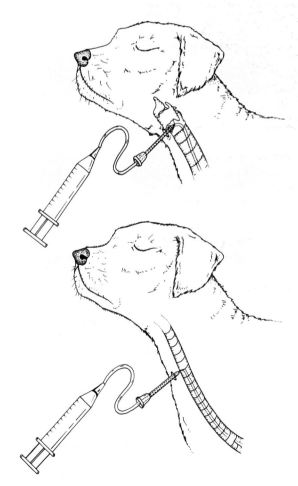

1.63 *Anatomical drawings illustrating the methods for translaryngeal (cricothyroid ligament) and transtracheal airway sampling.*

1.64 Skin punch biopsy

1. Adequate restraint (or sedation) of patient.
2. Clip the site and gently clean with 70% alcohol.

> The site must never be scrubbed or treated with antiseptics containing iodine.

3. Infiltrate around site with local anaesthetic (1–2 ml of 2% lignocaine).
4. Use biopsy punch to excise tissue, including underlying fat.
5. Take care to minimize trauma to specimen.
6. Usually multiple samples are taken.
7. Close biopsy site with simple interrupted sutures.

Bone marrow biopsy

Bone marrow biopsy is often indicated in the diagnosis of conditions affecting the lymphoid and myeloid systems. It may take the form of an aspirate or a core biopsy.

Indications

- Non-regenerative anaemia of undetermined cause
- Investigation for secondary immune-mediated haemolytic anaemia
- Staging and/or diagnosis of haemopoietic tumours
- Contraindicated where there is severe thrombocytopenia or coagulopathy.

Equipment

A disposable needle for bone marrow biopsy is shown in Figure 1.65. Ancillary equipment includes glass slides, a 20 ml syringe and EDTA collection tubes.

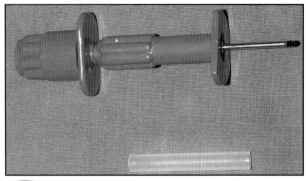

1.65 *A disposable bone marrow biopsy needle.*

Procedure

Sites for sample retrieval include the humerus, femur or iliac crest (Figure 1.66). The technique is described in Figure 1.67.

Lymph node aspiration

- Can normally be performed in conscious animal without sedation
- Uncooperative patients may need chemical restraint but infiltration of the biopsy site with local anaesthetic should be avoided because of tendency to cause tissue disruption of cells at biopsy site
- Try to avoid:
  - Largest node(s) (central necrosis likely)
  - Submandibular nodes (most dogs have gingivitis and/or periodontal disease, tends to lead to localized lymphadenopathy)

1.66 Bone marrow aspiration

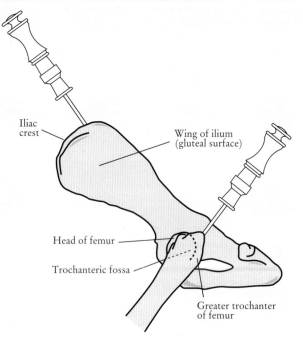

The iliac crest is the usual site for bone marrow aspiration.
Reproduced from the BSAVA Manual of Small Animal Clinical Pathology, *edited by M.G. Davidson, R.W. Else and J.H. Lumsden*

1.67 How to perform a bone marrow biopsy

1. Patient in sternal recumbency for iliac crest sample, lateral recumbency for femur sample.
2. Patient sedated; site clipped and scrubbed.
3. Site (including periosteum) infiltrated with local anaesthetic.
4. Stab incision in skin over biopsy site.
5. Bone marrow needle (Rosenthal needle with stylet in place) advanced into site and then introduced into bone in corkscrew fashion.
6. As needle passes into marrow space, may be pain reaction from dog (often indicates that needle is correctly placed).
7. Needle should be firmly in marrow space with no apparent wobble.
8. Stylet is removed; 10 ml syringe is attached to needle.
9. Bone marrow aspirated (may cause a few moments of pain) and smear made from contents of syringe.

Core sample

For core sample, use Jamshidi needle. The technique is usually performed under general anaesthesia. Carry out above procedure but, after aspirate has been retrieved:

10. Advance needle to obtain core sample
11. Rock needle back and forth after advancement to sever bone in needle from base
12. When needle is removed, use smaller wire obturator to retrograde biopsy material out of top of needle
13. Fix material in formalin for histopathology.

- Normal nodes contain at least 80% small lymphocytes
- Reactive node: variable numbers of small, medium and large lymphocytes together with plasma cells may be seen
- Cytological picture in lymphadenitis varies (many polymorphs if suppurative, macrophages if granulomatous)
- Metastasis from primary neoplasm gives cytological picture depending on parent tumour
- Cytological diagnosis relatively easy in some cases (e.g. mast cell tumours); others very difficult.

Equipment for fine needle aspirate biopsy

- Needle, 23 gauge or finer
- 10 ml hypodermic syringe
- Glass microscope slides.

Technique
The technique for fine needle aspiration biopsy is described in Figure 1.68.

1.68 Fine needle aspiration biopsy

1. Area over biopsy site is prepared aseptically.
2. Node to be biopsied is immobilized whilst the needle is advanced into it. Node should be fixed as close to surface of skin as possible.
3. Plunger is withdrawn rapidly six times, creating sufficient negative pressure in syringe to aspirate tissue sample. During procedure, needle may be repositioned several times without withdrawing it completely from tumour in order to obtain representative samples.
4. Slight negative pressure is maintained in syringe retaining tissue sample whilst assembled unit is withdrawn from tumour. Tissue often not apparent within syringe but adequate sample usually present in hub of needle.
5. Needle is removed and the syringe plunger withdrawn.
6. Needle is reattached to syringe.
7. Tissue aspirate is quickly expressed from hub of needle on to microscope slide; smear is prepared as for cytology sample.

Lymph node excisional biopsy
Although the aspirate is invaluable in assessment of diagnosis, only a complete excisional biopsy will give an indication of lymph node architecture.

- Requires general anaesthesia and surgical preparation of site over lymph node
- After surgical removal, node is sectioned lengthwise and impression smears are made
- Node and impression smear are fixed and sent for histopathological diagnosis.

Sampling the bleeding animal for a coagulation screen

- Sample should be taken with minimum of excitement as this may cause increase in platelet count and some of coagulation proteins
- Blood should be obtained with minimum probing of vessels
  - Ideally cephalic or saphenous vein should be used as haemorrhage is easier to control here
  - Blood should not be collected through catheter

- Preferred anticoagulant is 3.8% sodium citrate
- For most procedures, ratio of anticoagulant to blood is 1:9
- Submission of blood from normal individual of same species provides good control to rule out artefacts induced during sample processing and transportation.

Endoscopy

Care and cleaning of endoscopes
The nurse has a major role to play in the care and cleaning of endoscopes.

It is essential to transport endoscopes in their original case as the fibreoptic fibres are easily damaged by even minor knocks. However, when not in use it is important to hang flexible endoscopes vertically on a suitable hanger, permitting the insertion tube to remain straight. If the endoscope is kept in its case, the insertion tube will 'learn' a curved shape making future use difficult.

 The endoscope should never be exposed to autoclaving as the high temperatures would cause permanent damage.

When cleaning an endoscope it is important to use an aseptic technique to reduce contamination of the operator, equipment and environment. Remember that potentially zoonotic diseases may be present and personal safety is important. Ideally whenever possible an endoscope cleaning unit should be used, although a large basin can be used successfully.

Only modern endoscopes are fully immersible. They are recognized by a blue ring around the eyepiece and from data given in the instruction book. Only the insertion tube can be immersed in water on older endoscopes. If the latter endoscopes are immersed, permanent damage will occur.

Always follow the cleaning instructions provided by the manufacturer. In general the protocol in Figure 1.69 can be used to clean flexible endoscopes.

1.69 Cleaning protocol for endoscopes

1. Wash the endoscope in clean warm water with household detergent. Ensure all the biopsy channels are flushed through. Remove the red and blue buttons from the handpiece and wash separately.
2. Drain the detergent and lay the endoscope in a suitable endoscope disinfecting solution.

It is not acceptable to use any disinfectant, it must be approved for endoscopes. Failure to observe this rule may result in blockage of biopsy channels and damage to the endoscope lens system. Cidex, New Cidex and Dettol Endoscope Disinfectant are suitable. There are important Health and Safety regulations regarding the use of some of these solutions. Please read instructions carefully.

3. Following a suitable period of disinfection the endoscope should be rinsed in clean water before being reassembled, dried and hung back on the endoscope hanger.

Rhinoscopy

Rhinoscopy is the endoscopic visualization of the nasal passages.

- Rostral rhinoscopy examines the nasal cavity using an approach via the external nares
- Caudal rhinoscopy is used to evaluate the choanae and the nasopharynx via the oral cavity and pharynx.

Instrumentation

- Otoscope, and/or
- Rigid endoscope, and/or
- Flexible endoscope.

Patient preparation

- General anaesthetic required
- Patient usually in sternal recumbency.

Technique

Rostral rhinoscopy

- Rhinoscope is initially passed medially and then straightened to pass directly into the deeper nasal cavity (Figure 1.70)
- Assessment is made of the mucosa, the three primary meatuses and the choanae.

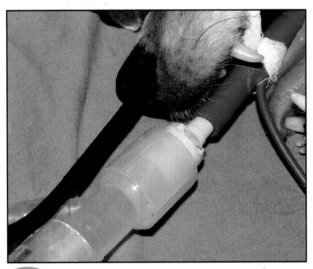

1.70 *Flexible rostral rhinoscopy in a dog.*

Caudal rhinoscopy

Best achieved using a small flexible endoscope.

- A mouth gag is placed
- The endoscope is passed via the oral cavity and retroflexed around the edge of the soft palate
- Assessment is made of the nasopharynx and choanae.

Tracheobronchoscopy

Indications

- Where direct assessment of the airways is required
- In differential diagnosis of lower airway causes of coughing
- Unexplained pulmonary changes on radiography
- Removal of foreign bodies.

Equipment

- Rigid bronchoscope (hollow bronchoscope for removal of foreign bodies or telescopic scope)
- Flexible bronchoscope (fibreoptic flexible endoscope)
- General anaesthesia
- Facilities for supplemental oxygen delivery (e.g. oxygen catheter)
- Biopsy/retrieval forceps.

Procedure

- On induction of anaesthesia there is careful examination of the larynx and a mouth gag is inserted
- The animal is positioned in sternal recumbency
- The bronchoscope is passed and there is sequential examination of:
  - Larynx: assessment of anatomy and function
  - Trachea: assessment of shape, dynamic changes associated with breathing, presence of oedema, mucus or haemorrhage, and colour of mucosa
  - Carina and mainstem bronchi: evidence of parasites (e.g. *Oslerus osleri*) and distortion of shape; enlarged bronchial lymph nodes (e.g. lymphosarcoma, tuberculosis) can cause pressure on main bronchi
  - Bronchial tree: assessment of lumen size, shape, presence of any mucosal changes (oedema, haemorrhage, mucus)
- Bronchoalveolar lavage or endoscopic biopsy may be performed using retrieval forceps
- Relatively safe procedure; complications not common but include those associated with anaesthetizing critically ill patient, haemorrhage and pneumothorax.

Upper gastrointestinal endoscopy

Upper gastrointestinal endoscopy refers to the examination of the pharynx, oesophagus, stomach and duodenum. The veterinary nurse plays an important role in the preparation of the patient and equipment for this procedure.

Patient preparation

The patient requires to be starved of food for 24 hours and of water for 4 hours if this is safe to carry out. This period of fasting is essential, especially if the patient has delayed gastric emptying, as endoscopy is impossible where food and water lie in the stomach.

Equipment

- The nurse should prepare the endoscopic equipment in advance of the patient's being anaesthetized to ensure that it is functioning normally. In addition to laying out the endoscope, it should be attached to the light source and air pump and their normal function confirmed. Biopsy forceps, pre-soaked card and bottles of formol saline should be made ready. A suitable lubricant should be available to assist in passing the endoscope.
- The nurse should lay out all equipment required for administration of general anaesthesia. This should include a mouth gag to prevent damage to the endoscope by the patient's teeth during the procedure.
- Once anaesthetized the patient should be placed in left lateral recumbency as this aids passage of the endoscope into the duodenum. The endotracheal tube should be tied to the mandible so allowing the endoscope to pass unobstructed along the hard palate and into the oesophagus.

Sample handling

During the procedure the nurse should assist with the collection of biopsy samples on to presoaked card and their careful transfer into formol saline bottles, which should be carefully labelled with the patient's details.

Colonoscopy

Equipment

The nurse should lay out the same endoscopic equipment as is required for upper gastrointestinal endoscopy. In addition suitable protective clothing and especially disposable gloves should be available to prevent personal contamination.

Patient preparation

- The importance of patient preparation for this procedure cannot be overemphasized. The continual movement of faecal material along the intestine makes complete emptying of the colon very difficult. Preparation is an important job for the veterinary nurse to carry out.
- Food should be withheld for 24 hours. An oral bowel cleansing agent such as Klean Prep® should be administered per os, up to 20 ml/kg, the day prior to the procedure. On the morning of the colonoscopy several warm water enemas should be administered.
- Once the enemas run clear, the patient may be finally prepared for endoscopy. Either sedation using a combination of acepromazine and buprenorphine can be used or general anaesthesia can be administered. The patient should be laid in left lateral recumbency for colonoscopy.

Hormone assays

Thyroid stimulation test (TSH test)

Although the measurement of basal T4 values in serum usually gives a good indication of thyroid function, it may occasionally fail to provide adequate information on which to base a diagnosis. In such cases the TSH (thyroid stimulating hormone) test is considered to be the most valuable test to perform. It is a dynamic test which assesses the pituitary–thyroid axis and is considered to be a definitive test of thyroid function. However, it is not routinely carried out in general practice because of the cost and difficulty in obtaining TSH. The protocol for the test is shown in Figure 1.71.

1.71 TSH test

1. Collect a resting clotted blood sample for T4 assay.
2. Slowly inject 0.1 IU/kg TSH i.v.
3. Collect a second clotted blood sample 6 hours later.

The nurse's role in assisting the veterinary surgeon to carry out this test includes:

- Preparing suitable blood tubes, syringes and needles for the test
- Correctly labelling the blood tubes, especially ensuring basal and 6 hour samples are not mixed up
- Clipping and preparing two veins for venepuncture
- Restraining the patient for venepuncture
- Centrifugation and separation of serum from samples, their packaging, and form completion for the laboratory.

Normal (euthyroid) animals will respond to injections of TSH by showing a rise of at least 1.5 times the basal T4 value, with the actual value being greater than 26 nmol/l.

Hypothyroid animals have a low basal T4 value and either fail to respond to TSH or respond poorly, with a value less than 26 nmol/l.

ACTH stimulation test

This is a simple test to perform and allows demonstration of excessive production of glucocorticoids by the adrenal cortex (Figure 1.72).

1.72 ACTH stimulation test

1. Collect 3 ml plasma to establish basal cortisol concentrations.
2. Inject 0.25 mg synthetic ACTH i.v. or i.m. (for dogs below 5 kg a dose of 0.125 mg should be used).
3. Collect a plasma sample at 30–60 minutes post-injection to measure cortisol levels.

In normal dogs, pre-ACTH cortisol levels are 20–250 nmol/l and post-ACTH values are 200–450 nmol/l. Post-ACTH levels > 600 nmol with associated clinical signs are strongly indicative of hyperadrenocorticism (Figure 1.73).

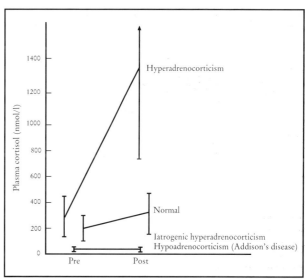

1.73 *Adrenocorticotropic hormone (ACTH) stimulation test. Interpretation of plasma cortisol concentrations determined before and after administration of synthetic ACTH.*
Reproduced from the BSAVA Manual of Small Animal Endocrinology, 2nd edition, edited by A.G. Torrance and C.T. Mooney

Low-dose dexamethasone test

This is reported to be a more reliable test for hyperadrenocorticism (Figure 1.74).

1.74 Low-dose dexamethasone test

1. Collect 3 ml plasma to establish basal cortisol concentrations.
2. Inject 0.01 mg dexamethasone/kg i.v.
3. Collect plasma 4 hours and 8 hours after dexamethasone injection.

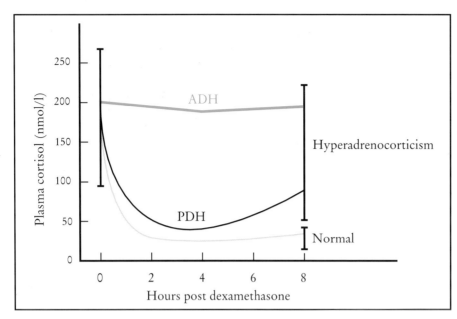

1.75
Low-dose dexamethasone suppression test. Interpretation of plasma cortisol concentrations determined during low-dose dexamethasone screening.
ADH represents the type of response seen in cases of adrenal-dependent hyperadrenocorticism.
PDH represents a possible response in pituitary-dependent cases.
Reproduced from the BSAVA Manual of Small Animal Endocrinology, 2nd edition, edited by A.G. Torrance and C.T. Mooney

A diagnosis of hyperadrenocorticism is confirmed if the dose of dexamethasone fails to suppress circulating cortisol in a patient with clinical signs (Figure 1.75).

High-dose dexamethasone suppression test
This test is used to differentiate between pituitary-dependent and adrenal-dependent hyperadrenocorticism. It has been used for many years but is becoming increasingly superseded by ACTH assays. The assay protocol is as for the low-dose test but the dose of dexamethasone is increased to 0.1 mg/kg. The high dose of dexamethasone inhibits pituitary ACTH secretion through negative feedback and thus suppresses cortisol levels. Adrenal tumours are not ACTH-dependent and are therefore not suppressed.

ACTH assay
This has largely superseded the high-dose dexamethasone suppression test. Samples are taken and cooled very quickly to 4°C. Plasma is quickly harvested and sent frozen to the laboratory. In dogs, high ACTH levels indicate pituitary-dependent disease; low levels indicate adrenal-dependent disease.

Other tests/procedures

Intradermal skin allergy testing
This test allows the identification of possible allergens causing allergic skin diseases (Figure 1.76).

Water deprivation test
The water deprivation test is used in the diagnostic approach to PUPD when common causes have been ruled out and diabetes insipidus is suspected. The technique (Figure 1.77) should always be used with caution.

1.76 **Intradermal allergen testing**

1. Initially, ensure that the patient will at least respond to intradermal histamine. Some patients on long-term therapy may not react to this test and so intradermal testing with potential allergens is not likely to yield beneficial results
   - Inject 0.05 ml of 1:100,000 histamine phosphate intradermally
   - A wheal 10–20 mm in diameter should be present 15–30 minutes after injection
   - If the wheal is < 10 mm, the test should be postponed.
2. A responsive patient should now be sedated. Alpha-2 agonists are suitable; acetylpromazine must *not* be used.
3. The skin over the lateral thorax is clipped but not chemically prepared.
4. Points where allergens are to be injected are marked with a felt-tipped pen, leaving 1.5 cm between points.
5. Dilutions of prepared allergens (e.g. preparations of house dust mite, house dust, mould, feathers, grasses) are injected using a 26 G needle. Water and histamine serve as negative and positive controls, respectively. The test is read 15–30 minutes post-injection.
6. Any wheal that develops is compared with the positive and negative controls and their diameters are measured.

1.77 **Water deprivation test**

1. Catheterize and empty bladder.
2. Determine urine specific gravity.
3. Record body weight.
4. Record urine and plasma osmolalities, PCV, total plasma protein and blood urea levels.
5. Withhold water and catheterize the bladder every 1–2 hours to repeat the above parameters.
6. The test is stopped when the patient has lost 5% of its body weight or the urine specific gravity exceeds 1.030. Failure to concentrate urine above 1.010 is highly suggestive of diabetes insipidus.

Bleeding time

Bleeding time is quick and easy to measure (Figures 1.78 and 1.79) and one of the best screening tests for von Willebrand's disease.

1.78 Mucosal bleeding time

1. Animal in lateral recumbency.
2. Strip of gauze held around maxilla to hold upper lip upwards.
3. Gauze held just tight enough to impede venous return, causing modest engorgement of mucosal surface.
4. Spring-loaded device used to make two 5 mm x 1 mm deep incisions in mucosal surface (site chosen where mucosa is devoid of visible blood vessels).
5. At exact time incisions are made, stopwatch is started.
6. Shed blood is blotted every 5 seconds with circles of filter paper placed against mucosal surface 1–2 mm below incision site.
7. Bleeding time endpoint is time from incision until filter paper fails to acquire red crescent when positioned near incision site.
8. Bleeding times for normal dogs 1.7–4.2 minutes (mean 2.6 minutes).

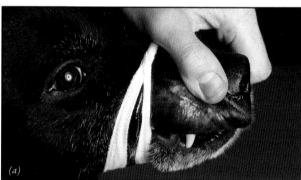
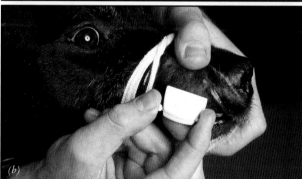
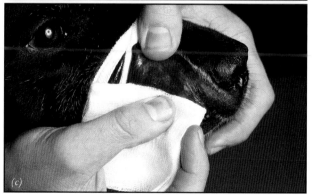

1.79 Mucosal bleeding time. (a) The upper lip is held upwards by gauze and the buccal mucosa exposed. (b) A spring-loaded device makes two small incisions. (c) Filter paper is applied to the mucosa near the incision site. A red crescent indicates that the tissue is still bleeding.

Electrocardiography

The electrocardiogram (ECG) is a graphical representation of the cardiac cycle and is an essential tool for the diagnosis of dysrhythmias. It can also provide useful information about the size of the heart and the possibility of any electrolyte disturbances (e.g. hyperkalaemia, hypokalaemia). ECG machines are common in general practice and the technique for performing the examination is outlined below.

Indications

- Assessment of patient with suspected cardiac disease
- Abnormal heart rate or rhythm detected on auscultation.

Technique

This is described in Figure 1.80.

1.80 How to take an ECG

1. Patient in right lateral recumbency on insulated surface
2. Electrodes are attached to loose skin on limbs. Plenty of gel applied to ensure good conductance.
   - RA (red) attached to right forelimb
   - LA (yellow) attached to left forelimb
   - LF (green) attached to left hindlimb
   - RF (black) attached to right hindlimb
3. Record calibration mark
4. Record a few complexes at 50 mm/s and then a longer strip (lead II) at 25 mm/s.

Interpretation

In the normal heart the recording will show a series of complexes (Figures 1.81 and 1.82). One complex represents the events in the complete cardiac cycle. Using these recordings the following can be assessed:

- Is the heart rate normal?
- Are there P waves?
- Are P waves associated with QRS complexes?
- Are complexes bizarre, wide or narrow?
- Are T waves normal?

Some examples of abnormalities are shown in Figures 1.83 and 1.84.

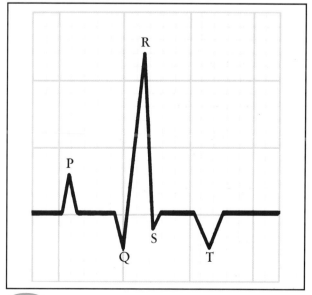

1.81 Normal canine lead II PQRST complex.

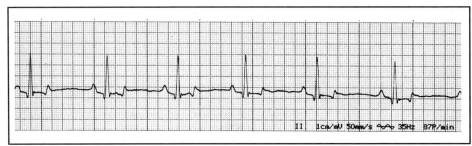

1.82

Normal regular sinus rhythm in a dog.
Reproduced from the BSAVA Manual of Small Animal Cardiorespiratory Medicine and Surgery, edited by V. Luis Fuentes and S. Swift

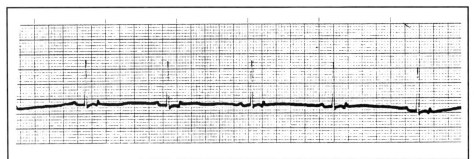

1.83

ECG from 13-year-old female Border Collie with sinus bradycardia (50/min) and first degree AV block (PR interval = 0.16 seconds) due to digoxin toxicity associated with renal failure. Lead II, 25 mm/s, 1 cm/mV.
Reproduced from the BSAVA Manual of Small Animal Cardiorespiratory Medicine and Surgery, edited by V. Luis Fuentes and S. Swift

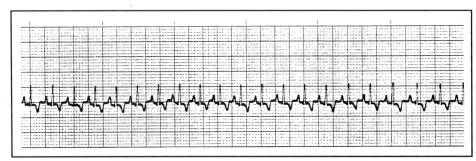

1.84

ECG from a 6-year-old neutered female Whippet with sinus tachycardia (200/min) associated with congestive heart failure. The bitch also had pleural effusion, which may explain the small R waves (0.6 mV). Lead II, 25 mm/s, 1 cm/mV.
Reproduced from the BSAVA Manual of Small Animal Cardiorespiratory Medicine and Surgery, edited by V. Luis Fuentes and S. Swift

An introduction to therapy

This section introduces the nurse to therapeutics. A small number of therapies have been selected from conditions described earlier in order to give an insight into the methodology of treatment.

Treatment of hyperthyroidism

Medical management
Medical management is not curative and is reserved for advanced cases with concurrent illness or where the owner does not wish surgery or radioactive iodine therapy. Medical management is also required for stabilization prior to surgery or in the short term for cats awaiting radioactive iodine therapy.

- Thioureylene anti-thyroid drugs (e.g. carbimazole) commonly used – provide reliable suppression of hormone production:
  - Dose of 5 mg per cat every 8 hours is initiated; normal T4 levels usually achieved within 7 days
  - For long-term medical management dose is reduced to 5 mg b.i.d. Once stabilization is achieved, patient has T4 checks every 3–6 months
- ß-Adrenergic blocking drugs (e.g. propanalol) are not used for bringing down T4 levels but are useful for controlling cardiac signs associated with hypertrophic cardiomyopathy.

Radioactive iodine

- Simple and safe method but requires specialist handling facilities
- Radioactive iodine is injected and concentrates in the thyroid gland; ß-particles emitted allow destruction of tumour tissue
- Cats require special housing facilities during treatment; often hospitalized 4–6 weeks
- Limited availability; waiting lists can be very long.

Surgery

- Thyroidectomy following preanaesthetic stabilization period using carbimazole ± propanalol for around 2 weeks
- Potential complications include postoperative hypocalcaemia (< 2 mmol/l) if parathyroid glands are removed or damaged
  - Manifests 1-5 days post surgery; clinical signs include anorexia and tetany
  - Emergency treatment involves intravenous administration of 10% calcium gluconate at 1.0–1.5 ml/kg over 10–20 minutes
  - ECG monitoring useful as infusion should be stopped in event of severe bradycardia, which can lead to cardiac arrest
  - Once over critical stage, calcium can be added to intravenous fluids
  - Some cats require oral maintenance therapy using calcium supplements and vitamin D preparations.

Protocol for management of status epilepticus

- Take baseline blood samples
- Intravenous diazepam to effect (2–4 infusions of 5 mg over several minutes). If no response by 15–20 mg, use alternatives. Do not exceed 15 mg in the cat
- Pentobarbitone (3–15 mg/kg i.v.) but watch for respiratory depression
- Intravenous catheter placement and fluid therapy
- If hypoglycaemia confirmed, administer dextrose (5% i.v.)
- Monitor vital signs
- If no underlying cause found, maintenance anticonvulsant therapy may be required.

Diabetes

Stabilization of the uncomplicated diabetic

- A detailed discussion with the owner is required to decide owner commitment, both emotionally and financially
- Introduce a consistent dietary and exercise regime. If owners can keep to this then it is possible that uncomplicated cases need not be hospitalized for the stabilization period
- A good starting point is to introduce single daily injections of an intermediate acting insulin (e.g. lente or NPH) alongside a daily diet of two equally divided meals (one fed at the time of injection and one fed 6–8 hours later)
- Start dose is 0.5–1.0 IU/kg s.c.
- Insulin doses are adjusted depending on single daily urine glucose estimation: three times daily urine glucose estimation or on daily blood glucose estimation (Figure 1.85). In the practice, rapid blood glucose measurements can be made using a portable glucose meter
- Most dogs will stabilize at 1.0–1.5 IU lente insulin/kg body weight per day. Dogs that require more than 2.0 IU/kg should be investigated for possible insulin antagonism
- After an initial stabilization period, some clinicians take serial blood glucose samples (every 2 hours) over a 24-hour period to create a glucose curve (Figure 1.86). This curve helps to determine whether a patient would benefit from twice-daily insulin or a longer-acting insulin.

1.85 Initial diabetic stabilization using single daily injections of lente insulin preparations

- Starting dose 0.5–1.0 IU/kg s.c.
- Feed evenly divided meals 6–8 hours apart with the first at the time of injection

Monitor urine glucose once daily
Measure urine glucose concentration just before the next injection and calculate insulin dose adjustments for the day.

Urine glucose concentration	Action
Negative	Reduce dose (10% or greater if clinical evidence of hypoglycaemia)
0.1–1%	Keep dose the same
>2%	Small increase in dose (10% or 0.1 IU/kg)

Monitor urine glucose three times daily
Measure urine glucose three times a day and calculate insulin dose adjustment. This method should protect against insulin-induced hyperglycaemia and can be performed by owners at home.

Urine glucose result at approximately:			Dose adjustment
7 hours post-injection (e.g. 3.30 p.m.)	13–14 hours post-injection (e.g. 10.00 p.m.)	Just before insulin injection (e.g. 8.00 a.m.)	
Negative	Negative	Trace	None
Positive	Positive	Positive	Increase by 10%
Negative	Negative	Negative	Decrease by 10%
Negative	Positive	Positive	Decrease by 20% (Somogyi 'overswing')
Negative	Negative	Positive	None
Negative	Positive	Trace	None

Monitor single daily (nadir) blood glucose
Requires access to in-house blood glucose analyser. A blood sample is obtained for glucose analysis when it is likely to be at its lowest (nadir) concentration. Using the single daily injection of intermediate-acting insulin and twice daily feeding schedule this is usually just before the second meal of the day.

Nadir blood glucose concentration (mmol/l)	Action
<3.5	Reduce dose
3.5–7.5	Keep dose the same
7.5–15	Small increase in dose (10% or 0.1 IU/kg)
>15	Large increase in dose (20% or 0.2 IU/kg)

- In all cases tabulate the insulin dose administered and the glucose results. Eventually, insulin doses will tend towards a mean dose which can be selected and adhered to for the first part of the maintenance period.

Reproduced from the BSAVA Manual of Small Animal Endocrinology, *2nd edition, edited by A.G. Torrance and C.T. Mooney*

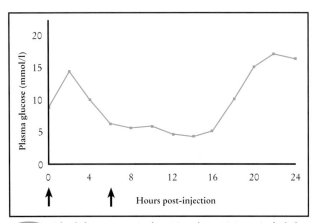

1.86 *Blood glucose curve (24 hour) in a dog receiving a single daily injection of lente insulin and two evenly divided meals (arrows). Note the early morning hyperglycaemia which is common in dogs receiving a single daily injection of intermediate-acting insulin. Reproduced from the BSAVA Manual of Small Animal Endocrinology, 2nd edition, edited by A.G. Torrance and C.T. Mooney*

Monitoring the diabetic patient

- Initial adjustments to insulin are made as described in Figure 1.85.
- Blood glucose estimations are then made weekly, then fortnightly and finally monthly.
- Daily urine glucose testing by the owner can be stopped after initial stabilization.
- Long-term glycaemic control can be estimated by laboratory measurement of plasma fructosamine. Fructosamine concentrations > 400 μmol/l suggest poor control. Fructosamine concentrations are independent of the time of day that the sample is taken.

Stabilization of the diabetic ketoacidotic patient

Ketoacidosis should be suspected when an animal is presented with a history of PUPD and polyphagia followed by a gradual deterioration in health, including weight loss, vomiting and anorexia. On presentation, these animals are often weak and depressed.

- Correct the dehydration and electrolyte deficits:
  - Intravenous normal saline (0.9%) is given to correct dehydration (i.e. replacement therapy) and supply maintenance fluid requirements. This is calculated in millilitres as [% dehydration/100] x body weight (kg) x 1000, plus 24-hour maintenance needs of 60–65 ml/kg/day, plus any other losses that may arise through vomiting or diarrhoea. If there is severe dehydration, then half of the estimated fluids can be given over the first 2–4 hours and the remainder over the following 20–22 hours
  - Infusion of fluids (and insulin) can make the patient severely hypokalaemic (resulting in weakness, anorexia, vomiting and cardiac dysrhythmias). In cats it can lead to cervical ventroflexion. In addition to hypokalaemaia there can be a concurrent hypophosphataemia, which can lead to Heinz body anaemia (especially in cats). Potassium is usually corrected once the dehydration has resolved (2 hours of fluid therapy) and is achieved using injectable 15% potassium solution containing 2 mmol potassium/ml. The amount given depends on the serum potassium levels (Figure 1.87). A rate of 0.5 mmol/kg body weight/hour should not be exceeded

- Severe hypophosphataemia requires intravenous phosphate administration. As a guide, 0.001–0.003 mmol phosphate/kg per hour for 6 hours is recommended for initial supplementation
- Administer 0.2 IU regular (soluble) insulin/kg i.m. and measure blood glucose hourly. Administer 0.1 IU insulin/kg i.m. hourly until the blood glucose is in the range of 10–15 mmol/l (4–8 hours).
- Once the glucose is in this range, the saline is replaced with a 5% dextrose or dextrose saline infusion until the animal stops vomiting or can eat normally
- Subcutaneous insulin is started (0.25–0.5 IU/kg) every 6 hours and the dose adjusted depending on response
- Once the patient is stable and eating, lente insulin can be started at the same dose as the subcutaneous soluble insulin.

1.87 **Potassium solution according to serum potassium level**

Serum potassium level (mmol/l)	Amount of potassium required (per litre of fluids at maintenance rate)
< 2.0	80 mmol
2.0—2.5	60 mmol
2.5—3.0	40 mmol
3.0—3.5	30 mmol
> 3.5	20 mmol

Protocol for management of severe thrombocytopenia and haemorrhage

- Blood is taken for analysis and intravenous access is established
- Intravenous dexamethasone is given as one dose of 0.2 mg/kg, followed by oral prednisolone at 2 mg/kg per day
- Intravenous vincristine is given as one dose of 0.5 mg/m². Vincristine, although it impairs platelet function to a small degree, increases platelet budding from megakaryocytes and can dramatically increase platelet counts over a 2–3-day period
- Fresh whole blood (platelet numbers and function decrease in stored blood) or platelet-rich plasma transfusion. In immune-mediated thrombocytopenia (ITP), the transfused platelets can be destroyed rapidly as well. The platelet count should be monitored closely.

Protocol for stable ITP patients

Prednisolone (2 mg/kg per day) orally, until the platelet count is adequate (2–4 weeks) ± azathioprine 2 mg/kg daily. Eventually, corticosteroids and azathioprine are given on an alternate-day basis. Azathioprine is kept at 2 mg/kg but the steroid dose is reduced by half every 2–4 weeks, as long as the platelet count remains adequate. The final maintenance dose of prednisolone is around 0.5–1 mg/kg every other day. Splenectomy may be considered in refractory cases.

Cancer chemotherapy

Introduction and definitions

Neoplastic disease is one of the most common clinical conditions seen in small animal practice. A *cancer* represents a population of cells that demonstrate a temporal unrestricted growth preference over normal cells, inhibition of differentiation and the tendency to invade tissues and metastasize.

At the turn of the twentieth century cancer was regarded as a disease that began locally and only at a very late stage spread to distant sites. Thus, initial attempts at disease control were confined to radical local excision or radiotherapy. Over time it became clear that many tumours metastasize early and patients may still die despite the primary tumour site remaining clear. It was therefore necessary to develop some form of systemic therapy.

Many of the cancer chemotherapy drugs used today stem from seminal experiments conducted from the 1940s onwards. Alkylating agents originated from research into chemical warfare and the antimetabolite class of drugs was born from research into nutrition and nucleic acid metabolism.

Considerations in using cytotoxic drugs

If owners of dogs and cats fear the word cancer, then they will fear the word chemotherapy even more. They frequently conjure up images of pain and suffering, very often from witnessing treatments in friends or relatives. It is imperative, when considering the use of such therapy in veterinary patients, that the following points are taken into consideration and explained to the owner:

- The usefulness of chemotherapy is often limited to very few tumour types (which is also true in human medicine)
- Doses are usually a compromise between efficacy and toxicity, and the potential toxic side effects of the drugs must be fully explained
- The owner must be counselled thoroughly, and must be committed to the treatment
- Quality of life is more important than quantity and very often the veterinary surgeon is not trying to cure the cancer but to give the patient a good quality of life for a reasonable amount of time.

The aims of chemotherapy can be threefold:

- Cure
- Palliation
- As an adjunct to another modality.

In human medicine chemotherapy is used in a more aggressive fashion in order to obtain a cure. This is often accompanied by high levels of toxicity, which require intensive medical care. In veterinary medicine this type of toxicity is unacceptable and so the doses used are much lower, thus aiming for maintenance of the disease rather than a cure.

Cellular targets for chemotherapy drugs

The cytotoxic drugs used in cancer chemotherapy can be broadly divided into the following six classes on the basis of their mode of action:

- Alkylating agents
  - Cyclophosphamide
  - Chlorambucil
  - Melphalan
- Antimetabolites
  - Cytarabine
  - Methotrexate
- Anti-tumour antibiotics
  - Doxorubicin
  - Epirubicin- Mitoxantrone
- Vinca alkaloids
  - Vincristine
  - Vinblastine

- Hormones
  - Corticosteroids
- Miscellaneous agents
  - Cisplatin
  - Hydroxyurea.

Most of the drugs work by inhibiting DNA replication or cell division in rapidly dividing tumours (Figure 1.88).

1.88 The cellular targets for cancer chemotherapy drugs

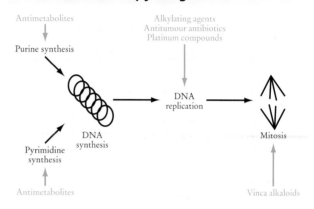

Calculating doses for patients

The therapeutic range for cytotoxic agents is very narrow and the dosage is therefore critical. The aim is to use the highest possible dose without causing significant toxicity to the host. The dose is usually calculated as a function of body surface area (in square metres). This is because the blood supply to the organs responsible for removal of the drugs (liver and kidneys) is more closely related to surface area than to body weight. Figures 1.89 and 1.90 are convenient conversion tables which remove the possibility of error when trying to calculate body surface area in a busy clinic.

1.89 Body surface area: dogs

Kg	m²	Kg	m²
1.0	0.10	26.0	0.88
2.0	0.15	27.0	0.90
3.0	0.20	28.0	0.92
4.0	0.25	29.0	0.94
5.0	0.29	30.0	0.96
6.0	0.33	31.0	0.99
7.0	0.36	32.0	1.01
8.0	0.40	33.0	1.03
9.0	0.43	34.0	1.05
10.0	0.46	35.0	1.07
11.0	0.49	36.0	1.09
12.0	0.52	37.0	1.11
13.0	0.55	38.0	1.13
14.0	0.58	39.0	1.15
15.0	0.60	40.0	1.17
16.0	0.63	41.0	1.19
17.0	0.66	42.0	1.21
18.0	0.69	43.0	1.23
19.0	0.71	44.0	1.25
20.0	0.74	45.0	1.26
21.0	0.76	46.0	1.28
22.0	0.78	47.0	1.30
23.0	0.81	48.0	1.32
24.0	0.83	49.0	1.34
25.0	0.85	50.0	1.36

Kg	m²	Kg	m²
2.0	0.159	3.6	0.235
2.2	0.169	3.8	0.244
2.4	0.179	4.0	0.252
2.6	0.189	4.2	0.260
2.8	0.199	4.4	0.269
3.0	0.208	4.6	0.277
3.2	0.217	4.8	0.285
3.4	0.226	5.0	0.292

Body weight is used to calculate the surface area by the following formula:

$$\text{Surface area (m}^2) = \{k \times [\text{body weight (kg)}]^{0.66}\} \times 10^{-4}$$

where the factor $k = 10.1$ for dogs and 10 for cats.

In most instances a combination of drugs is used to treat cancer, rather than a single agent. This is because a single agent will only affect those cells within a tumour that are sensitive to its actions and also may select for drug resistance. Combination protocols have been developed to contain drugs that:

- Affect various stages of cell division
- Have different modes of action
- Have no overlapping toxicity
- Do not interfere with each other's actions.

Timing and intervals between doses of drugs

The dose of drug to be administered is limited by the toxicity to normal tissues (myelosuppression and gastrointestinal toxicity). These tissues have enormous capacity for repair compared with the tumour and therefore a drug schedule is developed which allows the drug to be administered at intervals such that the normal tissue has time to repair without expansion of the residual tumour population (Figure 1.91).

The concept of induction and maintenance

The point was made earlier that in veterinary medicine the aim is control of disease rather than cure, because of the overwhelming toxicity of aggressive chemotherapy. In veterinary protocols the treatment begins with a short *induction* protocol, which uses moderately aggressive therapy to induce complete or partial remission. The animal is then introduced to a *maintenance* protocol, which may contain the same drugs but at lower doses or at longer intervals.

Safe handling and administration of cytotoxic drugs

Many cytotoxic drugs are carcinogenic, mutagenic or teratogenic. They can also be extremely irritant, producing harmful effects if they come into contact with the skin or the eyes. They should therefore be used with extreme care and respect. The major risks are as follows:

- Absorption via the skin or mucous membranes
- Aerosol formation when preparing liquid chemotherapy
- Inhalation
- Self-inoculation when administering injectable agents.

The use of a vertical laminar airflow hood for all drug handling is advised. However, access to these facilities is often limited to the major veterinary hospitals and so the following are guidelines for the safe handling of tablets and injectable agents in veterinary practice.

 Although these are guidelines, the practitioner should always, in addition, follow the safety regulations laid down by the individual country.

Handling and administration of tablets or capsules

- Tablets or capsules should never be divided, broken or crushed
- Disposable gloves should always be worn when handling or administering the drug (Figure 1.92)
- If tablets are provided in 'blister packs', then they should be dispensed in this form

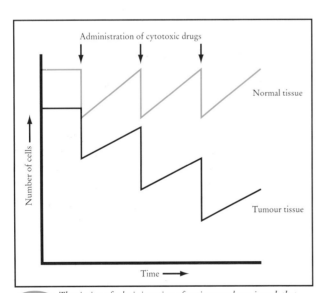

1.91 *The timing of administration of anticancer drugs is such that there is reduction in the tumour burden but sufficient intervals between doses to allow normal tissues (gut and bone marrow) to recover.*

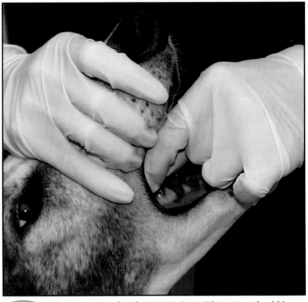

1.92 *Administration of oral cytotoxic drugs. The patient should have adequate restraint and the procedure should be carried out wearing gloves.*

- Staff and owners should receive clear instruction on administration
- Hands should be washed after administering drugs
- Excess or unwanted drugs should be incinerated in a chemical incinerator.

Handling and administration of injectable agents

- Most injectable cytotoxic drugs are administered via the intravenous route and an intravenous catheter should always be used for this purpose
- Locking syringe fittings are preferable to push connections
- Patients should be adequately restrained, and some may need to be sedated
- Protective clothing and gloves should be worn at all times (Figure 1.93)
- A laminar-flow fume cupboard should ideally be used when handling cytotoxic drugs (Figure 1.94).

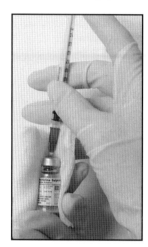

Drawing up cytotoxic drugs – care should be taken to prevent derosolization – by covering the syringe with a moistened swab.

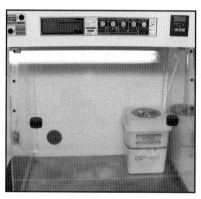

Ideally chemotherapeutic drugs should be handled in a laminar flow hood for protection of the operator.

Waste disposal

- Sharps should be placed in an impenetrable container, specific for chemotherapy, and sent for incineration
- Solid waste should be placed in labelled polythene bags and incinerated
- Disposal agents must be informed of the nature of the waste.

Drug spillage

In the event of drug spillage:

- Protective clothing should be worn
- The spillage should be mopped with absorbent disposable towels, which are then placed in polythene bags and disposed of
- Contaminated surfaces should be washed with copious amounts of water.

Chemotherapy toxicity

The major dose-limiting factor in chemotherapy protocols is drug toxicity, which can be broadly divided into immediate, delayed or late toxicity.

Immediate toxicity

- Anaphylaxis (e.g. doxorubicin infusion)
  - Can be prevented with pre-treatment with anti-histamines/corticosteroids
  - If it occurs, treatment should be stopped and the animal should be treated with intravenous fluids, corticosteroids, antihistamines
- Emesis
  - Can be reduced by premedication with anti-emetics
- Vasculitis/phlebitis (e.g. vincristine)
  - Can be prevented by using adequate restraint and intravenous catheters
  - In the event of perivascular injection, use local subcutaneous dexamethasone and cold compresses
- Tumour lysis syndrome (mainly a tumour-related complication).

Delayed toxicity

- Myelosuppression
  - Main dose-limiting effect of cytotoxic drugs used in veterinary practice
  - Most commonly the neutrophil count is affected, because these cells have the shortest life span
  - Occasionally platelet counts can fall and, rarely, red cell counts
  - Neutrophil counts reach nadir at 7–10 days and are usually recovered in 21 days
  - Neutropenia is serious side effect because of potential life-threatening infections; Figure 1.95 shows some management details for neutropenia in animals on chemotherapy
- Anorexia/vomiting/diarrhoea
  - For drugs that induce vomiting (e.g. cisplatin), metoclopramide can be used for management
  - Vomiting/diarrhoea occur through effects of drugs directly on gut; treatment is often symptomatic.

1.95 Neutrophil counts

Neutrophil count (x 10⁹/l)	Comment	Action
>3	Normal	Continue therapy
2-3	Some suppression	Reduce dose by 50%
<2	Severe myelosuppression	Stop treatment, monitor
<1	Severe risk of sepsis	Stop treatment + prophylactic antibiotics

Late toxicity

This category includes haemorrhagic cystitis (cyclophosphamide) and cardiomyopathy (doxorubicin). These effects are often individual to the particular drug.

The effect of chemotherapy on wound healing

Cytotoxic drugs affect rapidly dividing cells and therefore can have a deleterious effect on wound healing where chemotherapy is being combined with surgery or following a major biopsy procedure. In practice, most cytotoxic drugs can be used in the perioperative procedure where there is an indication to do so. Major problems can arise if the patient is extremely leucopenic and there is the possibility of wound infection, or if the patient is severely cachectic. In cases where wound healing may be a problem, the administration of vitamin A may reduce the effects of cytotoxic drugs on wound healing.

Reasons for treatment failure

Although chemotherapy is a useful modality of treatment for the small animal cancer patient, there are some circumstances when the treatment fails to yield a response. The main reasons for treatment failure include:

- Inappropriate tumour which is inherently resistant to chemotherapy
- Inappropriate selection of drugs
- Inappropriate selection of protocol and drug schedule
- Development of drug resistance.

Special nursing considerations

Animals undergoing cancer chemotherapy are usually housed on deep litter and a notice is placed outside the kennel stating that the patient is only to be handled by trained personnel. Any fractions patients should be sedated to prevent harm to themselves or to nursing staff while chemotherapeutic drugs are being administered.

For out-patients receiving single intravenous doses of drugs such as vincristine, the staff involved should be wearing adequate protective clothing as described.

In-patients receiving intravenous infusions of drugs such as cis platinum compounds can excrete active drug in their urine. Kennels should only be cleaned by trained personnel. Protective clothing (e.g. gowns, gloves and masks) should be worn to collect litter and to place it in polythene bags (double-tied) which will eventually go for incineration. Faeces and urine are considered hazardous and handled in the same manner. The kennel is cleaned with an appropriate detergent and washed with copious amounts of water. In specialized institutes, voiding kennels are often used to reduce the amount of handling of waste.

Further reading

Chandler EA, Gaskell CJ and Gaskell RM (eds) (1994) *Feline Medicine and Therapeutics*, 2nd edn. Blackwell Scientific Publications, Oxford

Davidson MG, Else RW and Lumsden JH (eds) (1998) *Manual of Small Animal Clinical Pathology*. BSAVA, Cheltenham

Ettinger SJ and Feldman EC (eds) (1999) *Textbook of Veterinary Internal Medicine*, 5th edn. WB Saunders, Philadelphia

Gorman NT (ed.) (1998) *Canine Medicine and Therapeutics*, 4th edn. Blackwell Science, Oxford

BSAVA Manuals covering relevant systems and disease in small animals, including:
Canine and Feline Nephrology and Urology
Companion Animal Nutrition and Feeding
Small Animal Endocrinology, 2nd edition
Small Animal Neurology, 2nd edition
Small Animal Oncology
Small Animal Diagnostic Imaging
Canine and Feline Gastroenterology
Canine and Feline Cardiorespiratory Medicine and Surgery

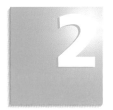

2 Advanced surgery and surgical nursing

Alasdair Hotston Moore and Cathy Garden

This chapter is designed to give information on:

- The roles of the members of the surgical team
- The principles of managing surgical supplies
- Certain advanced surgical procedures (their purpose, outline of the technique, and patient care)
- Certain minor surgical procedures with a view to being able to carry them out after further practical training

Introduction

The principles of surgical nursing and common surgical conditions were introduced in the *BSAVA Manual of Veterinary Nursing*. This chapter will discuss some major and less common surgical conditions and procedures. The care of such cases requires a team approach, and management of such a team and of the necessary surgical supplies will also be discussed. The Schedule 3 amendment to the Veterinary Surgeons Act (1966) allows registered veterinary nurses to undertake certain acts of minor veterinary surgery and some examples of these techniques will be covered in depth.

Theatre management

The surgical team

The surgical team includes every person in theatre at the time of a surgical procedure. Everyone has their own area of responsibility, but the common goal is to provide a safe environment, and to be concerned for the welfare of the patient. Normally a surgical team could be considered as: surgeon ± assistant surgeon, anaesthetist ± assistant, and nurse ± second nurse (if one is required to assist during surgery).

In veterinary surgery, frequently these roles are less well defined than indicated below, because of staffing limitations, but it is important that all members of the team understand their own roles to work efficiently.

Surgeon ± assistant surgeon

The lead surgeon is responsible for directing the operation and will carry out the majority of the surgery, particularly the core of the procedure.

The assistant surgeon assists during the procedure – for example, by swabbing the surgical field, applying lavage and

suction, providing retraction of tissues and cutting suture material as necessary. The assistant surgeon may be a veterinary nurse, veterinary surgeon or veterinary student. Veterinary surgeons in training positions or students may carry out the surgical approach and closure at the lead surgeon's direction and under supervision if appropriate. The assistant surgeon may also perform the role of scrub nurse if one is not present.

Anaesthetist ± assistant

The anaesthetist may be a veterinary nurse, veterinary surgeon or veterinary student. The anaesthetist is responsible for inducing, maintaining and supervising recovery from anaesthesia, with appropriate supervision or direction as necessary (veterinary nurses are not legally permitted to induce anaesthesia). Part of this role includes checking the equipment before use to ensure that all necessary supplies are present and in working order.

The assistant, if present, provides help as necessary – for example, by restraining the animal during induction and fetching supplies as needed.

Nurse ± second nurse

The nurse is responsible for preparing the theatre for surgery, in discussion with the surgeon. The nurse is usually also responsible for patient preparation and then assumes the role of a circulating nurse during the procedure, attending to non-sterile items (surgical suction machine, electrosurgery control units, power supply units) and providing wrapped surgical supplies as necessary.

There may also be a scrub nurse who prepares and manages the instrument trolley, handing instruments to the surgeon and receiving back those not in use. The scrub nurse should keep the instruments clean during surgery by wiping or rinsing in sterile saline as necessary and keep account of disposable items such as swabs, needles and suture packs.

Policies and procedures in theatre

There is a direct correlation between the number of people in the operating theatre, the activity of these people, and the number of airborne bacteria. This is due to the number of skin particles (some of which are microbes) shed from a normal skin. An increase in the number of people in the operating room increases the number of organisms shed; the activity of these personnel within the operating room encourages the organisms present to become airborne and therefore increase the risk of contamination to the surgical site. With this in mind it is pertinent to minimize the number of people present in the room during surgery and the movement of personnel in and out of the operating room.

The theatre suite should have aseptic areas, where instrument trolleys are set out and gowning and gloving are performed, and other areas where instruments are cleaned and packed ready for sterilization. All personnel in theatre should be aware of the 'clean' and 'dirty' areas and of the movement of personnel between these areas (Figure 2.1).

It is useful to have policies and procedures written out for new staff or visitors to the department. These should:

- Be regularly updated
- Have the support of all staff
- Be enforceable

- Contain guidelines for visitors and new staff with reference to personnel traffic control
- Contain safety regulations
- Provide guidelines on theatre protocol.

Some theatres may also require protocol to be written out for other techniques:

- CPR
- Care and cleaning of specialized equipment
- Handling of surgical specimens.

Stock levels and rotation of stock

- Stock levels of supplies will be influenced by the type and number of surgical cases seen at the clinic
- There should be adequate stock of all surgical supplies to cover busy periods, with enough supplies left to cover emergencies until the next order can be delivered
- Records of orders should be kept to enable stock levels to be monitored, to make repeat orders easier and to check on delivery
- It is advisable to keep an address book with the contact details of all suppliers or contacts made when ordering stock and buying or repairing equipment. This enables all staff to deal with ordering new or repeat stock items.

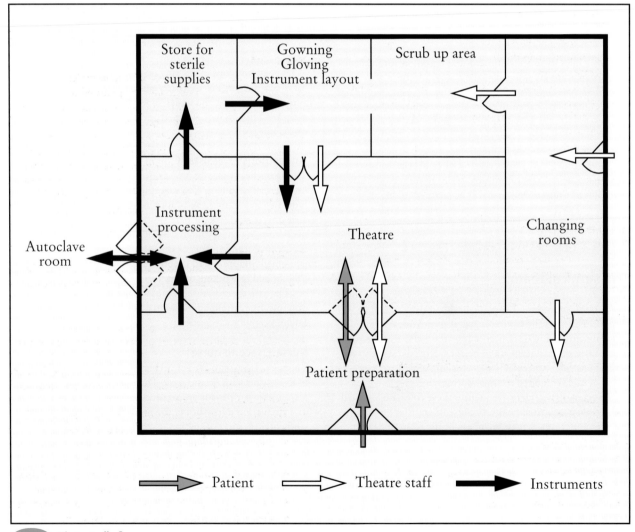

2.1 *Theatre traffic flow.*

Shelf life of sterile supplies

It could be said that any package, once sterilized, should be considered sterile until it is opened for use, provided the package has not obviously been damaged or become wet during storage.

Damage to the package or damp conditions during storage may not always be immediately obvious. To ensure sterility of items when used they should be checked regularly and resterilized if necessary.

For easy reference all items should be marked with the date of sterilization. It is usually easiest to write this on the outside of the pack itself. It is also helpful to include the contents of the package and the packer's initials on the label. Different methods of packaging and storage of equipment affect the length of suitable storage time. As a general rule infrequently used items should be checked and resterilized approximately every 6–8 weeks if they have not been used recently. Any item where the sterility is in question should be assumed to be non-sterile.

Consider the following points when wrapping and storing equipment:

- Double wrapping using linen drapes has been shown to increase storage time by 3 weeks
- Double wrapping also provides an extra safety margin when opening the package
- An outer layer of water-resistant material, such as paper or disposable drape material, will further increase storage time
- Open shelf storage allows up to 10 times more contamination on the outside of the pack than closed storage, and therefore reduces storage time
- Unnecessary handling of wrapped instruments, vibration or changes in atmospheric conditions may cause contamination of a surgical pack and so should be minimized.

Advanced surgical techniques

Thoracic surgery

Surgery of intrathoracic structures is commonly performed in referral centres and larger practices. Many of the specialized techniques involved in management of these cases relate to anaesthesia and are covered in Chapter 3. Other considerations will be dealt with here. The commoner surgical procedures undertaken are listed in Figure 2.2.

2.2 Common thoracic surgical procedures

- Lung lobectomy
- Bronchotomy
- Transthoracic oesophagotomy
- Pericardectomy
- Ligation of patent ductus arteriosus
- Division of vascular ring obstructions of the oesophagus
- Ruptured diaphragm repair[a]

a Although the surgical approach is transabdominal in most instances, similar considerations apply as for transthoracic procedures.

Intra- and postoperatively, the availability of certain instruments and equipment is helpful for these procedures (Figure 2.3).

2.3 Specialized equipment for thoracic surgery

- Long-handled instruments (dissecting scissors, dressing and rat-tooth forceps, haemostatic forceps)
- Surgical staplers (for lung lobectomy)
- Oscillating saw (for median sternotomy)
- Thoracic retractors (e.g. Finochietto and paediatric rib spreader)
- Vascular forceps (e.g. Satinsky's)
- Vascular snares
- Ligature passing forceps (e.g. Debakey's)
- Aneurysm needles
- Pott's scissors
- Chest drain tubes, connecting tubes and connectors
- Underwater trap or 'Pleurovac'
- Heimlich valve
- Surgical suction
- Surgeon's headlamp
- Sterile endotracheal tubes and a sterile anaesthetic circuit, or connections to allow use of a non-sterile circuit outside the surgical field
- Long-acting local anaesthetic agent (e.g. bupivacaine solution)

Teamwork

Since these patients are potentially unstable under anaesthesia, the surgical team must be prepared to overcome any problems that arise. Immediately before induction of anaesthesia the surgeon and assistant should scrub up and prepare their trolley, so that they can carry out an emergency thoracotomy should the patient suddenly deteriorate at induction. Similarly the anaesthetist, whether a veterinary surgeon or a veterinary nurse, must ensure that all equipment and drugs that may be required are readily available, prepared and in full working order before the induction of anaesthesia.

Patient preparation

The patient must be thoroughly assessed before surgery. In addition to the usual clinical examination the following are carried out:

- Good quality thoracic radiographs are taken
- Preoperative blood tests are performed and the patient is stabilized
- Pre-existing pleural gas or fluid accumulations are drained before induction of anaesthesia. Analysis of this fluid may give further information
- The animal must be treated for shock and life-threatening injuries before anaesthesia is undertaken if there is a history of prior trauma
- Pain may well be present and analgesia will help to overcome this and improve the animal's ventilation, despite the potentially depressive effects of some of these agents. Stress will exacerbate the animal's condition and it must be handled with sympathy and without excessive manual restraint: sedation, used cautiously, is usually helpful in all but the most placid patients

- To minimize the duration of anaesthesia, the surgical site should be prepared immediately prior to induction as far as possible, if this can be done without distressing the patient. Anaesthesia is often induced in theatre, again to minimize the delay before surgery and so that any emergency procedures can be carried out at once
- Oxygen supplementation may be given (for example, by face mask) prior to induction, again if this can be done without distress.

Intraoperative care
Most points of interest are covered in Chapter 3. However, it is worth emphasizing that anaesthetic management is critical for success in thoracic surgery. Other issues that must be addressed include:

- Development of intraoperative hypothermia. During thoracotomy a large surface area of core body tissues is exposed and heat loss is rapid. This is particularly important in relatively small patients. To counteract this, the theatre should be kept warm (between 18 and 22°C). Steps to minimize heat loss in other ways must also be explored:
  - ensuring that fluids given intravenously or used for lavage are at body temperature
  - using a heat/moisture exchanger in the anaesthetic circuit
  - placing a heat pad under the patient
  - wrapping the patient in insulating material
- Intravenous fluids. These are given as a matter of course during thoracic surgery. The type of fluid will depend on any pre-existing fluid or electrolyte imbalances
- Recovery from anaesthesia. This can be prolonged (because of the development of hypothermia, use of opiate analgesics and postoperative sedation) and fluid therapy is continued throughout this period.

Postoperative care
The following steps are important.

Radiography
Thoracic radiographs are taken routinely after thoracic surgery. The first are taken immediately after surgery to check placement of the drain and to assess the amount of pleural accumulations present. Radiography is repeated later if continuing drainage occurs and prior to removal of the chest drain.

Chest drain placement
A chest drain is almost invariably placed during surgery and maintained for upwards of several hours. This allows removal of any air or fluid that remains in the thorax after closure or that develops subsequently. Occasional exceptions are very small patients, particularly cats, when chest drains seem to be excessively uncomfortable and a decision may be made to remove any pleural accumulation at the end of surgery by catheter thoracostomy rather than an indwelling drain.

Chest drain care
The drain is sealed by an underwater seal, gate valve, three-way tap or Heimlich valve (Figures 2.4 and 2.5). These may allow continuous drainage (underwater trap or Heimlich valve) or require periodic suction. In either case gentle suction is applied to the drainage tube as frequently as necessary to remove pleural accumulations. In most cases the majority of air is removed within the first hour after surgery: continued drainage of air suggests an ongoing leak or technical problem with the drain. After the first hour, if there is little being removed by the drain, suction may be

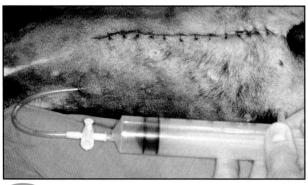

2.4 *Thoracic drain in place.*

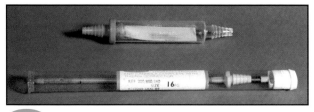

2.5 *Heimlich valve and thoracic drain.*

used hourly for 4 hours and thereafter every 4 hours. Otherwise suction is applied as frequently as necessary.

Chest drain removal
The chest drain is removed after 12 hours or so (usually the morning after surgery) if there are no complications. This can usually be done without anaesthesia or sedation.

Antibiotic therapy
This is used at the discretion of the veterinary surgeon – presence of a chest drain in itself is not an indication for its use.

Analgesia
Pain after thoracic surgery has a limiting effect on the animal's ventilation pattern. Analgesics should be used as necessary to allow uninhibited breathing. Combinations of systemic opiates, NSAIDs, epidural agents and local anaesthetics are particularly effective.

Sedation
Chemical restraint may be necessary to prevent patient interference with the chest drain and connecting tubes if an underwater seal is used.

Bandaging
In all cases, the chest drain and valve must be carefully bandaged to prevent damage or displacement by the animal, which could lead to a fatal pneumothorax (Figure 2.6).

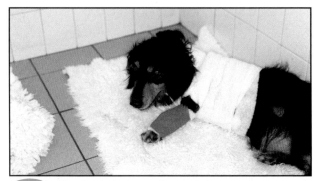

2.6 *Chest bandage to protect thoracic drain.*

Transsthoracic oesophagotomy

Transthoracic oesophagotomy (TTO) is indicated for the removal of oesophageal foreign bodies when other techniques have failed. Generally forceps retrieval under endoscopic or fluoroscopic control is preferred to surgery. Candidates for this surgery are frequently dehydrated because of oesophageal obstruction and complications such as aspiration pneumonia and oesophageal perforation may also have developed. Patient preparation should include:

- Fluid therapy to replace fluid deficits due to loss of voluntary intake and exceptional losses due to pleural effusion
- Prophylactic intravenous antibiotics immediately before surgery and continued after surgery if perforation is present
- Chest drainage as necessary
- Radiography – commonly the foreign body is lodged in the caudal thoracic oesophagus, but its position and the site of incision are determined from preoperative radiographs (Figure 2.7).

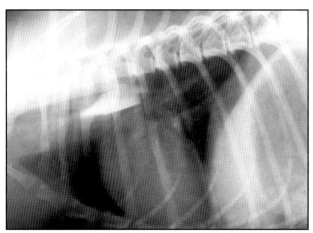

2.7 *Radiograph of dog with intrathoracic oesophageal foreign body (ingested bone).*

Surgical technique

- Lateral intercostal approach, immediately over the position of the foreign body
- Lungs are reflected from over the oesophagus and the area is isolated by packing swabs moistened with sterile saline around the intended site of the oesophagotomy incision
- Oesophageal wall is incised longitudinally over or cranial to the foreign body, which is then removed, and the oesophageal lumen is inspected before closure
- If there is a pre-existing perforation, this is also closed
- Packing is removed
- Pleural space is lavaged
- Chest drain is placed before the intercostal incision is closed.

In addition to the usual postoperative care after thoracotomy, other steps are necessary, as follows.

Dietary management

In most cases, if the surgeon is confident that a satisfactory closure of the oesophageal wall has been made, oral fluids are offered from 12 hours after surgery. If these are ingested and no complications arise, liquid or soft foods are offered thereafter.

In cases where oesophageal closure is tenuous, it may be elected to withhold oral food and fluids for 7–14 days. These animals must then be provided with fluidsand nutrition by another route. Nasogastric or pharyngostomy tubes that cross the area of repair are contraindicated. Gastrostomy tube feeding is the preferred route, and this tube is conveniently placed under the same anaesthetic as the TTO. Such a tube can also be placed postoperatively if evidence of leakage at the suture line becomes apparent and oral feeding must be stopped. Management of tube feeding is discussed in the *BSAVA Manual of Veterinary Nursing*.

Antibacterial therapy

Antibacterial therapy is continued postoperatively if perforation or aspiration pneumonia was present before surgery or gross contamination of the tissues occurs at surgery. Given the mixed population of organisms present in the obstructed oesophagus, a combination of agents effective against anaerobes and aerobes is appropriate – for example, intravenous amoxycillin–clavulanate and metronidazole.

Oesophageal strictures

Strictures can occur in these patients postoperatively, and so a transition to soft food is made within a few days if the animal is recovering normally. This is intended to encourage stretching of the oesophagus during healing, to prevent the occurrence of narrowing as scar tissue is produced. Frequent small meals are given initially.

Drain removal

The drain is removed if there is no continuing drainage from the chest tube once oral intake has restarted, or after 24–48 hours if the animal is kept *nil per os*.

Patent ductus arteriosus ligation

Patency of the embryonic ductus arteriosus (PDA) persisting into postnatal life will result in congestive heart failure. Surgery to occlude this vessel is usually recommended in affected animals. Non-surgical methods to close the vessel have not been widely used in veterinary medicine. If possible, the surgery should take place before heart failure has developed; or, if this has already happened, heart failure should be treated medically in an attempt to stabilize the animal before surgery.

Surgical technique (Figures 2.8 and 2.9)

- Left lateral thoracotomy, usually at the fourth intercostal space
- Underlying cranial lobe of the left lung is displaced caudally to reveal the PDA covered by the mediastinal pleura
- Following sharp incision of the pleura, the PDA is isolated by a combination of sharp and blunt dissection. This is the most hazardous part of the procedure, since the wall of the vessel is often fragile and easily torn. If haemorrhage results, it is often profuse and can be fatal within a few minutes
- Two or more lengths of a permanent suture (e.g. silk) are placed loosely around the vessel
- Ligatures are slowly tightened to occlude the vessel. Systemic blood pressure often rises markedly as this is done and may be accompanied by a bradycardia. Usually these resolve gradually and the vessel can be completely ligated but sometimes a vasodilator drug must be given to restore homeostasis

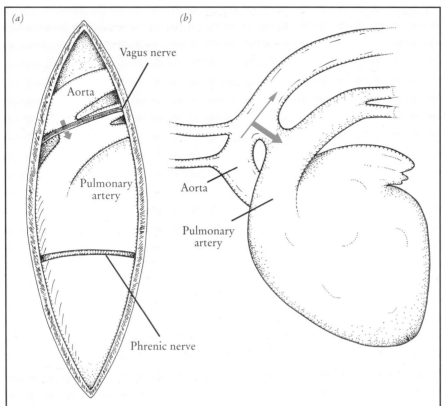

(a)

Vagus nerve

Aorta

Pulmonary
artery

Phrenic nerve

(b)

Aorta

Pulmonary
artery

2.8

(a) View of a patent ductus arteriosus
(PDA) seen at left lateral thoracotomy.
(b) The aortic blood flow is divided between
that descending to the trunk and that passing
through the PDA. This results in reduced
systemic blood flow and pulmonary
congestion.

↓ PDA

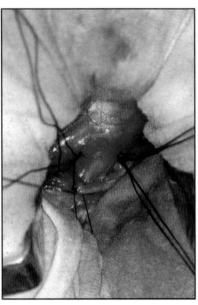

2.9

Intraoperative view of
aorta, PDA and
pulmonary artery, with
ligatures placed around
the PDA.

aortic arch (PRAA) and in these patients the oesophagus
becomes constricted between the ligamentum arteriosum and
the base of the heart (Figure 2.10). Typically, signs of
regurgitation develop soon after weaning. If diagnosis is
delayed, the animals can become markedly malnourished and
aspiration pneumonia can develop. These complications must
be managed before surgical treatment.

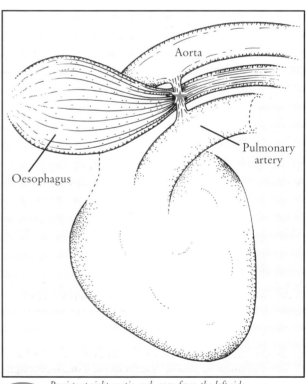

- Once the ligatures are tied, a chest drain is placed and the
  thorax is exited routinely
- Chest drains may not be placed if the patient is small
  (under 3 kg), in which cases pleural air is removed by
  needle or catheter thoracostomy.

  Peri- or postoperative antibiotics are not necessary unless
any surgical complications are encountered.

  The chest drain is usually removed after 12–24 hours if
drainage has ceased.

Division of a vascular ring

Vascular ring anomalies result from abnormal development of
the great vessels. The commonest type is a persistent right

Aorta

Oesophagus

Pulmonary
artery

2.10 *Persistent right aortic arch, seen from the left side.*
★ *Ligamentum arteriosum*

Steps to consider in presurgical management include:

- Fluid therapy to correct pre-existing dehydration due to failure of voluntary intake
- Treatment of aspiration pneumonia. Parenteral antibiotic therapy, fluid therapy, physiotherapy and nebulization may all be used
- Tube feeding to reduce the protein and energy malnutrition present in severely affected animals. A gastrostomy tube is often appropriate. In less severely affected animals, introduction of a liquid diet and postural feeding may be sufficient.

Surgical technique

- Left lateral thoracotomy is carried out at the fourth or fifth intercostal space
- Cranial lung lobe is reflected and the dilated cranial portion of the oesophagus is identified beneath the mediastinal pleura. In cases of PRAA, the ligamentum arteriosum is present overlying the oesophagus at the point where it is constricted
- Ligamentum is isolated, doubly ligated and transected. Any remaining fibrous bands constricting the oesophagus are dissected free and transected. It is often helpful to pass a large oesophageal tube at this point to identify areas of restriction
- Thoracotomy is closed routinely. A chest drain may not be placed if the animal is small (see PDA, above).

Particular points in peri- and postoperative care include the following.

Antibiotic therapy
Antibiotics are justified perioperatively because of the debilitated condition of affected animals and are continued postoperatively in selected cases (those with aspiration pneumonia or severe malnutrition).

Avoidance of hypothermia
These patients are particularly at risk of intraoperative hypothermia, because of the thoracotomy itself and because of their small size, lack of body fat and immaturity. Particular care must be taken to prevent this as much as possible and facilities for gentle postoperative rewarming should be available (e.g. an incubator).

Persistent regurgitation
Postoperatively, the animal may continue to regurgitate. Postural feeding is a useful nursing measure to reduce this. Persistent regurgitation is a poor prognostic indicator but some animals are sufficiently improved to tolerate postural feeding and dietary manipulation. Overall, the outcome after treatment is around 50% success in terms of animals becoming acceptable house pets.

Lung lobectomy
Removal of one or more lung lobes is indicated in a variety of conditions. Animals tolerate removal of several lobes, or the entire left lung, without excessive respiratory compromise. Common indications include:

- Primary lung tumours (in the absence of gross metastasis)
- Lobar pneumonia (including abscesses and inhaled foreign bodies not amenable to endoscopic retrieval or bronchotomy)

- Lung lobe torsion
- Pneumothorax due to trauma or ruptured bullae not responsive to conservative management
- Severe trauma to a lung lobe.

Surgical technique

- Lobectomy is usually carried out through a lateral thoracotomy on the affected side, with the incision based over the hilus of the affected lobe (judged from preoperative radiographs)
- Alternatively, a ventral midline approach (median sternotomy) can be used. This approach is usually chosen when there is a need to inspect all of the lung lobes and particularly if a refractory pneumothorax is present and the site of leakage cannot be determined before surgery. Although sternotomy can be performed with hand instruments (hand saw, sternotomy knife, osteotome), power tools (an oscillating saw) greatly facilitate the surgery in larger patients
- Lobe of interest is identified and isolated. To identify the site of any air leakage it may be helpful to fill the thorax with sterile saline and look for bubbles escaping from any pulmonary or bronchial lesion
- Lobe is freed from any adhesions to surrounding lobes, pleura or mediastinum and the lobar vessels and bronchus are identified
- Vessels and bronchus are either ligated and oversewn by hand, or a surgical stapler (Figure 2.11) may be used to close all of these structures at once
- Stump is examined to check for leaks of blood or air before the chest is exited routinely.

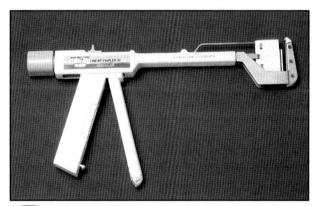

2.11 *Surgical stapler, suitable for pulmonary lobectomy.*

Perioperative antibiotics are given because of the risk of tissue contamination when the bronchus is severed, but need not be continued after surgery in most cases. The chest drain is removed after 12–24 hours if no complications are apparent.

Bronchotomy
Bronchotomy is occasionally indicated to inspect the lumen of a bronchus at surgery. The commonest indication is probably removal of an inhaled foreign body, if endoscopic retrieval has failed. Such foreign bodies (typically grass seed heads in dogs) can usually be retrieved by experienced endoscopists and this is the treatment of choice in most cases (Figure 2.12). If the foreign body is wedged in one bronchus and the pulmonary parenchyma is not judged to be irreversibly infected, a thoracotomy can be carried out to allow access to the bronchus.

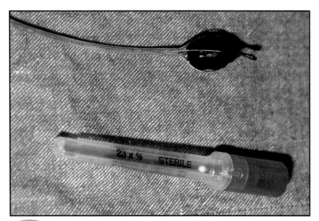

2.12 *A bean removed endoscopically from the trachea of a puppy.*

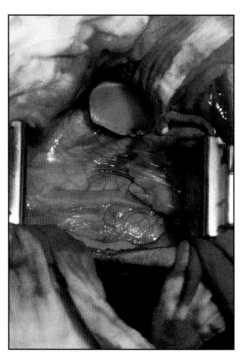

2.13 *Intraoperative view of pericardial sac of a dog undergoing pericardectomy. The phrenic nerve can be seen crossing the surgical field.*

Surgical technique

- Lateral thoracotomy approach over the hilus of the affected lobe (based on preoperative radiographs)
- Incision is then made in the bronchus and the foreign body is grasped and removed. During this procedure, ventilation of the patient is interfered with because of leakage of inspired gas through the bronchotomy. In most cases, this can be managed by intermittently closing the hole in the bronchus to allow ventilation. Less commonly, it may be necessary to introduce a long endotracheal tube to allow selective ventilation of the contralateral lung
- Bronchotomy is closed and the site checked for leaks prior to routine closure.

Antibiotic therapy and postoperative care are the same as following pulmonary lobectomy.

Pericardectomy

Excision of the pericardium is carried out in animals with pericardial disease. The commonest indication is pericardial effusion which causes heart failure, usually in large or giant breeds of dog. Heart failure occurs due to pressure of fluid accumulating in the pericardial sac, constricting the ability of the heart chambers to fill. Drainage of the pericardium percutaneously (pericardiocentesis) relieves the problem, but often the fluid reforms and the problem recurs.

The aim of the surgery is to remove the pericardial sac so that any fluid that forms is dispersed into the pleural space, where its volume is less significant. Surgery also allows the surgeon to inspect the pericardium and heart for any identifiable cause of fluid accumulation: tumours can be the underlying cause in some cases. The surgeon aims to excise as much pericardium as possible – typically, all the pericardium ventral to the phrenic nerves (which are attached to it) is removed (Figure 2.13). This can be done via a lateral thoracotomy or median sternotomy, at the surgeon's preference. The chest is closed routinely over a chest drain.

Perioperative antibiotics may be given, particularly if the surgery is prolonged or an infectious cause of effusion is suspected. The chest drain is removed after 12–24 hours if no complications arise.

Ruptured diaphragm repair

Although not strictly speaking a thoracic surgical procedure in most cases, similar considerations apply as for the above conditions and so the surgical treatment is included here. The preoperative care of these patients and the timing of surgery are critical.

Preoperative care

Most affected animals are presented within 24 hours of the inciting cause (road traffic injury, fall or other blunt thoracic trauma). However, the perioperative mortality is greater within the first 48 hours after injury than if surgery is delayed until after this period. Exceptions are animals with other complications (e.g. concurrent abdominal injuries) and those with displacement of the stomach into the thorax (gastrothorax). Gastrothorax can lead to gastric dilation and rapid deterioration in respiratory function and so early surgical exploration is indicated. During the period of stabilization before surgery the following are important:

- Fluid therapy to treat for shock
- Pain control with appropriate analgesics
- Gentle handling and sedation to minimize patient distress. Careful selection of diagnostic and other procedures and sympathetic handling are critical. Struggling with the patient to obtain thoracic radiographs may precipitate decompensation and death.

Perioperative care

Anaesthesia can destabilize the patient; therefore as much preparation as possible should take place prior to induction of anaesthesia.

- Clipping: the ventrum of the animal from manubrium to pubis and the lateral thorax on the side into which the abdominal organs are displaced should clipped. The animal must be handled to minimize distress, and clipping postponed if it causes distress
- Preparation of the surgeon and instrument trolley: the surgical team should scrub up and prepare the trolley so that surgery can commence immediately if the animal destabilizes at induction
- Patient positioning: during further preparation after induction, the animal is kept as much as possible in lateral recumbency, with the side into which the organs are displaced underneath.

Surgical technique

- Cranial abdominal midline approach is chosen in most cases. This allows inspection of the abdominal viscera for any concurrent injuries and access to the entire diaphragm, and can be extended cranially with a sternotomy if necessary
- Intermittent positive pressure ventilation will be necessary once the abdomen is opened
- Abdominal retractors (e.g. Balfour's) are helpful to maintain exposure
- Tear in the diaphragm is identified and the displaced organs are retracted into the abdomen. This is usually straightforward, but in chronic cases organs may have become incarcerated within the hernia ring or have formed adhesions to thoracic tissues. In such cases the tear in the diaphragm may have to be enlarged or a sternotomy carried out
- Entire abdomen is inspected for concurrent injuries prior to closure
- Chest drain is placed through the lateral thorax before the diaphragmatic tear is closed. Preplacement of sutures may make closure of the tear easier
- Abdomen is closed routinely
- Air remaining in the pleural space is removed via the chest drain after surgery: the lungs should *not* be forcefully inflated prior to diaphragmatic closure to achieve this. Forceful inflation of the lungs is associated with significant postoperative complications (pulmonary oedema).

Antibiotics are given perioperatively if incarcerated organs are returned to the abdomen. In such cases, rapid and short-acting corticosteroids (e.g. hydrocortisone) may also be helpful to overcome the toxaemia occasionally encountered in these cases. The chest drain is removed after 12–24 hours if no complications arise.

Cardiac surgery

Other than ligation of PDAs (above), cardiac surgery is rarely carried out in the UK, even in referral centres. A number of procedures have been described and used in dogs and cats, but their use has been restricted. In many cases, a limiting factor has been the availability of bypass technology. This is required to enable most surgery that involves actually entering the heart chambers.

Airway surgery and respiratory obstruction

This section will consider the special requirements of patients with respiratory obstruction and those undergoing surgery of the pharynx, larynx and trachea. The common diseases of this area have been outlined in the *BSAVA Manual of Veterinary Nursing* (Chapter 6).

Management of acute respiratory obstruction

Animals with obstructive dyspnoea are often critically affected and can rapidly deteriorate and die. Obstruction results from a variety of disease processes and can also follow surgery of the pharynx, larynx or trachea. A similar approach can be used in all these cases (Figure 2.14).

Bypassing the obstruction

If attention to the steps outlined in Figure 2.14 is unsuccessful in improving the situation, attempts can be made to bypass the area of obstruction. This can be done by corrective surgery (e.g. for laryngeal paralysis), induction of anaesthesia and intubation (e.g. for pharyngeal obstruction) or tracheotomy

2.14 Management of acute respiratory obstruction

Complication	Impact	Treatment
Patient distress	Animals with obstruction become excited and and distressed. Oxygen demands are increased, and increased respiratory efforts worsen the cause of obstruction	Allow the patient to settle before further procedures. Comfort the patient. Sedate the animal: the beneficial effects of sedation outweigh concern over respiratory depression in these cases
Hypoxia	Low blood oxygenation will prove fatal. Providing supplementary oxygen can be helpful in improving this, but may be done without further distressing or overheating the patient	Oxygen mask: effective but may distress the patient. Oxygen cage: reduces access to patient and can produce hyperthermia if not carefully controlled. Nasal oxygen tube: well tolerated once in position. Oxygen hood: placing clear plastic over an Elizabethan collar allows local oxygen supply. Well tolerated but beware of hyperthermia and hypercapnia
Hyperthermia	Core temperature often rises during airway obstruction. Increases oxygen consumption and increases respiratory efforts in an attempt to pant. Hyperthermia can be fatal if severe	Move patient to a cooler environment. Use fans to circulate air around the patient. Apply tepid water to the paws and ears. Clip excess hair. Apply tepid water to the skin. Place ice packs around the patient. Monitor temperature carefully to avoid hypothermia
Local inflammation	Swelling of tissues at the site of obstruction occurs as a result of increased air flow around them. Surgery also causes tissue swelling	Drug therapy: rapidly acting corticosteroids (intravenous hydrocortisone or dexamethasone)

(e.g. after surgery for brachycephalic obstruction syndrome). In emergencies, placing a large-gauge needle through the skin into the trachea can provide an alternative airway.

Tracheotomy

Indications

- Airway obstruction producing marked hypoxia and not amenable to conservative management or definitive treatment
- Intraluminal surgery of the upper airway
- Extensive oral or pharyngeal surgery to improve surgical access
- After airway surgery when severe swelling and worsened postoperative obstruction is anticipated (e.g. after surgery for brachycephalic obstruction syndrome in small breeds).

Surgical technique

- Can be done under sedation with local anaesthesia, but preferably induce general anaesthesia and intubate the patient if possible
- Prepare the surgical site (ventral midline of neck, immediately below larynx)
- Extend the neck
- Midline incision through skin and divide muscles in midline
- Hemicircumferential incision between tracheal rings
- Introduce tracheostomy tube (Figure 2.15) between rings (it may be helpful to place stay sutures around the proximal and distal rings to allow manipulation of the trachea should the tube need to be replaced)
- Suture tube to skin to secure (tape ties are unreliable)
- Alternative technique is the use of a needle tracheotomy kit (available commercially).

Tracheostomy tube care

- Have suction equipment available and ready for use
- Use suction tubing that is of a suitable diameter to remove any mucus or discharge but will not block the entire diameter of the trachea
- Use small amounts of sterile saline if necessary to unblock the tube. Have the suction ready and use immediately to clear the airway
- The equipment used to place the tube (Figure 2.16) must remain at hand in case the tube becomes displaced or blocked.

Removal of the tracheostomy tube

- Tube is removed once airway is patent
- Timing can be difficult and tube may have to be removed and replaced if patient remains unacceptably dyspnoeic
- Incision is usually left to heal by second intention, since it is invariably contaminated.

Special considerations for airway surgery

Particular concerns are pre-existing dyspnoea, ability to manage the airway during surgery and postoperative dyspnoea. The animal must be handled carefully and attention paid to the features of obstructive dyspnoea (above). To facilitate postoperative care, surgery should be planned for the early part of the day.

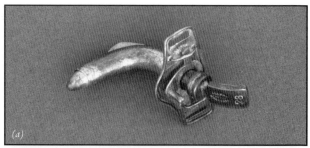

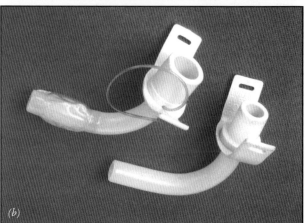

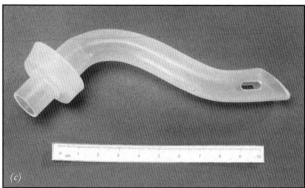

2.15 *Various types of tracheostomy tubes. (a) Silver tube. Similar tubes with separate inner and outer parts are useful since they are easily cleaned in situ. This tube has an obturator, which facilitates replacement. (b) Disposable plastic tubes. Cuffed types are sometimes preferred for anaesthesia. (c) Silicon tube designed specifically for dogs. The curve improves retention within the trachea.*

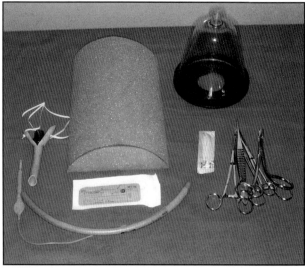

2.16 *Equipment used for tracheotomy. A homemade emergency tracheostomy tube is shown.*

2.17 Provision of an airway during intraluminal surgery

Method	Advantages	Disadvantages
Brief period of extubation	Straightforward	Limited to brief procedures Cannot provide ventilation Does not guard the airway
Tracheotomy intubation	Allows full control Tube removed from surgical site	Complicates postoperative care
Sterile ET tube placed at surgical site	Surgeon controls access Useful during tracheal reconstruction Allows full control	Surgeon has to work around tube

Intraoperative care

The prime concern during surgery is to maintain a safe airway. During extraluminal surgery (that is, when the procedure does not involve surgery within the airway itself), such as laryngoplasty ('tie-back'), this is relatively straightforward. Nonetheless, provision must be made to remove and replace the tube if the surgeon requires this. A laryngoscope should be at hand, with a variety of endotracheal tubes. In some cases, an armoured endotracheal tube (one that is resistant to kinking) may be necessary.

During intraluminal surgery, maintenance of the airway is more difficult. A variety of techniques (Figure 2.17) can be used and they should be available at the time of surgery in case they prove necessary.

Postoperative care

Concerns in the postoperative period include:

* *Obstruction* – Airway surgery may provoke sufficient swelling that the airway is more severely compromised in the first few days after surgery than it was before. Preoperative treatment with corticosteroids is often used to reduce this complication. The animal must be closely observed during the first few hours to detect worsening dyspnoea. Animals showing evidence of distress or cyanosis are managed as above. Equipment for tracheotomy and for oxygen supplementation should be immediately available (Figure 2.18)
* *Coughing* – Excessive coughing after surgery is distressing to the patient and can worsen inflammation and place undesirable stress on the surgical site. It should be managed with sedation or anti-tussive treatment (the opiate analgesics provide both actions)
* *Dysphagia* – Particularly after laryngeal or pharyngeal surgery, the ability to swallow and prevent aspiration may be compromised. Food is usually withheld for 12 hours after surgery. After this, a soft but not flaky food is advised for the next 4–6 weeks. Complete tinned foods often fulfil this need. Milk should not be given and swimming must stopped. Postoperative antibiotics are continued for 10–14 days to prevent secondary infection (aspiration pneumonia).

Neurological surgery

Surgery of the nervous system encompasses a variety of techniques, including repair of peripheral nerves, intracranial surgery and spinal surgery. The most commonly performed of these in veterinary surgery involve spinal surgery and most attention will be given to this area. Repair of peripheral nerves is rarely carried out. Nursing aspects of such cases largely relate to

2.18 Equipment requirements for tracheotomy

* Anaesthetic machine, circuits and range of ET tubes
* Laryngoscope
* Oxygen mask
* Surgical pack
* Self-retaining (e.g. West) or handheld retractors
* Sutures (e.g. monofilament nylon)
* Positioning aids (sandbags, wedges, etc.)
* Tracheostomy tubes

the specific neurological defect involved. For example, an animal with paralysis of a limb arising from nerve severance will benefit from physiotherapy to maintain muscle tone and mobility of the limb prior to surgical repair and in the recovery phase.

Intracranial surgery

Surgery of the intracranial central nervous system (brain) is carried out in a few specialist centres. Successful outcomes depend on careful preoperative assessment, careful surgical technique using the correct instrumentation and excellent postoperative care.

Preoperative assessment includes the use of advanced imaging techniques (MRI or CT scan) and this has been a limiting factor in the availability of this type of surgery. As access to these imaging techniques increases, intracranial surgery will become more widely used.

Postoperative care is demanding: alterations in intracranial pressure must be monitored and addressed as necessary. Patients are often neurologically depressed for several days after surgery and are at risk of seizures, which can have a devastating effect. For these reasons, round-the-clock observation and nursing care must be provided for at least the first 3–5 days postoperatively. During this time, general nursing care will also have to be provided: assisted feeding, physical therapy and encouragement and support from both nursing staff and owners. Excellent communication with the animal's owners is particularly important in these cases.

Spinal surgery

Surgery of the spine is the commonest type of neurological surgery performed. The indications for this type of surgery include:

* Intervertebral disc disease (degeneration and prolapse)
* Congenital malformations of the vertebrae
* Discospondylitis (infection of the intervertebral disc)
* Neoplasia affecting the spinal cord (arising in adjacent tissues, the vertebrae or within the cord itself)
* Trauma resulting in instability of the vertebrae or compression of the cord.

Of these, the commonest are disc disease and congenital malformations – including the 'wobbler syndrome' (a disease of certain large and giant breeds of dog – notably Great Dane and Dobermann – in which malformation of the cervical vertebrae leads to spinal cord damage and gait abnormalities or neck pain).

Management of these cases depends critically on the selection of animals likely to benefit from surgical rather than conservative or medical treatment and the choice of the most appropriate surgical technique. These decisions are based on:

- Careful history taking
- Clinical (including neurological) examination
- Imaging of the spine, including plain radiography, contrast radiography (myelography and epidurography) and, increasingly, advanced imaging techniques (MRI and CT scans)
- Ancillary tests such as cerebrospinal fluid analysis and electrodiagnostic procedures (e.g. electromyography, EMG).

Preoperative care

The urgency of spinal surgery varies. In some cases, in the face of a severe neurological abnormality (such as loss of pain sensation in the feet) or a rapid deterioration in neurological function, surgery must be carried out within 12–24 hours for optimum success. In other cases – for example, in animals with congenital lesions and non-progressive signs, or in older animals where there is spinal pain but minimal neurological deficits – the need for surgery is less urgent and the surgeon may wait to assess the result of medical management before undertaking surgery.

The preoperative care of spinal patients depends on the severity of their signs and the area of the spinal cord affected.

Patients with little neurological dysfunction and no spinal instability

No specific nursing care is required except for maintaining cage rest and minimal exercise. This aims to reduce movement of the spine, which will reduce pain and limit the progression of disease. Typical cases are those with cervical intervertebral disc prolapse. Nonetheless, care must be taken to limit the movement of such cases. Cage rest and analgesia will often encourage them to move more freely, but this must be restricted: for example, they must not be allowed to jump up, climb steps or take exercise off the lead. A harness may be more suitable for restraint than a collar and lead.

Patients with instability of the vertebral column

Steps to reduce the mobility of the vertebrae are indicated: in addition to cage rest, splints to reduce movement of the affected area may be used. One example is atlantoaxial subluxation, seen in young small-breed dogs. These animals have a congenital malformation of the atlantoaxial joint (between the first and second cervical vertebrae). This results in instability of these structures and a tendency for compression of the spinal cord at this point. A neck collar may be used in these dogs to prevent flexion of the neck, which causes the compression. Cases like this with spinal instability must be handled carefully to limit movement of the affected vertebrae. This is particularly the case when under anaesthesia, since the loss of muscle tone makes the vertebrae more mobile.

Patients with significant neurological deficits

Greater nursing care is required. This can be challenging, particularly with large-breed dogs and with animals in pain that may resent handling. Paraplegic animals (those with hindlimb weakness) require assistance to walk, but walking is encouraged both as physiotherapy and for toilet purposes. Small dogs can be supported manually by one person but large paraplegic dogs need two or more people to carry them out and support them. A large towel can be used as a sling under the abdomen to support the hindquarters.

Quadriplegic animals

By definition, these are usually unable to rise and must be nursed in recumbency. To prevent hypostatic pneumonia in the lower lung they must be turned every 4 hours. They are prone to pressure sores and decubital ulcers. The incidence of these is minimized by turning the patient regularly, nursing on a soft surface (e.g. foam bed), cleanliness and dryness of the skin and supporting surface, and adequate nutrition. The limbs must be massaged to promote muscle tone and circulation and range of movement exercises used to maintain muscle strength and limb mobility (see Chapter 4).

Patients with urinary retention

This is not uncommon, particularly in quadriplegic patients. It can be the result of an unwillingness to urinate because of an inability to posture (also seen in paraplegics and with severe hindlimb injuries) or because of disruption to the nerve supply of the bladder or urethra. Urinary retention must be actively managed to prevent further complications: chronic overfilling of the bladder can result in permanent dysuria. When the bladder becomes distended, urine will tend to leak from the urethra (urinary retention and overflow, URO) but this is not an indication of the ability to urinate normally and will result in damage to the bladder. Drugs can be used in such patients to relax the urethra and increase tone in the bladder, but usually other measures are more appropriate to allow emptying of the bladder:

- Gentle compression of the bladder through the abdominal wall. This will allow expression of the urine, particularly in more chronic cases. As the patient recovers, this compression will often prompt automatic contraction of the bladder and the animal will void the remaining urine without further help
- Urethral catheterization. In other cases, particularly soon after an acute injury, bladder compression is ineffective: excessive force must not be used, since there is a risk of bladder rupture. In these animals the bladder must be emptied by catheterization. This can be done by repeated passage of a catheter as necessary or by placement of an indwelling catheter. The choice of approach will be made by the veterinary surgeon. Indwelling catheters carry a greater risk of ascending infection but are less traumatic than repeated catheterization and can make nursing care more manageable, particularly in large dogs. Indwelling catheters should be connected to a closed collection system (a custom-made unit or a giving set and empty fluid bag), which helps to keep the patient clean and dry as well as reducing the risk of ascending urinary infection (see Chapter 4).

Intraoperative care

- *To avoid exacerbating the injury*, the anaesthetized animal must be moved with particular caution. This may include use of a rigid stretcher, avoiding excess flexion or extension (particularly of the neck), and careful manipulation during radiography

- *Myelography* may be carried out during the same anaesthetic, and if so the animal's head may have to remain elevated during anaesthesia and recovery
- *Hypothermia* must be minimized. Spinal surgery, particularly if radiography is carried out at the same time, can be lengthy and efforts must be made to minimize heat loss. Radiography is often performed in a relatively cool environment and there is also potential conductive loss to the table; these effects can be reduced by covering or wrapping the patient in insulating material and placing such material between the animal and table. If this overlies the cassette it must be radiolucent and clean
- *Careful positioning* in theatre is critical to maximize surgical access. A variety of positioning aids are helpful – for example, a roll of firm support to place under the lumbar area if a lateral approach to the lumbar spine is used. This prevents a tendency for the spine to sag and helps to open up the intervertebral spaces on the upper side. For cervical surgery from a ventral approach, moderate extension of the cervical spine is necessary: a cradle with a cervical step may be used to achieve this
- *Specialized instrumentation* is used in spinal surgery. This includes hand instruments such as laminectomy rongeurs and picks to enter and explore the spinal canal, and power instruments such as compressed air burrs which facilitate removal of overlying bone. In addition, if spinal instability is present, instruments for placement of internal fixation devices (screws, washers, Kirschner wires and plates) will be required. Whenever power tools are used, saline must be available to lavage the tissues to prevent the build-up of excessive heat and to remove bone fragments. Surgical suction is often helpful to remove saline lavage and to clear the field of haemorrhage. Bipolar diathermy is useful to control haemorrhage from surrounding tissues
- *Haemorrhage* is a potential problem during spinal surgery, and can be difficult to control if it arises from the venous sinuses within the spinal canal. In some cases it can be controlled by surgical suction, packing and application of bone wax but it can be severe enough to require transfusion of whole blood or packed cells. This is particularly the case when a ventral slot procedure is used in cervical surgery in large dogs
- *Perioperative antibiotics* are given if the surgical procedure is prolonged or internal fixation is carried out.

Postoperative care

On-going nursing considerations are generally an extension of preoperative care and are addressed above. In addition, if a myelogram has been performed there is a risk of adverse reactions (particularly seizures) during recovery from anaesthesia. During this time, the animal is kept with the head slightly elevated (a foam wedge large enough to place the whole animal on, in lateral recumbency, is useful) and close observation is necessary during the first 12 hours. The intravenous catheter is kept in place during this time and diazepam for injection should be available for treatment of seizures, should they occur.

Once the animal is ready for discharge from the clinic, the owners may need instructions on how to nurse the animal at home, particularly if it is still unable to walk or if bladder control has not returned. Since the nurses have been responsible for this care until now, they are often the most appropriate staff to demonstrate this to the owners. After discharge the owners will need support, advice and encouragement to rehabilitate their pet and will need to maintain contact with the practice, often via the nursing staff, who must be familiar with the care procedures and the likely progress of the animal. Staff should seek advice from the surgeon on the expected prognosis and time course of recovery so that they can communicate effectively with the owners.

Animals with moderate or severe limb weakness are unable to exercise sufficiently to maintain or restore muscle bulk. These cases in particular benefit from hydrotherapy during rehabilitation, in the form of whirlpool baths or swimming, with appropriate supervision.

Major orthopaedic surgery

The definition of major orthopaedic surgery is somewhat arbitrary. This section will include extensive internal fixation, external fixation using Kirschner–Ehmer and similar apparatus, and hip replacement. Other orthopaedic surgery is covered in Chapter 6 of the *BSAVA Manual of Veterinary Nursing*.

Preoperative care

The preoperative care of animals undergoing orthopaedic surgery is largely dealt with in the *BSAVA Manual of Veterinary Nursing*. The degree of care required will depend on the nature and severity of the animal's disease.

- *Young animals undergoing elective surgery for angular limb deformity* need no special preoperative preparation
- *Animals requiring repair of injuries sustained in major trauma* (for example, road traffic accidents or big dog/ little dog confrontations) need extensive preoperative assessment and treatment of concurrent injuries before definitive treatment of their orthopaedic injuries
  - These patients frequently have other injuries that must be identified and managed before or concurrently with their bone injuries – for example, shock, thoracic trauma and abdominal trauma. These are usually investigated prior to anaesthesia: for example, abdominal and thoracic radiographs are often taken as part of the initial assessment
  - In many cases, repair of fractures is not an emergency procedure and other life-threatening injuries can be dealt with as a priority initially
  - Exceptions to this are some spinal injuries and open fractures: in the latter case the prognosis for effective repair is better if surgery is carried out within a few hours of injury
- *When surgery is delayed*, the animal is managed in such a way as to not worsen the injury
  - In some cases a bandage or splint may be used to immobilize the limb but in many cases confinement to a cage will suffice
  - During this time, the animal may require fluid therapy, analgesia and attention to toilet needs (access to a suitable area or urinary catheterization)
- *Animals undergoing elective major orthopaedic surgery* should be in as good a state for surgery as possible
  - Their body weight can be manipulated by changing their dietary regime so that they are neither excessively fat nor thin at the time of surgery. Excess body weight may worsen recovery from surgery and poor body condition may slow wound healing or make postoperative infections more likely

– Any remote infections should be treated and eliminated before elective extensive orthopaedic surgery. Common sites of infection include the skin (pyoderma), mouth (particularly dental disease) and urinary tract. Infections at any of these sites can seed to cause infections at the site of orthopaedic repairs

– When skin infection is not present, the patient should still be as clean as possible before surgery and bathing with a mild cleansing shampoo on the day before surgery may be helpful

– As a matter of course, animals should not be hospitalized before elective surgery, since their skin will rapidly be colonized by the hospital population of bacteria, which are more likely to be resistant to commonly used antibiotics

– Similarly, the hair should not be clipped until immediately before surgery, since this will inevitably lead to some epithelial damage and a resulting increase in skin bacterial numbers.

Intraoperative care

Intraoperative care is largely limited to that generally required for major surgery.

• *Hypothermia* during prolonged procedures must be guarded against

• In some instances there is a risk of *significant haemorrhage*, and fluid therapy must be planned with this in mind. Following recent trauma, there may already have been significant blood loss, externally or into the tissues, and the effect of this must be considered

• *Perioperative antibiotic therapy* is routine in extensive orthopaedic procedures, since there is a significant risk of infection around any implants used. This is particularly important when marked soft tissue damage, including skin perforation, is present or when surgery is prolonged

  – The most appropriate regime is to give intravenous antibiotics during patient preparation (i.e. 30 minutes before the skin incision is made) and again at appropriate intervals to provide effective antibacterial levels during the first 12 hours after surgery

  – A drug that is effective against common skin bacteria (which are the commonest cause of wound infections in this instance) is chosen (e.g. cephazolin or clavulanate–amoxycillin)

  – Antibacterial therapy may be continued after surgery, particularly if there was an open fracture or a break in aseptic technique during surgery.

Postoperative care

Postoperative care depends on the type of disease and the method of repair.

• Often after limb surgery a *dressing* will have been applied – to offer further support to a repair, to protect the wound from contamination, or to reduce the tendency for postsurgical swelling. A Robert Jones or similar dressing is used to provide support and this may be left in place for some days if no complications develop. Light dressings are commonly removed or replaced after 24–48 hours

• The degree of *exercise restriction* required will vary from case to case

  – In some instances the surgeon may wish to encourage early exercise to minimize joint stiffness and muscle atrophy after surgery. In these cases, swimming may be a useful way to provide this without excessive weightbearing

  – In other cases, cage confinement may be necessary or the surgeon may apply a bandage to restrict limb use (a Velpeau or Ehmer sling)

• In all cases, *analgesia* should be continued after surgery as necessary: it is rarely appropriate to discourage activity by withholding pain control.

Internal fixation

Various methods are used to repair bone defects (fractures, osteotomies and ostectomies) in small animals (Figure 2.19). These techniques may be used as single methods but often they are used in combination to produce a satisfactory repair. External fixators (see below) may also be used with methods of internal fixation. A large selection of instruments is available for such surgery. The nurse must be familiar with the appearance, use and care of instruments available in each establishment.

2.19 Methods of internal fixation

• Intramedullary pinning[a]
• Lag screw placement[a]
• Cerclage wiring[a]
• Interfragmentary wiring[a]
• Kirschner wire placement[a]
• Bone plating
• Intramedullary nailing[b]

a See BSAVA Manual of Veterinary Nursing *Chapter 6*
b *A rarely used technique; not described here*

Some instrument sets are intended for use with particular implant systems. An example is the Association for the Study of Osteosynthesis/Association for the Study of Internal Fixation (AO/ASIF) system. This system includes plates and screws of a wide variety of types and sizes and instruments to apply them. Generic types of similar equipment are also available, as well as implants that are not part of a larger system.

In most cases, the surgeon will select the system to be used but the theatre nurses are usually responsible for ensuring that the stock of implants is maintained. Whichever system is used, it is important that only implants from the same source and intended to be used together are selected: incorrectly matched implants will lead to poor results due to mismatching of sizes and chemical reaction between metals of different types. Figure 2.20 indicates the typical equipment requirements for internal fixation and the size of implants needed when the AO/ASIF equipment is used for repair of long bones.

Implants are often not removed once the fracture has healed. This is particularly the case with older animals. In younger animals the surgeon more frequently elects to remove the implants. This is because they may interfere with bone growth. Implants are also removed if complications such as infection become apparent, although it may be possible to delay removal until after the fracture has healed. Following removal, the implants must be disposed of: with the exception of clamps from external fixators (see below), implants are not designed for reuse and are at risk of breaking if this is attempted.

External fixation

An alternative to the use of implants that are buried within the body to repair bone defects is the use of external fixators. These use thin pins or wires, placed through the skin and anchored into bone, that are then secured to frames or scaffolding placed alongside or around a limb. Common examples are the Kirschner–Ehmer apparatus (Figure 2.21) and the Ilizarov fixator (Figure 2.22).

2.20 Typical equipment requirements for internal fixation

Typical equipment for placement of bone plates

- Variety of plates, screws and washers
- Hand or power drill
- Plate-holding and bone-holding forceps
- Reduction forceps
- Countersink
- Handheld retractors (e.g. Hohmann)
- Self-retaining retractors (e.g. West's)
- Plate-bending irons
- Tap sleeve
- Drill bits
- Drill guide
- Screwdriver
- Tap (for non-self-tapping systems)

Typical equipment for placement of intramedullary pins, cerclage and Kirschner wires

- Variety of pins and wires
- Power-driven chuck
- Pin-holding forceps
- Drill bits
- Jacob's chuck and key
- Pin or wire cutters
- Hand or power drill

Selection of implant size for internal fixation of long-bone fractures

Animal size	Implant size
Large/giant dogs	4.5 mm AO set
Medium/large dogs	3.5 mm AO set
Small dogs/cats	2.7 mm AO set
Miniature dogs and cats	2.0 mm AO set (Miniplate)

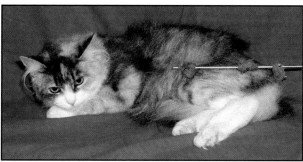

2.21 *External fixator (Kirschner–Ehmer apparatus) in place to repair a femoral fracture in a cat.*
Courtesy of Dr J Innes

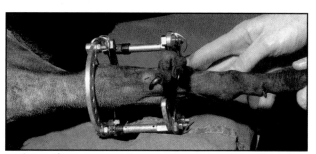

2.22 *Ilizarov apparatus in use to correct a congenital malformation in a puppy.*
Courtesy of Dr J Innes

In some cases, the surgeon may decide to improvise a similar system, particularly in unusual cases such as fractures in unusual species or the repair of mandibular fractures. In these instances the external frame is replaced by quick-setting plastics, for example.

One particular instance when external fixators are of great use is the management of fractures with extensive local soft tissue trauma or infection. Internal fixation of these is often unsatisfactory because infection is perpetuated around the implants. External fixation allows implants to be placed away from the immediate area and also allows access for open wound management, if necessary, whilst providing stability for healing of the fracture.

Aftercare of animals with external fixators includes the following.

Daily adjustment

Some external fixators allow the movement of bone fragments after their placement. These can be particularly useful in the treatment of angular limb deformities and malunions. If this is necessary, the surgeon may instruct the nurse or owner on how this is to be done.

Dressing

Following placement of the fixator, occasionally a compressive (modified Robert Jones) bandage is applied and changed or removed after 2–3 days. After this, no further dressing of the limb may be required but the fixator is commonly covered in bandaging material to prevent the sharp ends damaging the patient or owner. Although the fixator can have an alarming appearance to the owner, it is usually well tolerated by the animal.

Pin tract care

Commonly there is some discharge from the skin when the pins enter (pin tracts). The surgeon will advise on whether any care for this is necessary: in many cases it will dry to a crust and no attention to it is necessary or desirable.

Re-examination after discharge

The animal is commonly discharged after a few days. The animal will be re-examined periodically to evaluate healing and check that the pins or fixator have not loosened. If healing is satisfactory, parts of the apparatus may be removed to increase the loading on the healing repair ('scaling down' of the fixator). Once the surgeon is satisfied that the repair is stable and adequately strong, the fixator will be removed entirely.

Total hip replacement (THR)

This procedure is performed at veterinary schools and some referral practices. It is essentially restricted to use in dogs and the primary indication is hip dysplasia. Case selection is important: the decision for surgery is based on the response of the dog to conservative and medical management and consideration of alternative surgical treatments (excision arthroplasty, triple pelvic osteotomy, intertrochanteric osteotomy, pectineal myotomy). Details of these techniques can be found in other texts.

Total hip replacement is essentially the removal of the components of the native joint (acetabulum and femoral head and neck) and their replacement by synthetic prostheses (Figure 2.23). Several integrated systems are available, consisting of the implants and the specialized instrumentation required. These systems may be modular: that is, include interchangeable acetabular cups, femoral heads, femoral necks and femoral shaft inserts so that the optimum combination

Advanced surgery and surgical nursing | **55**

can be selected at the time of surgery. The most commonly used systems are cementable – the implants are fixed in position with bone cement (methylmethacrylate) – but systems that do not require cement are under development.

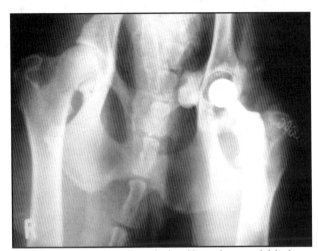

2.23 *Postoperative radiograph of total hip replacement, left limb. Courtesy of Dr J Innes*

Preoperative care
The most critical element here is to ensure that the animal is in the optimum condition for surgical recovery:

- Elimination of concurrent infections
- Attention to body condition
- Treatment of concurrent problems (including other orthopaedic conditions).

Intraoperative care
The nurse must be familiar with the instrumentation so that the surgeon can be assisted efficiently. The surgeon, nurse and assistant may choose to review the equipment before it is sterilized. The majority of the equipment is supplied as a set dedicated to the particular implant system chosen. Additional requirements may include an oscillating saw and blades, power drill and retractors. Infection will prove disastrous because of implant loosening and particular care must be taken to avoid intraoperative contamination.

Postoperative care
The animal is confined to a kennel for 48 hours after surgery and for the first week the animal must be supported whilst walking on any slippery surfaces. Increased lead exercise is introduced over the following 6 weeks. Postoperative checks are carried out at 10 days, 3 months, 6 months and annually thereafter.

Schedule Three procedures

The Veterinary Surgeons Act allows registered veterinary nurses to carry out minor acts of veterinary surgery on small animals at the direction of a veterinary surgeon. The range of techniques has not been defined, except that it excludes surgeries involving entry into a body cavity (including castration). The Act places emphasis on the ability of the individual nurse to carry out these operative procedures and the directing veterinary surgeon must ensure that the nurse has received the necessary further training. Since the Act has not defined a list of suitable procedures, the authors cannot provide more than general guidance, but certain nurses may be in a position to undertake the following, given suitable guidance and experience:

- Minor surgery, including wound closure and skin mass removal
- Dental scaling
- Dental extraction
- Abscess treatment
- Aural haematoma treatment.

Minor surgery

Principles of instrument handling for wound closure and other minor surgery

Towel clips
Towel clips are used to secure drapes to the skin. The two common types in use are crossover and Backhaus. Crossover clips have a spring action and do not have ring handles. Backhaus clips are ringed instruments and have a locking action. Both types have curved tips.

- The tips are placed downwards towards the tissue
- The tips are placed across the corner of the draped area close to the edge of the drape
- One tip is placed on each drape and the tips pushed down on to the drape and underlying skin as the handles are closed (Figure 2.24)
- Once the clip is placed, the handles can be tucked under one of the drapes.

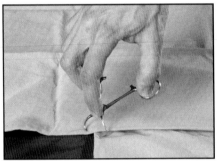

2.24 *Securing the drapes with towel clips.*

Scalpel
The scalpel is most commonly used in minor surgery to cut the skin. The scalpel is preferred to scissors for this purpose since it is generally sharper and cuts the skin without crushing. Generally a No.10 blade (semi-curved) is used for this.

The veterinary nurse must be able to place and remove the disposable scalpel blade on the handle without danger of self-injury; this can be done with forceps or by the correct manual technique. If done manually, the blade is kept directed away from the palm so that if the fingers slip the hand is not cut. The forceps technique is safer.

For skin incisions the scalpel is held in a pencil grip by most surgeons, although a palm grip is one alternative. Most importantly the scalpel must be held positively and firmly so that it is used with firm controlled pressure (Figure 2.25).

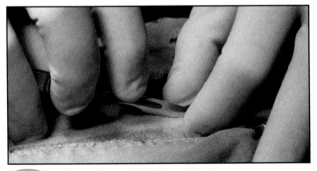

2.25 *Making a skin incision with a scalpel.*

The skin incision:

- The curved part of the blade, not the tip, is used to cut the skin
- Skin is kept under tension during incision, by stretching it with the fingers of the non-dominant hand, so that it gapes open as the cut is made
- The blade is held perpendicular to the skin so that the cut edges of the skin are at right angles to the surface
- The skin should be cut firmly so that the full thickness is incised at one stroke
- It is best to cut the full length of the intended incision in one stroke, or without lifting the blade, so that a single smooth cut results.

Occasionally a scalpel is used to make a stab incision through the skin, for example to lance an abscess. For this the blade is turned over and the tip is used. A No.11 blade may be preferred. The skin is kept tense and the fingers used to ensure that the blade penetrates no deeper than intended.

Thumb forceps

The two types of thumb forceps commonly used in minor surgery are the rat-toothed tissue forceps ('rats') and the atraumatic or dressing forceps. The latter are distinguished by the lack of hooks at the tips and the presence of serrated tips. Rat-toothed forceps are used to manipulate tough tissue such as the skin – atraumatic forceps are used to hold other tissues. In some cases, holding the tissues with the fingers or with fine rat-toothed forceps may be preferable to excessive use of atraumatic forceps. The forceps are held in a pencil grip, balanced across the hand. Whichever forceps are used, they potentially damage the tissue so they should be used as gently and infrequently as possible.

Tissue forceps

Other tissue forceps are occasionally used in minor surgery. Allis tissue forceps are traumatic to tissue because of their crushing action. However, they can be clamped on to tissue to prevent repeated grasping by thumb forceps. This is most applicable to holding tissue that is to be excised, such as a skin mass. They are occasionally used to hold skin edges but in that case should be applied to the dermis rather than the skin surface.

Scissors

Scissors are used to cut tissue and suture material. Ideally, separate scissors should be used for each purpose since suture material will blunt the blades. The common types of scissors in use are Mayo and Metzenbaum. Mayo scissors are the 'standard' type and are relatively heavy in design. They are usually made with two round-tipped blades (blunt–blunt). They are used for cutting dense tissue and suture material. Metzenbaums are lighter in construction, with longer handles and finer blades, again usually blunt–blunt. They should only be used for cutting fine tissue. Both types can be curved or straight.

Use of scissors:

- The scissors are held in the right hand with the thumb and fourth finger in the rings. The finger should only go through up to the first joint. The index finger rests along the blade and the third finger wraps around the ring (Figure 2.26).

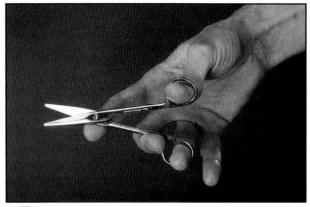

2.26 *Holding scissors.*

- Scissors can be used for cutting or blunt dissection
- For blunt dissection, the blades are pushed closed into the tissue and then opened to tear and separate. In this way large vessels and nerves are avoided
- Cutting is usually done in several small strokes but the tissue should be cut smoothly, not sawn through
- The tips of the blades are used for cutting tissues
- Suture material is cut with the parts of the blades nearest the hinges.

Artery forceps (haemostats)

Artery forceps are used to occlude blood vessels. Several types are available and the smallest appropriate should be chosen. Artery forceps can be applied to vessels before they are cut or once the tissue has been incised and a bleeding point is seen.

Use of artery forceps:

- The tips of the instrument should be used to pick up the blood vessel or bleeding point with the minimum of additional tissue (Figure 2.27)
- Curved forceps are useful to reach difficult areas
- Once clamped, bleeding vessels can be dealt with in various ways:
- very small vessels will not bleed if the forceps are removed after 2 minutes
- vessels smaller than 3 mm in diameter can be occluded by twisting and pulling until the tissue is pulled away
- larger vessels should be ligated using 2 or 3 metric gauge absorbable ligature. Three square knots are tied around the tissue in the tips of the forceps.

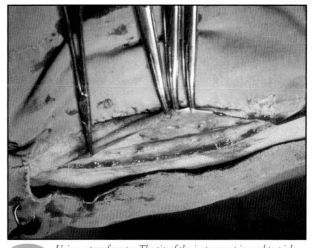

2.27 *Using artery forceps. The tip of the instrument is used to pick up a blood vessel.*

The tips of artery forceps are also sometimes used for blunt dissection, particularly for the isolation of vessels before clamping and division.

Needle holders

The common types in use are Mayo, Kilner, MacPhail, Olsen–Hagar and Gillies. The last two types combine needle holders and suture scissors. Gillies vary from the other patterns in that they do not have locks to hold the needle in place: the surgeon must keep the handles closed to hold the needle. This makes them less suitable for intricate suture placement.

The Mayo, Kilner and Olsen–Hagar needle holders are held in the same way as scissors: with the thumb and fourth finger. Gillies have a large ring for the thumb and a smaller one for the fourth finger. Exceptionally, Gillies are available in a left-handed pattern. MacPhail needle holders are held in the palm of the hand.

Needle holders are used to grasp the suture needle and pass it through the tissue. Suture needles are designed to be gripped in the region between one third and one half of the length from the eye: this area is flattened for this purpose (Figure 2.28).

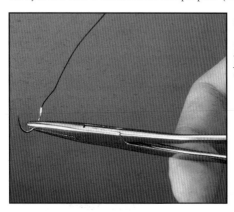

2.28

Needle holders grasping the flattened region of a suture needle.

Several principles aid the effective use of needle holders and needles:

- Hold the needle in the region between half way along its length and two thirds towards the eye. This region is slightly flattened to allow gripping by the needle holders
- Use appropriate sized needle holders: wide jaws will damage curved needles
- Do not handle the tip of the needle with needle holders or forceps: these will blunt the tip
- Pass the needle through the tissue in a smooth curve that follows the shape of the needle. Use the wrist to roll the needle along its curve. Failure to do so is the commenest cause of the needle bending
- Do not attempt to straighten a bent needle; the needle will be further weakened and is likely to break
- Discard blunt needles!

Choice of suture material for closure of wounds and minor surgery

A variety of suture materials is available (see *BSAVA Manual of Veterinary Nursing*, Chapter 7). Often the selection is a matter of personal preference and practice policy, but some guidelines are suggested:

- Use absorbable suture material for buried patterns (subcutaneous and subcuticular sutures and all ligatures)
- Use non-absorbable for exposed skin sutures and plan removal at the appropriate time (7–10 days)
- Use non-reactive materials in preference to those known to provoke tissue reaction
- Use material of a gauge appropriate to the tissue strength.

Figure 2.29 gives a guide to the selection of suture material for minor surgery.

2.29 Selection of suture material for minor surgery

Type	Characteristics	Indications	Suggested gauge
Monofilament nylon (polyamide) Monofilament polypropylene	Non-reactive Permanent Fair handling/knot security	Suture of choice for exposed skin pattern	1–2 metric for cats and thin skin in small dogs 3 metric for thick skin in dogs
Multifilament or braided nylon	More reactive than above Good handling and knot security	Second choice for skin Preferred by many because of handling characteristics	1–2 metric for cats and thin skin in small dogs 3 metric for thick skin in dogs
Polyglactin 910 Polyglycolic acid	Absorbable Multifilament Non-reactive in the absence of contamination	Subcuticular Subcutaneous Muscle Mucous membranes Not recommended for exposed skin patterns	1–3 metric
Polyglactin 910 (rapid absorption)	Strength lost in 7–10 days	Occasionally used for skin to eliminate need for suture removal	2–3 metric
Poliglecaprone	Absorbable Monofilament Fair to good handling	Subcuticular Subcutaneous	1–2 metric
Chromic catgut	Absorbable Natural and reactive synthetic alternatives generally preferable Relatively inexpensive	Subcuticular Subcutaneous Muscle Not recommended for exposed skin patterns	1–3 metric
Silk	Non-absorbable Natural and reactive Excellent handling and soft	Occasionally used for exposed patterns in the skin, particularly around the face	1–3 metric

Suture patterns

Sutures are placed in different patterns to achieve a variation in the way in which tissue edges are apposed. In most cases in minor surgery the aim is simply to appose the edges, that is to bring the tissue together so that the layers are aligned. In other instances suture patterns are chosen that tend to *invert* (fold the edges inwards) or *evert* (roll the edges out).

Suture patterns may be:

• Continuous, in which all of the length of a wound is closed by a single length of suture with a knot at either end

• Interrupted, where the wound is closed by a number of separate stitches with individual knots.

The choice of interrupted or continuous is made on assessment of these factors in each case (Figure 2.30). Most surgeons favour interrupted patterns in the skin because of the possible risk of patient interference and wound disruption but in patients that are unstable under anaesthesia, and for long wounds, a continuous pattern can be worthwhile. Suture patterns are summarized in Figure 2.31 and illustrated in Figure 2.32.

2.30 Interrupted versus continuous sutures

	Advantages	Disadvantages
Interrupted	More secure since one stitch may be lost without incision disrupting	Slower to place More suture material required More material left is used in buried position
Continuous	Placed more rapidly Less suture material used Less buried suture left Allows spread of tension along suture line Produces better seal	Theoretically less secure

2.31 Suture patterns

	Description	Features	Typical applications
Interrupted			
Simple interrupted appositional (SIA) (Figure 2.32a)	Individual stitches placed as simple loops across the wound	The standard pattern Produces good apposition	Skin closure Midline closure Visceral closure
Horizontal mattress (Figure 2.32b)	Placed as loops with a bite on each side of wound parallel to wound edge	Produces some eversion Resists effects of tension more than SIA	Skin, especially in presence of tension
Cruciate mattress (Figure 2.32c)	Similar to horizontal mattress but strands cross over wound	Less eversion than above Resists effects of tension more than SIA Faster than above	Skin, especially in presence of tension
Vertical mattress (Figure 2.32d)	Placed as loops with a bite on each side of wound perpendicular to wound edge	Produces some eversion Resists effects of tension more than SIA Interferes with blood supply less than horizontal mattress	Skin, especially in presence of tension Most commonly used interspersed with SIA to resist effects of tension
Continuous			
Simple continuous (SC) (Figure 2.32e)	Running stitch	Rapidly placed Prone to patient interference if used in skin Theoretically insecure	Fascia, including midline Muscle Viscera
Ford interlocking (Figure 2.32f)	'Blanket stitch'	Rapidly placed Better apposition than SC Slightly more secure than SC Effective seal	Long skin wounds
Intradermal/ subcuticular (Figure 2.32g)	Buried continuous stitch to close skin	Slower than other skin patterns Resists tension Avoids patient interference Does not require removal	Skin Presence of tension Sites prone to interference (e.g. castration)

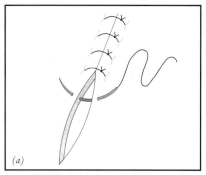

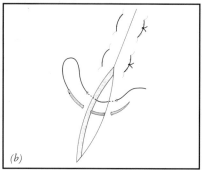

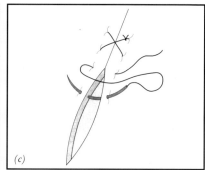

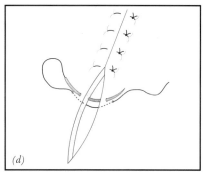

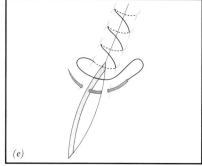

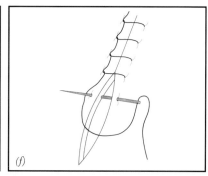

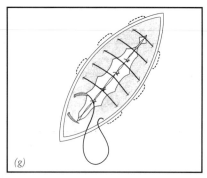

(a) *Simple interrupted suture.* (b) *Horizontal mattress pattern.* (c) *Cruciate mattress pattern.*
(d) *Vertical mattress pattern.* (e) *Simple continuous suture.* (f) *Ford interlocking suture.*
(g) *Subcuticular closure.*

Reproduced from Williams J (1992) Exam help: Suturing. Veterinary Practice Nurse, *4 (4),
pp. 13–19, with the permission of the author and publisher.*

Placement of skin sutures

The aim of skin suturing is to bring the edges together
into anatomical alignment, with no inversion, minimal
eversion and no overlapping. The *simple interrupted
appositional* (SIA) suture (see Figure 2.32a) is particularly
useful for this. It is suitable for closure of the skin in
almost all circumstances and produces good apposition
if placed correctly. If used in the presence of tension it
may cause necrosis of the skin edges and in these cases an
alternative pattern may be preferred or tension-relieving
stitches can be placed in addition to the SI pattern. A
typical example would be the use of vertical mattress
stitches placed to reinforce SI sutures during skin flap
surgery.

Skin edges should be handled gently to prevent tissue
damage and delayed healing or patient interference. The most
commonly used devices for skin handling are fine rat-toothed
forceps or the finger tips.

SI sutures are usually placed using a curved cutting needle,
needle holders and rat-toothed forceps (Figure 2.33).
Placement with a hand-held straight cutting needle has some
advantages but is less widely used.

2.33 Placement of simple interrupted skin sutures

1. Forceps are used to stabilize the far skin edge and the
   needle passed in a rolling action through the skin
   thickness. As a general rule, the size of the bite (from
   the edge to where the suture enters the skin) should be
   equal to the skin thickness, but experience is necessary
   to judge the placement for best apposition.
2. The needle is grasped by the needle-holders, fingers or
   rat-toothed forceps and pulled through the skin.
3. The near skin edge is stabilized and the needle brought
   through to exit the skin surface. The same thickness of
   tissue and depth of bite should be included on each side
   of the wound.
4. The suture is tied with three or four square knots. The
   first knot is usually placed with a double throw (to
   make a 'surgeon's knot'). Usually an instrument tie is
   used for speed and economy (hand ties tend to be
   slower and use more suture material).
5. The knot is tied so that the skin edges are apposed but
   without crushing the skin. The suture should be
   slightly loose so that if the skin swells it does not
   become strangulated.

- Most wounds can be sutured from one end towards the other (usually left to right or top to bottom)
- Irregularly shaped and curved wounds are often better closed by placing a few sutures along the wound and then interspersing the remainder between these initial sutures. One technique is to place the first stitch in the middle of the wound and then place further stitches in the middle of each remaining segment until closed.

Alternatives to skin sutures

The commonly used alternatives to the use of sutures for the skin are staples and tissue adhesives (cyanoacrylate glue). The latter is useful for small incisions under little tension (and to replace skin sutures that the patient removes prematurely). The glue is applied to the surface of the skin as the edges are held together.

Staples are a rapid method of closure but are relatively expensive. The skin edges are held together whilst the staple gun is held centrally over the wound. It is pressed gently down while the handle is squeezed to discharge one staple. The handle is released and the stapler moved away.

Adhesive strips which are commonly used to close small skin wounds in human patients have not been successful in animals.

Michel clips are a type of staple used occasionally in large animals but they have not been widely used in small animals.

Wound closure

General wound management is covered in the *BSAVA Manual of Veterinary Nursing*, Chapters 1 and 5. A critical decision in wound management is when and whether to close a wound or leave it to heal by second intention. Figure 2.34 is a guide to this decision.

The timing of wound closure is presented in Figure 2.35.

Wound closure is undertaken once tissue contamination has been reduced or eliminated. Clean and clean–contaminated wounds should be closed as soon as possible to avoid further contamination or devitalization. Wounds with greater degrees of contamination or infection require treatment as open wounds before closure, or can be excised as a whole and the fresh incision treated as a clean wound.

Skin mass removal

Veterinary nurses planning this type of surgery need an understanding of the background to the techniques, including

2.34 Decision making in wound management

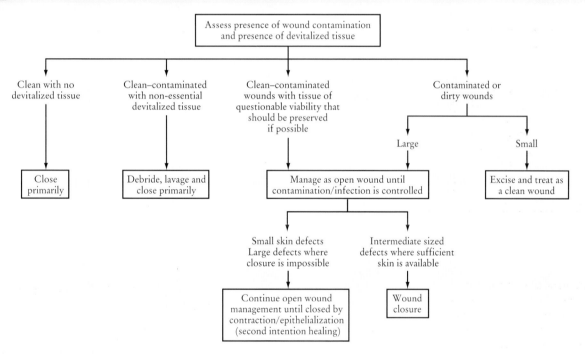

2.35 Wound closure timing

Closure method	Application	Definition
Primary closure	Clean or cleaned wounds No skin tension	Immediate closure of skin edges (usually with sutures)
Delayed primary closure	Contaminated wounds Unknown tissue viability Skin tension present	Wound debrided and lavaged Closed after 2–5 days treatment
Secondary closure	Contaminated or dirty wounds	Closure delayed until 5 days or more after injury Granulation tissue and skin edges excised at time of closure
Second intention healing	Large skin defects with extensive tissue devitalization Used when closure is not possible	Healing by granulation, contraction and epithelialization

the differential diagnosis, principles of surgical oncology, simple surgical techniques and possible complications.

Differential diagnosis of skin masses

Swellings affecting the skin and subcutaneous tissues can originate from a variety of processes and each of these should be included in the differential diagnosis initially. These swellings can be divided into those that are and those that are not associated with the skin/subcutis itself. Swellings not associated with these tissues include lymph nodes, hernias and normal anatomical features. It is important to be aware of the position of these so that inappropriate treatment is not started.

Swellings arising from diseases of the skin/subcutaneous tissues include:

- Abscesses
- Haematoma/seroma
- Inflammatory/degenerative lesions
- Benign tumours
- Malignant tumours.

Figure 2.36 gives further details.

Aids to diagnosis

A number of clinical and laboratory tests are useful to aid in the diagnosis of skin masses.

Position

A knowledge of the position of lymph nodes (which may or may not be palpable in the normal animal) and the predilection sites of pathological lesions (calluses, perianal adenomas, etc.) is necessary.

2.36 Differential diagnosis of skin masses

Non-neoplastic skin masses

Skin mass	Treatment	Prognosis
Callus	Conservative or excision	Guarded: persist or recur
Hygroma	Conservative, drainage or excision	Guarded: persist or recur
Epidermal or dermal cysts	Excision	Excellent
Calcinosis circumscripta	Excision	Excellent
Infection: Staphylococcal pyogranuloma, atypical mycobacterium infection (feline leprosy), actinomycosis, etc.	Excision if discrete and single; systemic and topical antibiotics if extensive or multiple	Guarded if not completely excised Require prolonged medical therapy
Non-septic inflammation: nodular panniculitis, acral lick granuloma, etc.	Conservative or excision	Guarded if not excised or if cause cannot be identified
Miscellaneous causes, e.g. nodular dermatofibrosis	Variable	Variable

Common skin neoplasms (*not* an exhaustive list)

	Incidence	Treatment	Prognosis
Epidermal origin			
Basal cell tumours	Uncommon	Excision	Excellent
Papilloma	Rare	Conservative (usually regress with age)	Excellent
Squamous cell carcinoma	Relatively common	Excision with margins or radiotherapy	Fair if completely excised
Sebaceous adenoma	Common	Excision	Excellent
Perianal adenoma	Common	Excision and castration (hormonally responsive growth)	Excellent
Perianal adenocarcinoma	Rare	Excision	Guarded: local recurrence and metastasis occur
Mesenchymal origin (i.e. deeper layers)			
Soft tissue sarcoma	Common	Excision with wide margins (amputation of limbs appropriate)	Guarded: local recurrence common unless wide margins taken
Lipoma	Common	Excision	Excellent
Haemangiopericytoma	Uncommon	Excision with wide margins (amputation of limbs appropriate)	Guarded: local recurrence common unless wide margins taken
Haemangiosarcoma	Rare	Excision with wide margins	Guarded: metastasis not uncommon
Mast cell tumour	Common	Excision with wide margins or medical therapy (corticosteroids)	Guarded: recurrence and metastasis common
Histiocytoma	Uncommon	Excision or conservative	Excellent: usually regress with age
Lymphoma	Rare	Medical therapy	Poor: usually recur even if respond initially
Melanoma	Uncommon	Excision	Poor: usually metastasize

Appearance
Although the physical appearance may be useful in diagnosis, it is notoriously unreliable.

Palpation
The relation of a mass to overlying skin or underlying tissues (e.g. fixation) may be helpful but may be misleading. Whilst some malignant tumours display fixation, this may not be detectable early in their development. The texture of the swelling itself may be of interest: lipomas have a soft rubbery consistency, but this must not be considered to be diagnostic.

Patient's age, breed and sex
Certain conditions occur more commonly in certain types of animals. For example, perianal adenomas are most common in older entire male dogs and lipomas are most common in obese middle-aged dogs, but these features are not completely reliable.

Blood tests
Occasionally these may be of benefit in diagnosis, but more commonly they are used as a presurgical 'health screen'. Whether this is considered necessary is a matter of practice policy.

Radiography
Radiographs of the chest and abdomen, as a check for metastases, are indicated prior to the removal of masses confirmed to be malignant on histopathology or where the size or position of the mass would require reconstructive surgery.

Biopsy
Laboratory examination of excised tissue should be carried out in almost all cases. This step should be presented to the owners as an integral part of the operation, rather than an optional extra. Biopsies are required to allow a proper prognosis to be given to the owner and to assess the outcome of initial treatment and to plan further treatment.

Biopsy of skin masses
Biopsy samples can be obtained at two stages in treatment: before excision or after excision. When a small skin mass is found, in a location where simple excision without reconstruction is practical, and the animal is otherwise well, the mass should be excised and submitted as an excisional biopsy to the laboratory.

A pre-excisional biopsy should be taken in the following instances:

- When a mass cannot be excised simply, because of its size or position or because of the patient's health
- When a conservative approach is considered (e.g. a possible lipoma)
- When a malignant or widespread disease is suspected (presence of multiple masses, enlargement of local lymph nodes, etc.).

Pre-excisional biopsies can be taken in several ways, as follows.

Fine-needle aspirate biopsy (FNAB)
A hypodermic needle and syringe can be used to collect small tissue samples from a mass by aspiration. These samples (often consisting of a few cells within the needle) are blown on to a slide and smeared. This technique is recommended as a first step if a fluid-filled mass is suspected, and is also particularly valuable in the diagnosis of mast cell tumours, which have a very characteristic cytology. Often neither sedation nor local anaesthesia is required.

Core needle biopsy (e.g. Trucut)
A Trucut or similar needle can be used to obtain a cylinder of tissue from a solid mass. Local anaesthesia and sedation are often required.

Incision biopsy
A slice of tissue, which should include the margin of abnormal and normal tissue, can be collected with a skin biopsy punch or a scalpel. This will require sedation and local anaesthesia or general anaesthesia, but offers the best chance of obtaining a reliable pathology report. Samples obtained by incisional or core biopsy are fixed in formal saline and processed at the laboratory for histopathology, which is often more worthwhile than cytology.

Culture of biopsy samples
In some cases, biopsy samples should be submitted for bacterial culture as well as cytology or histopathology. Frankly purulent FNAB samples should be sent for culture, preferably by sending the fluid in a sterile pot, or by squirting some on to a transport swab. Incisional biopsies from possible inflammatory or infected lesions should also be submitted. The biopsy sample is split in half. One part is placed in normal saline and the other is wrapped in a sterile saline-soaked swab and submitted in a sealed sterile container.

Rationale for skin mass removal
Reasons for suggesting the removal of a skin mass include:

- Aesthetics – often the owner requests removal because the mass is unsightly. This is particularly the case if ulceration occurs, and these lesions are also unpleasant to the animal because of irritation
- Interference with function – large masses can be disabling because of their size
- Danger to life – masses of a malignant or inflammatory nature may be life threatening of themselves and so treatment is advisable.

One common question is when to excise a mass. A prognosis cannot be offered in the absence of a definitive diagnosis and owners should not be dissuaded from surgical treatment of a mass in an otherwise healthy animal, even if aged. When a mass is first noticed, it is not possible to predict its subsequent behaviour. A wait-and-see approach may allow the mass to increase in size, complicating surgery, or allowing the spread of a malignancy. A definitive diagnosis should be made as soon as possible and for most small skin masses an excisional biopsy is the best approach.

Excision of simple skin masses
Veterinary nurses are likely to excise two types of skin masses: those involving the subcutaneous tissues, and those involving the skin itself or the skin and underlying subcutaneous tissue. If there is any doubt as to whether adjacent tissue is involved it should be included in the excision. In all cases, careful planning of the procedure beforehand is worthwhile, to ensure that the full extent of the lesion is appreciated and that the most appropriate type of approach is made.

Excision of a subcutaneous mass (e.g. lipoma)

- Use a scalpel to make an incision in the skin over the mass
- Use blunt and sharp dissection with scissors to separate the mass from surrounding tissues. Hold the tissue to be excised with rat-tooth or tissue forceps

- Subcutaneous tissue in most sites (particularly over the trunk and proximal limbs) is present in excess and can be boldly excised without concern for skin closure or loss of function
- Deal with any haemorrhage as appropriate. There is often one or more large vessels supplying lesions of this type entering from the deeper tissues. An attempt should be made to identify and clamp these with the *tips* of haemostat forceps before cutting through them
- Close the 'dead space' left by the removal of the mass from the subcutaneous tissue with an absorbable suture in a simple continuous pattern using rat-tooth forceps and needle holders
- Close the skin in an appropriate fashion. Most commonly, simple interrupted skin sutures of a non-absorbable material are used.

Excision of a mass involving the surface of the skin

- Use a scalpel to make an elliptical incision around the lesion. To allow a neat closure, this should be three to four times as long as it is wide
- Include a border of apparently normal tissue around (and below) the lesion (the 'margin of excision'). The optimum size of the margin will be determined by the precise pathological diagnosis. Generally, in the absence of a diagnosis, it should be at least 1.5 cm. This should ensure complete excision (that is, failure to regrow) of most locally recurrent lesions. A narrower margin is acceptable when a pre-existing diagnosis allows this and on the rare occasions when a clinical diagnosis is obvious. The outstanding example here is the sebaceous adenomas seen commonly on older dogs and appearing as 'warts', which require only a narrow margin
- Following excision, deal with any haemorrhage and close the defect as above.

Simple surgical techniques in skin surgery

Skin incision
The way in which the initial skin incision is made will greatly affect the end result. Skin should be cut only with a scalpel, since the crushing effect of scissors will impair wound healing. It is easier to achieve neat closure if straight incisions are made and elliptical incisions have sides of equal length.

Subcutaneous dissection
Following the skin incision, the tissue to be excised has to be separated from the surrounding tissue. During excision try to handle abnormal tissue as little as possible and avoid cutting into it: this will reduce the risk of spreading the disease into the tissue that remains. Allis tissue forceps can be helpful for this. The tissue to be removed is separated from surrounding tissue by a combination of sharp (cutting) and blunt dissection, using scissors. Cutting causes less trauma to remaining tissue but blunt dissection can make it easier to control and isolate a discrete firm mass. In blunt dissection, tension is used to separate layers of tissue. This can be done by splitting tissue between the finger tips, 'wiping' with a swab or opening the points of scissors to tear tissue.

Haemostasis
During excision a degree of haemorrhage is inevitable. This must be controlled to ensure that wound healing is not delayed.

Subcutaneous closure
It is important to obliterate the hole (dead space) left following excision of a subcutaneous mass, to reduce the accumulation of fluid at the site postoperatively (seroma formation). This will also help to control any continuing haemorrhage. Dead space can be reduced by the use of drains, but suturing of the subcutaneous tissue is more likely to be used in this instance. A simple continuous suture of an absorbable material (chromic catgut, polyglactin or polydioxanone, for example) is used to pull the subcutaneous tissue gently together to either side of the defect. Subcutaneous tissue (fat or muscle) holds tension poorly and the suture should only be tight enough to appose the tissue.

Skin closure
To promote rapid healing, the skin edges should be neatly held together with the surfaces closely apposed. Infolding of the skin edges or a step in height across the wound should be avoided. Some outfolding (eversion) of the edges can be acceptable. The edges should be able to be brought together without excessive tension. When this is not possible, it may be possible to loosen the skin by using blunt dissection to 'free up' skin edges by undermining them.

The skin edges can be held together during healing with sutures, staples or skin adhesive.

Bandaging
Simple wounds resulting from excised skin masses rarely need bandaging. However, these can be useful to reduce postoperative swelling or where haemorrhage continues after skin closure. Surgical wounds on the limbs often fall into this group and a firm pressure bandage, including the foot, may be useful on the extremities. A non-adherent contact layer is usually chosen. The bandage is removed or changed after 2–3 days.

Antibiotic use
There is probably no requirement for antibiotics for this surgery, if asepsis is observed, unless another surgery, especially dentistry, is carried out at the same time.

Postoperative complications

Haemorrhage
Slight postoperative haemorrhage is usually easily managed with pressure bandaging. Significant bleeding is unlikely after this type of surgery but if it is seen the veterinary surgeon should be informed, and pressure bandaging applied until further advice is available.

Swelling
Most commonly, postoperative swelling is due to seroma formation, and no treatment is required if the wound is otherwise apparently healthy. It is worth considering whether a change in technique might prevent the problem in future (use of a drain or bandage, for example). Large seromas are sometimes drained, but this can introduce infection. Less commonly, swelling may be due to infection, resulting in inflammation or abscessation. Treatment of these may include reopening the incision to allow flushing, antibiotic treatment and application of warm compresses.

Dental care

The assessment of patients with dental disease is covered in Chapter 6 of the *BSAVA Manual of Veterinary Nursing*. This section will concentrate on the treatment of periodontal disease and removal of diseased teeth. For more detail on these procedures, consult publications listed in the section on further reading.

Treatment of periodontal disease

The processes resulting in periodontal disease are:

- Accumulation of debris and bacteria (plaque) at the tooth/gum interface
- Associated inflammation (gingivitis), with swelling, redness, pain and fragility of the gums
- Mineralization of the plaque to form calculus
- Enlargement of the crevice at the root/gum margin with formation of a periodontal pocket (periodontitis)
- Recession of the gum margin and later of the alveolar bone.

Steps in the management of periodontal disease:

- Preventive therapy (home care)
  - Tooth brushing
  - Mouth washes
  - Avoidance of sticky foods
- Systemic investigations to rule out underlying or concurrent disease
- Dental hygiene (scaling)
- Surgical treatment (extraction and gingival surgery).

Scaling is the removal of plaque and calculus from the tooth surface, above and below the gingival margin. Manual, ultrasonic and sonic equipment is in use.

Patient preparation

- Investigation of systemic disease, as directed by the veterinary surgeon (optional)
- Presurgical antibiotic or antiseptic treatment, to reduce gingival inflammation (optional)
- Perioperative antibiotics, used in the presence of systemic disease, when other surgery is carried out concurrently and in animals with congenital heart disease
- General anaesthesia with endotracheal intubation and pharyngeal packing. Effective treatment cannot be carried out in the sedated patient.

Equipment

Suitable equipment makes the task less traumatic, quicker and more effective. It must be maintained properly – for example, servicing of powered tools and sharpening of hand instruments.

- Operator protection must be used (face mask, gloves and goggles)
- Irrigation and suction are helpful – and essential with power tools
- A variety of hand instruments (scalers, probes and curettes) must be available
  - Ultrasonic scalers greatly improve the results of the procedure and speed the process. The nurse should be given instructions in the correct use and maintenance of these instruments
  - Sonic and rotosonic scalers are in less common use
- Following scaling, the tooth surfaces must be polished with an appropriate handpiece, prophylactic cup and paste.

Dental extraction

Teeth beyond salvage should be extracted. The criteria for extraction versus conservation are not clear-cut and will reflect practice policy, the owner's wishes and the ability of the owner to provide home care, but the following is a guide when taking decisions in favour of extraction:

- Advanced periodontal disease (loosening of roots, gingival pockets more than 5 mm deep)
- Caries or feline neck lesions where restorative techniques are not available or when insufficient tooth remains for practical repair
- Retained deciduous teeth
- Tooth trauma with pulp exposure or necrosis, when restorative treatment is not available
- Malocclusion causing damage to the soft tissues of the mouth, when orthodontics are not available.

Extraction techniques

Teeth selected for extraction must be removed without damage to surrounding tissues and without leaving remnants of tooth root in the socket. Several techniques are available and choice is based on the affected tooth and the equipment available.

Elevation and extraction

Used for single rooted teeth with straight roots (incisors and deciduous canines):

- Use an appropriately sized root elevator to disrupt the periodontal ligament around the circumference of the root
- Use repeated controlled pushes to do this without fracturing the root or alveolus
- Continue until the tooth is loose and can be extracted by traction with extraction forceps placed at the root–crown junction.

Fragmentation

Suitable for small teeth (especially cats, except the canines):

- Use a dental burr to destroy all of the tooth material within the alveolus (the firm dental tissue can be differentiated from the soft alveolar bone as the burr is used)
- Finish by flushing the socket.

This technique is also used in larger teeth after amputation of the crown, again with the burr or saw.

Root division

Multi-rooted teeth are most easily extracted after separation of the root into its parts:

- Use a burr or saw to cut through the crown to the furcation of the roots
- Elevate each root individually, using an elevator around the root and gentle leverage between the tooth fragments.

Gingival flap elevation

Used for the carnassials (with root division) and the permanent canines. Elevation of a gingival flap on the buccal surface over the root allows removal of the alveolar bone and the tooth can then be lifted out:

- Use a scalpel and periosteal elevator to raise the gingiva in a flap over the lateral wall of the alveolus
- Use a burr to remove the alveolar bone and expose the root
- Use an elevator to loosen the tooth by disrupting the periodontal ligament on the rostral, caudal and medial surfaces of the root
- Lift out the tooth, avoiding pressure on the medial alveolar wall
- Flush the socket and remove any protruding bone
- Replace the flap and suture into place (e.g. 2 metric absorbable suture on a cutting needle)

For complications of tooth extraction, see Figure 2.37.

Complications of dental extraction

Complication	Comments	Avoid by
Fracture of jaw	Commonest in older animals with advanced periodontal disease	Careful technique with minimal force
Root retention	Follows root fracture	Full elevation before traction
Oronasal fistulation	Commonest after maxillary canine extraction Follows fracture of medial alveolus	Careful technique (e.g. gingival flap formation)
Haemorrhage	Profuse haemorrhage occasionally follows extraction Rarely, there may be an underlying haemostatic deficiency (haemophilia, thrombocytopenia, von Willebrand's disease)	Packing of socket usually arrests the bleeding Attempts to suture the gingiva over the socket are usually futile
Dry socket	Failure of alveolus to fill with granulation tissue after extraction Rare in animals	Curettage of alveolus after extraction

Abscess treatment

Subcutaneous abscesses are common in small animals. Veterinary nurses may play a large part in the management, both in the clinic and in advising owners about aftercare. Prior to treatment, consideration should be given to the likely cause, since this may affect the management of such a case.

- In *cats*, the majority of abscesses result from bite injuries. Common sites include the base of the tail, head and neck and sometimes the limbs. Involvement of underlying structures must be considered, particularly the joints and the veterinary surgeon will assess the case in the first instance
- In *dogs*, a wider variety of causes are commonly encountered (Figure 2.38).

- In *rabbits*, facial abscesses are a particular problem. Most are associated with underlying dental and/or nasolachrymal duct disease. Prognosis is guarded because of this, unless the underlying problem can be resolved.

Steps in abscess management

- The abscess must be opened before antibiotics are given. Failure to do so may result in the formation of a cold or sterile abscess (pocket of pus in the absence of inflammation)
- Diagnosis may be confirmed by aspiration of pus (use a 20G needle and syringe) and examination of the specimen cytologically and bacteriologically
- When lanced, the abscess should be 'pointing' (thinning of tissues over abscess and softening of a superficial area): encourage by the use of warm compresses

Causes of cutaneous abscesses in dogs

Abscess	Location and comments	Treatment
Malar abscesses	Commonly develop in region of zygomatic arch Associated with disease of maxillary teeth, especially upper carnassial	Teeth must be closely examined and radiographs may be taken Treatment of dental disease (often extraction) necessary to resolve
Para-aural abscesses	Develop on side of face, in region of horizontal canal of external ear	Ear canal must be examined and radiographs of middle ear are usually indicated Treatment of ear disease (often ear canal ablation) necessary to resolve
Anal sac abscess	Concurrent anal sac impaction and infection	Managed by local care (warm compresses, lavage) until inflammation is resolving Anal sacculectomy often necessary in longer term
Interdigital cyst	Arise within interdigital web May be due to presence of a foreign body (grass seed) Often no foreign body present but due to dermatitis	Managed by incision and poulticing Recurrent cases may benefit from excision of webs
Penetrating wounds	Various wounds (including surgical interventions and bites) can result in abscess formation Requires significant contamination and tissue damage to have occurred	
Foreign bodies	Various foreign bodies can result in abscesses Many possible sites Consider as possible cause if abscess fails to heal after local treatment	

- During this process, the abscess may burst spontaneously
- Lance at soft point. This may require sedation, or local or general anaesthetic. Clip hair from the area and surgically prepare the skin. Lance with bold stab incision, typically with a number 11 scalpel blade
- Express pus
- Flush the cavity with sterile saline or antiseptic solution. Extend stab incision as necessary
- Continue to flush until all pus is cleared. Digitally explore the cavity to break down any pockets present. Flush again
- Topical antibiotics are not usually indicated and may perpetuate inflammation
- Systemic antibiotics are often unnecessary in the absence of gross local inflammation
- Occasionally, a drain (e.g. Penrose) may be inserted into the cavity
- Provide aftercare: continue to flush cavity daily until filled with granulation tissue or contracted. It may require bathing with warm antiseptic solution to loosen and remove exudate at incision.

Aural haematoma

This is the commonest disease of the pinna in dogs. Blood accumulates within the thickness of the auricular cartilage and is most obvious on the concave (inner) aspect. Sometimes it results from trauma, such as head shaking due to otitis externa, but often there is no evidence of other ear disease and an immune-mediated cause has been suggested in these cases.

Treatment

- Examine for signs of otitis externa (including foreign bodies in the ear canal) and treat as necessary
- Many cases of aural haematoma are treated by surgical drainage; several techniques have been described and all seem to be useful

- In all cases and techniques, an incision is made through the skin on the hairless (concave) surface of the pinna to evacuate the haematoma
- Continued postoperative drainage is achieved by placing a drain (Penrose or teat cannula) into the cavity or by excising an ellipse of skin
- If an ellipse of skin is excised, this is often made in an S shape orientated along the length of the pinna, to reduce the effects of contraction during healing
- A series of large mattress sutures may be placed full thickness through the pinna to eliminate dead space. The sutures are orientated along the length of the pinna and the auricular blood vessels are avoided. They must not be placed tightly or ischaemic damage will result
- The ear is usually bandaged postoperatively to prevent patient interference, protect the drain or wound, reduce dead space and prevent the adverse effects of head shaking. The bandage is changed after 3 days
- The drain is removed after 3–5 days and any sutures after 7–10 days
- Alternative treatment methods are conservative (which may result in scarring and distortion of the pinna) and medical (needle drainage of the haematoma, followed by injection of a corticosteroid).

Further reading

Crossley DA and Penman S (1995) *Manual of Small Animal Dentistry*, 2nd edn. BSAVA, Cheltenham

Slatter D (1993) *Textbook of Small Animal Surgery*, 2nd edn. WB Saunders, Philadelphia

Swaim SF and Henderson RA (1997) *Small Animal Wound Management*, 2nd edn. Williams and Wilkins, Baltimore

Theilen GH and Madewell BR (1987) *Veterinary Cancer Medicine*, 2nd edn. Lea and Febiger, Philadelphia

Williams J, McHugh D and White RAS (1992) Use of drains in small animal surgery. *In Practice* **14**, 73–81

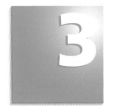

3 Advanced anaesthesia

Garry Stanway

This chapter is designed to give information on:

- Some of the more advanced anaesthetic techniques used in general practice
- Interactions between anaesthetic drugs and disease
- Combinations of anaesthetic drugs and their use in a safe and targeted manner

Balanced anaesthesia

What is balanced anaesthesia?

General anaesthesia is often considered to be a single entity. Anaesthetic drugs induce anaesthesia and the depth of anaesthesia varies with dose. Patients that are too lightly anaesthetized will respond to painful stimuli; patients that are too deeply anaesthetized will show signs of anaesthetic drug overdose, including low blood pressure, slow respiratory rate and low heart rate.

This is a useful concept but it is too simplistic. It is better to consider the three components that make up 'general anaesthesia':

- Narcosis or unconsciousness
- Muscle relaxation
- Analgesia or suppression of reflex responses to surgical stimulation.

These three components are known as the triad of anaesthesia (Figure 3.1).

Balanced anaesthesia is the term used to describe the anaesthetic technique that uses several specific agents to provide these three components of anaesthesia. For example:

- A volatile anaesthetic agent to provide narcosis (unconsciousness)
- A neuromuscular blocking agent to provide muscle relaxation
- A short-acting opioid analgesic to provide suppression of reflex responses to surgical stimulation.

Consider a routine bitch spay procedure. Although the animal appears to be anaesthetized adequately, its heart and respiratory rates increase when tension is applied to the ovarian ligament. This is not a conscious reflex: the bitch is not aware of the surgery – it is a reflex response to the pain of surgical stimulation.

A common response to this situation is to increase the vaporizer setting. This works but it is not an ideal solution to the problem. Inhalation anaesthetic agents are good narcotics (good at inducing unconsciousness), reasonable muscle relaxants but poor analgesics and therefore poor suppressors of reflex responses to surgical stimuli. Increasing the vaporizer setting in this situation has the desired effect, but at a cost: it increases the less desirable cardiovascular effects of the volatile agent.

By applying the triad of anaesthesia, the response to this situation can be much more specific. In the spaying example above, administering a rapidly acting analgesic agent such as fentanyl would be just as effective as increasing the vaporizer setting but without producing the undesirable side effects. (The use of analgesics during anaesthesia may appear unnecessary as the patient is anaesthetized and so, by definition, cannot feel pain. However, pain is still detected and, although the animal is not 'aware', its body still reacts to these painful stimuli. Analgesics are given to anaesthetized patients to suppress these reflex responses.)

Although all patients benefit from balanced anaesthetic techniques, it is those patients at higher risk that benefit the most. They are more susceptible to the cardiovascular depressant effects of the inhalation anaesthetic agents.

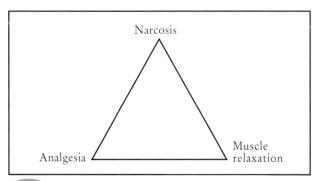

3.1 *Triad of anaesthesia.*

Drugs used in balanced anaesthesia

Drugs used in balanced anaesthesia can be grouped as follows.

- Drugs inducing narcosis (volatile anaesthetic agents)
  - Halothane
  - Enflurane
  - Isoflurane
- Analgesics
  - Morphine
  - Pethidine
  - Methadone
  - Fentanyl
  - Alfentanyl
  - Local anaesthetic agents
  - (NSAIDs)
- Muscle relaxants (neuromuscular blocking agents)
  - Curare
  - Alcuronium
  - Vecuronium
  - Atracurium
  - Pancuronium
  - Suxamethonium.

Drugs inducing narcosis

The inhalation anaesthetic agents commonly used in practice are all good at inducing narcosis. All are suitable for use as part of a balanced anaesthetic technique. They have the advantage that all anaesthetists are familiar with their effects. This is significant if neuromuscular blocking agents are used, as these abolish the signs traditionally used to monitor the 'depth' of anaesthesia.

Inhalation anaesthetic agents

Halothane

- Relatively low solubility produces a more rapid recovery from anaesthesia when compared with older volatile anaesthetic agents such as methoxyflurane and ether
- Produces a dose-dependent fall in cardiac output and blood pressure as well as depressing respiration
- Sensitizes the heart to the dysrhythmic effects of adrenaline. High levels of adrenaline often occur following a stressful induction of anaesthesia; in these circumstances, fatal cardiac dysrhythmias may be seen. This situation is made even worse if thiopentone has been used as the anaesthetic induction agent.

Enflurane

- An isomer of isoflurane; has very similar properties to isoflurane but is less popular
- Produces seizure-like electrical activity in the brain and should be avoided in patients suffering from epilepsy.

Isoflurane

- Less soluble than halothane and therefore produces even more rapid induction of and recovery from anaesthesia
- Can be used as both induction and maintenance agent
- Very useful for anaesthetic induction in exotic mammals
- Produces less severe myocardial depression than halothane but overall fall in blood pressure is similar, due to more profound peripheral vasodilation
- Does not sensitize the heart to adrenaline as much as halothane, therefore fewer cardiac dysrhythmias.

Analgesics

Mechanism of action of opioid analgesics

Opioid analgesics exert their effects through receptors in the spinal cord. When these receptors are occupied, they block the transmission of pain up the spinal cord to the higher brain centres. These receptors have been classified and named. They include the μ (mu), δ (delta) and κ (kappa) receptors. The μ receptors are particularly associated with the relief of pain. Opioid analgesics occupy these receptors and produce analgesia.

There are two categories of opioid analgesic:

- The pure μ agonist opioids (such as morphine, methadone, pethidine, fentanyl and alfentanyl) occupy these μ receptors, producing analgesia. At higher doses, more receptors are occupied and the amount of analgesia produced is greater
- The partial μ agonists (such as buprenorphine and butorphanol) behave in a peculiar manner. At low doses they produce analgesia but, as the dose increases, the amount of analgesia produced reaches an upper limit. If the dose is increased beyond this, the analgesic effect actually starts to fall.

This odd property of the partial μ agonists limits their usefulness. If they are given to a patient that is in pain but the degree of pain relief produced is inadequate, a top-up dose cannot be given as it is likely that further doses will result in a reduction in the amount of analgesia produced.

Furthermore, partial μ agonists should not be given after pure μ agonists because the partial μ agonist will displace some of the pure μ agonist from the μ receptor. Again, this will reduce the amount of analgesia experienced by the patient.

Because of their long duration of action, their limited analgesic properties and the fact that they cannot be combined with the more useful pure μ agonist opioids, partial μ agonist opioids are not used as part of a balanced anaesthetic regime.

Analgesic agents

Morphine

- Pure μ agonist
- Useful component of balanced anaesthesia when given before surgery
- Cannot be given by intravenous route, as this can induce release of histamine
- Less suitable for use during anaesthesia, due to slow onset of action.

Pethidine

- Pure μ agonist
- Shorter acting than morphine (1–2 hours in the dog)
- Cannot be given by intravenous route
- Useful if given before surgery.

Methadone

- Pure μ agonist
- Similar to morphine
- Will provide some of the analgesic component of balanced anaesthesia if given before surgery
- Should not be given by intravenous route.

Fentanyl

- Pure μ agonist
- Short acting (about 20 minutes, depending on route of administration)
- Does not affect blood pressure when given intravenously
- Produces brief period of apnoea following intravenous injection
- Frequently used as part of balanced anaesthetic technique: rapid onset and short duration of action mean that (within reason) can be given to effect throughout anaesthesia
- Can be used in anaesthetized cats as long as last dose is given at least 20 minutes before end of anaesthesia.

Alfentanyl

- Pure μ agonist
- More rapidly effective than fentanyl but produces longer period of apnoea following intravenous injection
- Can induce severe brachycardia when given intravenously, therefore often mixed with atropine before injection
- Cumulative, so subsequent doses may need to be reduced.

NSAIDs

- In general, cannot be given to patients that are to be anaesthetized – risk of renal damage associated with this practice; therefore most NSAIDs unsuitable for use as part of balanced anaesthetic technique
- Carprofen an exception and licensed for this purpose.

Local anaesthesia

- Can totally block transmission of pain from site of surgery, so can be usefully applied to technique of balanced anaesthesia for certain surgical procedures
- Epidural anaesthesia, for example, can be used as part of balanced anaesthetic technique for surgery on perineum of dogs.

Neuromuscular blocking agents (NMBAs)

Neuromuscular blocking agents provide a much greater degree of muscle relaxation than can be achieved using the more conventional anaesthetic agents. They act at the neuromuscular junction (Figure 3.2) to block the transmission of nerve impulses to the muscles and so prevent muscle contraction.

Mechanism of action of neuromuscular blocking agents

When a nerve impulse travels to the end of a motor nerve, it stimulates the release of acetylcholine into the neuromuscular junction. This acetylcholine attaches to specific receptors on the surface of the muscle fibre. When enough of these receptors are occupied, the muscle fibre contracts. The neuromuscular junction contains cholinesterase, which breaks down the acetylcholine.

Neuromuscular blocking agents are structurally similar to acetylcholine and they compete with the acetylcholine for places on the receptors. If the neuromuscular blocking agent occupies enough of the receptors, the release of acetylcholine into the neuromuscular junction will not result in contraction of the muscle fibre.

There are two classes of neuromuscular blocking agent:

- Non-depolarizing NMBAs simply occupy the acetylcholine receptor, preventing the acetylcholine from attaching and so preventing a muscle contraction
- Depolarizing NMBAs attach to the acetylcholine receptor and stimulate it, resulting in a brief contraction of the muscle fibre. They then prevent the acetylcholine from attaching and stimulating any further contractions.

NMBAS as part of a balanced anaesthetic technique

Without muscle relaxation, many surgical procedures would be difficult. The volatile anaesthetic agents do produce some muscle relaxation but only at relatively high doses. NMBAs are included as they allow a reduction in the dose of the conventional anaesthetic agents.

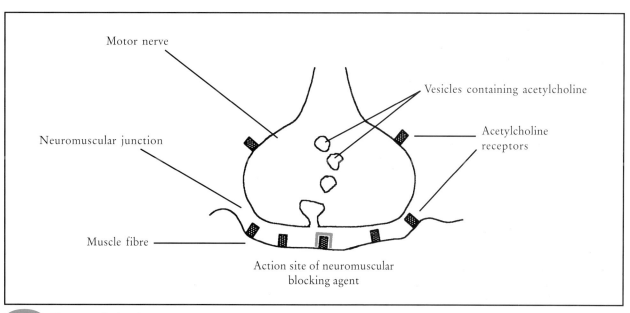

3.2 *Neuromuscular junction.*

NMBAs produce paralysis of all muscles – including the muscles of respiration; therefore it is imperative that facilities for intermittent positive pressure ventilation are available.

Non-depolarizing NMBAs

Curare

- Needs 2–3 minutes to take effect
- Duration of action 35–40 minutes
- Mainly of historical interest.

Alcuronium

- Duration of action around 35–40 minuts
- Return to spontaneous respiration followed by prolonged period of partial paresis, making 'reversal' with anticholinesterase drugs obligatory (see section below for details on reversal of NMBAs); difficult to reverse this drug if more than one dose given.

Vecuronium

- Duration of action around 20 minutes
- Found to be very little placental transfer when used in humans
- Hepatic insufficiency can greatly increase duration of action
- Non-cumulative.

Atracurium

- Deteriorates slowly at room temperature, so must be stored at 4°C
- Spontaneously breaks down in plasma at physiological temperatures and pH; therefore duration of block is not affected by renal or hepatic disease.

Pancuronium

- No significant side effects
- Partially excreted unchanged by kidneys, so must be used with care in animals with impaired renal function
- Duration of action prolonged in animals with impaired biliary excretion.

Depolarizing NMBAs

Suxamethonium

The only example of a depolarizing NMBA is suxamethonium, which causes a transient stimulation that leads to twitching. Because of the mode of action of this drug, substances that antagonize the non-depolarizing blocks (anticholinesterase type drugs) potentiate the depolarizing block.

- Associated with postoperative pain in ambulatory patients in human studies
- Duration of block varies between species (6–8 minutes in horse, 15–20 minutes in dog)
- Classically described as being used to provide good intubation conditions in cat and pig but otherwise not used in veterinary anaesthesia.

When to use neuromuscular blocking agents

As well as being an essential component of balanced anaesthesia, neuromuscular blocking agents are indicated for several other procedures:

- Surgical access to the cornea is greatly enhanced if the eye is centrally positioned. During conventional anaesthesia, the eye is usually rotated ventrally. NMBAs improve surgical access by relaxing the muscles of the eye
- Joint luxations are easier to reduce when NMBAs are administered
- NMBAs do *not* make fracture reduction any easier
- The use of NMBAs can make the removal of oesophageal foreign bodies easier in dogs, as their oesophagus contains a significant amount of striated muscle
- Relaxed intercostal muscles are not as severely damaged during thoracic surgery. This can significantly reduce the pain resulting from thoracic surgery as well as improving surgical access.

Monitoring anaesthetic depth during neuromuscular blockade

Many of the signs that are used to assess the 'depth' of anaesthesia are controlled by striated muscle (e.g. jaw tone, eye reflexes, eye position, voluntary movement). When NMBAs are used, these important signs are abolished. Instead, signs such as heart rate and blood pressure must be used as indicators of depth of anaesthesia.

It is also possible for the patient to be aware of the pain of surgery without showing any of the usual signs, such as gross movement or alterations in respiratory rate and rhythm. This makes it imperative that the anaesthetist ensures the patient is insensible to pain and fear throughout the duration of anaesthesia. This is most easily achieved if the anaesthetist becomes familiar with the actions of all of the anaesthetic agents used before combining them with NMBAs.

Signs of inadequate anaesthesia during neuromuscular blockade

- Heart rate increases
- Blood pressure increases
- Mucous membrane pallor
- Lacrimation
- Voluntary movement not always completely abolished when NMBAs used – any voluntary movement must be taken as a warning that anaesthesia is inadequate.

Monitoring the degree of neuromuscular blockade

As with all drugs, the exact effects of a given dose of NMBA in an individual patient cannot be predicted precisely. In one individual the dose may produce 20 minutes of paralysis; in another the blockade may last significantly longer. It is important for the anaesthetist to know what effect a given dose of NMBA is having on the patient. This allows the anaesthetist to judge:

- The correct time to give supplemental doses if the blockade needs to be prolonged
- When the blockade has worn off sufficiently for the patient to be weaned off the ventilator
- When it is safe to reverse the blockade using anticholinesterase type drugs (see later in this chapter for more details on the reversal of NMBAs).

The degree of paralysis is measured by electrically stimulating a superficial motor nerve and watching for any evidence of muscle activity. For example, electrodes can be placed over the ulnar nerve: when the nerve is stimulated electrically, the animal's digits twitch.

'Train of four' stimulation

It has been found that stimulating a muscle fibre repeatedly in quick succession provides more information about the degree of blockade than a single stimulation on its own. Consequently, it is usual to stimulate the nerve electrically four times over 2 seconds. This is known as a 'train of four' stimulation (Figure 3.3).

Interpreting 'train of four' stimulation

The responses to 'train of four' electrical stimulations of the ulnar nerve given at different stages are as follows.

- *Normal response*: digits twitch four times; each twitch will be of the same strength
- *Response seen immediately after giving NMBAs*: no twitching of the digits (indicating that the patient is completely paralysed)
- *Response seen once effects of NMBA start to wear off*: some movement of the digits. At first, the digits only twitch in response to the first of the four stimulations. As the effects of the NMBA decline further, all four twitches can be seen, but the first twitch of the four is strongest and the last twitch is weakest (this progressive weakening of the twitches with each stimulation in the 'train of four' is called 'fade', explained below)
- *Response seen once effects of NMBA have worn off completely*: four digit twitches of equal strength (indicating that the patient is no longer affected by the NMBA).

In a clinical situation, the electrodes are placed over the ulnar nerve before any NMBAs are given and the nerve is then stimulated. This is done in order to confirm that the electrodes are correctly positioned and that the nerve stimulator is working correctly. After the NMBA has been administered, the nerve is stimulated every few minutes and the response from the digits is monitored.

A single digit twitch in response to the train of four indicates that the neuromuscular blockade is starting to wear off. At this point, a further dose of NMBA may be given to prolong the blockade. When the fourth twitch returns, the blockade may be reversed using anticholinesterase type drugs.

Explanation of the cause of fade in 'train of four' nerve stimulations

When the motor nerve depolarizes, acetylcholine is released into the motor end plate. This acetylcholine stimulates the muscle fibre to contract. There is only a limited amount of acetylcholine available in the end of the nerve. If more acetylcholine is not brought down from the nerve fibre to replenish supplies, subsequent depolarizations will release less and less acetylcholine and so produce weaker and weaker muscle contractions.

- In the normal animal, the release of acetylcholine stimulates not only muscle contractions but also the movement of more acetylcholine down into the end of the motor nerve ready for the next depolarization
- As well as blocking the acetylcholine receptors responsible for muscle contractions, NMBAs block the acetylcholine receptors responsible for this preparatory mobilization of more acetylcholine into the end of the motor nerve

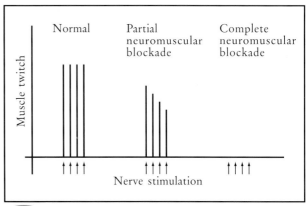

3.3 *'Train of four'*.

- As the effects of the NMBA start to wear off, the muscle contractions return before the replenishment mechanism has recovered, resulting in the progressive weakening of muscle contractions known as fade.

Reversing the effects of NMBAs

It is often desirable to reverse the effects of a neuromuscular blocking agent. This is mainly to ensure that the patient is capable of effective spontaneous respiration during the recovery period.

Acetylcholine released from the motor fibre competes with the NMBA within the motor end plate for acetylcholine receptors on the muscle fibre. The released acetylcholine is normally broken down rapidly by cholinesterase.

Anticholinesterase drugs prevent this rapid breakdown, resulting in more acetylcholine being available to compete with the NMBA, and so producing an effective reversal of the neuromuscular blockade.

Anticholinesterase drugs

Neostigmine and pyridostigmine

- Administered with atropine to block the muscarinic effects of the anticholinesterase
- Combination given in small incremental doses until all of the neuromuscular blockade has been reversed
- Effects are not immediate: 4 minutes should be allowed between doses for full effect to be seen
- Effectiveness of this reversal can be measured using nerve stimulator described earlier
- Full reversal indicated by return of four equal-strength muscle contractions in response to 'train of four' nerve stimulations.

Intermittent positive pressure ventilation (IPPV)

Intermittent positive pressure ventilation is essential in any situation where the patient is not able to ventilate itself adequately:

- Thoracic surgery where the chest cavity is open to the atmosphere
- When neuromuscular blocking agents have been given to the patient

- During any periods of apnoea, such as those following the induction of anaesthesia with thiopentone or propofol or resulting from the intravenous injection of fentanyl
- During respiratory arrest
- As part of cardiopulmonary resuscitation (CPR).

Anaesthetic gas and vapour are pushed into the patient's lungs by squeezing the reservoir bag on the anaesthetic breathing circuit. Manual IPPV (Figures 3.4 and 3.5) allows the anaesthetist total control of the patient's ventilation and in some cases this can be an advantage. Mechanical ventilators (Figure 3.6) free the anaesthetist from the task of bag squeezing but they are not essential. Because it is very difficult to use mechanical ventilators on cats and small dogs, manual IPPV is preferred in these cases.

3.4 How to perform manual IPPV

How much and how often does the bag need to be squeezed?

When carrying out IPPV, the aim is to produce slight hyperventilation.

- The ventilatory rate should be slightly more than the normal respiratory rate of the patient when it is conscious (during CPR this rate should be increased to 40–60 breaths per minute)
- The patient's chest movement should be slightly more obvious than during normal respiration
- During thoracic surgery, watch the lungs inflate and not the chest movement. If lung tissue protrudes beyond the surgical wound during inspiration, the lungs are being overinflated. (Because lung expansion is not restricted when the thoracic cavity is open, it is easy to damage the lungs by overinflation.)

3.5 IPPV with individual circuits

With a T-piece

1. Occlude the open end of the reservoir bag with the fingers of one hand
2. Allow the bag to fill and then inflate the patient's lungs by applying gentle hand pressure to the reservoir bag
3. Release the bag and the open-ended tube and allow the patient to exhale.

With a Bain

1. Gently squeeze the reservoir bag whilst watching the chest inflate
2. Let go of the bag and the patient will exhale
3. The pop-off (adjustable pressure limiting, APL) valve may have to be partially closed to achieve this
4. If the bag becomes overly full during the expiratory pause, the pop-off (APL) valve should be opened a little.

With a circle circuit

1. Close the pop-off (APL) valve
2. Squeeze the reservoir bag to inflate the patient's lungs
3. Release the bag and open the valve to allow the patient to exhale.

3.6 IPPV with mechanical ventilators

The two most common types of ventilator in veterinary practice are bag squeezers (often used in equine anaesthesia) and minute volume dividers.

- *Bag squeezers* replace the breathing bag on either a circle or a Bain breathing circuit. The respiratory rate and inspiratory volume can be altered. On many, there is also a control to alter the inspiratory to expiratory ratio
- *Minute volume dividers* (such as the Manley and the Minivent) store the gases coming from the anaesthetic machine and deliver them as individual breaths. Only the inspired volume and the inspiratory flow rate can be altered. The actual number of breaths given to the patient in 1 minute is controlled by varying the total fresh gas flow rate and the inspired volume. Minivent type ventilators need to be fitted to a Magill or Lack breathing circuit. The Manley Ventilator is a breathing circuit in its own right.

As with manual IPPV, the aim is to slightly overventilate the patient.

Typical canine respiratory values

Tidal volume:	10–20 ml/kg body weight
Respiratory rate:	15–30 breaths/minute
Minute volume:	200 ml/kg body weight/minute

Bag squeezers

1. Set the tidal volume and respiratory rate to suit the patient
2. Replace the reservoir bag of the breathing circuit with the pipe from the ventilator and close the pop-off valve on the circuit
3. Switch on the ventilator
4. Watch the movement of the patient's chest
5. The ventilator should slightly overexpand the patient's chest
6. Reduce the tidal volume if the patient's chest expansions are too great.

Minute volume dividers

1. Set the tidal volume to suit the patient
2. Adjust the fresh gas flow to equal the patient's minute volume
3. Switch the ventilator to 'Ventilate' (or connect the ventilator and the patient to the circuit)
4. Adjust the tidal volume control until the patient's chest is slightly overexpanded with each inspiration.

Returning to spontaneous respiration

Respiration is stimulated by a build-up of carbon dioxide within the patient's tissues. IPPV reduces the patient's carbon dioxide level and so removes the stimulus necessary for spontaneous respiration. At the end of IPPV, the ventilatory rate must be reduced to allow carbon dioxide levels to build up again. This increased carbon dioxide tension then stimulates the return of spontaneous respiration.

- Switch the ventilator to spontaneous respiration or disconnect the ventilator from the circuit and *open* the pop-off valve

- Manually ventilate the patient at a low respiratory rate (3–4 breaths/minute) to allow carbon dioxide levels to build up whilst watching for the return of spontaneous respiration
- Ideally, monitor oxygenation concurrently.

Local anaesthesia

In large animals, where general anaesthesia is a high risk procedure, local anaesthesia is used to carry out a variety of surgical procedures. The demeanour of cattle is such that abdominal surgery can be carried out under local anaesthesia (with or without mild sedation).

Small animals, however, will not lie still without the aid of chemical restraint. This, and the fact that general anaesthesia is a relatively safe procedure in small animals, means that the use of local anaesthesia is restricted to providing postsurgical analgesia and the analgesic component of balanced anaesthesia.

Local anaesthetic agents

Procaine

- Slow onset of anaesthesia
- Poor penetration of moist mucous membranes.

Lignocaine

- The most commonly used local anaesthetic agent in veterinary practice

- Rapid onset
- Effective when applied topically to moist mucous membranes
- Very rapidly removed from tissues. Adrenaline is added to some preparations in order to slow down this absorption and so prolong the activity of this local anaesthetic solution.

Mepivacaine

- Used to perform local nerve blocks for diagnosis of equine lameness.

Bupivacaine

- As stable as lignocaine and can be repeatedly autoclaved
- Onset of action similar to that of lignocaine but much longer acting
- Most usefully used to provide analgesia following surgery.

Local anaesthetic techniques

Local anaesthetic techniques include:

- Topical
- Local infiltration
- Regional analgesia
- Intravenous regional analgesia
- Epidural analgesia
- Subarachnoid analgesia.

These are described in Figure 3.7, along with examples.

3.7 Local anaesthetic techniques

Technique	Description	Example
Topical	Local anaesthetic can be applied directly to moist mucous membranes. Absorbable gel containing local anaesthetic available for use on skin	Applied to the eye to facilitate ocular examination. Local anaesthetic cream can be placed over site of intended venous puncture, making it much less traumatic for patient
Local infiltration	Site of surgery is infiltrated with local anaesthetic	Typically used to suture small wounds
Regional analgesia	Nerves innervating region where surgery is to be performed blocked by injecting local anaesthetic into tissues that surround them where they run close to skin surface	Cornual nerve block used to desensitize horn buds of calves prior to disbudding
Intravenous regional analgesia	Tourniquet placed around limb and local anaesthetic introduced into one of distended veins distal to it. Local anaesthetic then blocks conduction of nerves that run in close proximity to veins. Results in extremely good analgesia of distal portion of limb for as long as tourniquet remains in place	Used to allow surgery on feet of cattle and occasional limb surgery in dogs
Epidural analgesia	Local anaesthetic can be introduced into fat that surrounds spinal cord. Local anaesthetic blocks nerves as they leave spinal canal. Results in loss of sensation and motor activity in region of body supplied by affected nerves	Very useful for providing analgesia to anus, perineum and hindlimbs of animals undergoing surgery
Subarachnoid analgesia	Local anaesthetic can be deliberately introduced into cerebrospinal fluid surrounding spinal cord	Rarely used, because of high risks associated with this technique

Anaesthesia of the at-risk patient

General considerations

Anaesthetists are particularly concerned about the following organ systems:

- Brain (the target organ of anaesthetic drugs and particularly sensitive to the effects of hypoxia)
- Heart (pumps oxygenated blood around the body; sensitive to depressant effects of anaesthetic agents)
- Liver and kidneys (important for elimination of many anaesthetic drugs from the body)
- Lungs (vital for gas exchange).

Anaesthesia affects these organ systems more than others. Most anaesthetics depress the myocardium, reduce renal and hepatic blood flow and depress respiration.

Equally, disease will alter the way that anaesthetic drugs affect the patient. In the sick patient, the anaesthetist must try to predict the interactions between the disease and the anaesthetic and try to avoid any drugs that, because of disease, are likely to be unsafe.

For example, in animals with liver disease, where the patient's ability to metabolize drugs may be limited, the duration of action of most drugs is increased. Short-acting anaesthetic drugs are chosen, as any increase in the duration of action of short-acting agents will not be as dramatic as the increase in duration of action of longer-acting drugs.

The choice of anaesthetic agent is often based on the fact that it causes fewer adverse effects than other available drugs. For example, acepromazine may be chosen over an alpha-2 agonist for the sedation of a patient with mild heart disease as it has fewer effects on the cardiovascular system.

The character of the animal presenting for surgery has a large bearing on the kind of anaesthetic used. One common indication for thoracic surgery in young dogs is for the surgical correction of a patent ductus arteriosus. Although their cardiovascular system is compromised by their disease, they can be very excitable animals. Heavy sedation with high doses of acepromazine is not desirable, but a traumatic induction can cause the animal's oxygen requirement to exceed the heart's ability to supply oxygenated blood. In this case it may be necessary to compromise and use some form of sedation to avoid the risks associated with overexcitement.

ASA Risk Assessment

The American Society of Anesthesiologists (ASA) has categorized patient risk according to disease and life expectancy (Figure 3.8).

It is unusual to need to perform emergency surgery on critically ill patients. There is often time available to stabilize the patient using fluid therapy, for example. This will usually significantly reduce the risks associated with anaesthesia.

Complications are much more likely in sick patients, and preparations should be made to deal with those complications which, because of the condition involved, are most common. For example, in cases of gastric dilation and volvulus syndrome, ventricular premature contractions are sometimes seen. These may occur frequently enough to require treatment with lignocaine. The dose of lignocaine can be pre-calculated in order to save time in the event that it is needed. A collection of equipment and drugs that may be needed during anaesthetic crises or other emergencies can be collected in a

---

3.8 ASA risk assessment

Level	Description	Example
I	Healthy	Routine bitch spay
II	Mild systemic disease	Grade II/VI heart murmur with no clinical signs
III	Severe systemic disease	Grade IV/VI heart murmur with clinical signs of heart failure
IV	Severe systemic disease which is a constant threat to life	Pyometra
V	Patient unlikely to survive 24 hours with or without surgery	Bleeding splenic haemangiosarcoma

3.9 Contents of crash trolley

Equipment
- A range of endotracheal tubes (4–12 mm diameter)
- A range of tracheotomy tubes
- Laryngoscope
- Stethoscope
- A range of syringes (2–20 ml)
- A range of needles (16–22 g, 12.5–50 mm length)
- Two urinary catheters (for intratracheal drug delivery and suction of the tracheobronchial tree)
- Intravenous catheters (18, 20 and 22 g)
- Surgical spirit
- Clippers
- Resuscitation bag ('Ambu' bag)
- Small surgical pack and rib retractors

Drugs
- Adrenaline (1:1000)
- Atropine (0.6 mg/ml)
- Dobutamine (250µg/ml)
- Lignocaine (20 mg/ml)
- Dexamethasone (100 mg/ml if possible)
- Atipamazole
- Frusemide (50 mg/ml)

'crash trolley' ready for use (Figure 3.9). Drugs used in anaesthetic emergencies are listed in Figure 3.10 along with suggested doses.

Anaesthetic drugs should be administered carefully to very sick patients. In many cases, there will be a significant delay between intravenous injection and the onset of action of the drug. It is better to titrate intravenous drugs to effect rather than giving them as large boluses.

Anaesthetic monitoring for the at-risk patient

Good patient monitoring is vital for any anaesthetized patient. It is even more important with the at-risk patient. The patient's parameters should be constantly monitored and recorded on anaesthetic record sheets.

Electronic monitoring aids are very useful when anaesthetizing the at-risk patient. Oxygen saturation should be measured using a pulse oximeter wherever possible and the patient's ECG recorded.

Drugs used in anaesthetic emergencies

Drug	Action	Indication	Suggested dose
Adrenaline (epinephrine)	Increases cardiac output by increasing heart rate and cardiac output	Cardiac arrest Unresponsive hypotension	0.05–0.1 mg/kg 1 ml of 1:1000 solution per 10 kg i.v., intratracheal or intracardiac
Atropine	Vagolytic	Bradycardia	0.02–0.05mg/kg 1 ml of 0.6 mg/ml solution per 15 kg
Dobutamine	Increases cardiac output	Hypotension	1–5 µg/min
Lignocaine	Stabilizes myocardium	Used to treat ventricular premature contractions and ventricular tachycardia	Dogs: 1–6 mg/kg 1 ml of 2% solution per 10 kg Cats: 0.25–1.0 mg/kg 0.1 ml of 2% solution per 4 kg cat
Dexamethasone	Anti-inflammatory	Often used after successful CPR	1–2 mg/kg
Atipamezole	Alpha-2 antagonist	Used to reverse the sedative effects of alpha-2 agonists	Dogs: 0.05–0.2 mg/kg i.m. Cats: 0.5 mg/cat i.m.
Frusemide	Diuretic	Used to treat cerebral oedema – a common consequence of CPR	2 mg/kg i.v./i.m.

For some procedures, certain parameters require closer attention. For example, blood oxygen saturation levels should be carefully monitored during thoracic surgery as they will reflect any inadequate ventilation.

Ten rules of thumb

There are ten 'rules of thumb' for anaesthesia in at-risk patients:

1. *Stick with what you know*
   It is probably better for anaesthetists to use drugs they are familiar with (provided that the drugs are not absolutely contraindicated) rather than trying something different for the first time with a sick patient.

2. *General anaesthesia*
   A well thought-out and carefully managed anaesthetic is a lot less detrimental to a patient than a badly considered heavy sedative.

3. *Intraoperative fluids*
   All anaesthetized patients should be given intravenous maintenance fluids such as Hartmann's throughout anaesthesia at a rate of 5–10 ml/kg/hour (this rate may need to be higher in the at-risk patient).

4. *Acepromazine*
   Do not use in patients that are in physiological shock or have suffered blood loss.

5. *Nitrous oxide*
   Do not use in any situation where there may be a *closed* air-filled space within the body (e.g. pneumothorax or gastric dilation and volvulus syndrome).

6. *Halothane*
   This can cause cardiac dysrhythmias in combination with circulating catecholamines.

7. *Propofol*
   Propofol's main advantage is that it is very short acting. It has very similar cardiovascular depressant effects to thiopentone.

8. *Morphine/methadone*
   Do not use in cases of head trauma where there is a risk of cerebral oedema, as they may make the oedema worse.

9. *Diazepam or midazolam*
   These are safe sedatives in sick patients but they tend to make fit healthy patients unmanageable.

10. *Alpha-2 agonists*
    Do not use in compromised patients.

Anaesthetic considerations for specific cases

Caesarean section (Risk Level IV)

Considerations

- This is emergency surgery and so the patient will not have been starved (but periparturient animals are unlikely to have a full stomach)
- There is a risk of drug toxicity to the neonates. Use drugs that are least likely to affect neonates
- Analgesia, as with all surgical procedures, is very important but be sure that any analgesics given will not adversely affect the neonates
- Some analgesics (e.g. opioids) are excreted in milk and can affect the neonates after parturition.

Premedication
Provided that the patient is calm and easily handled, sedative premedication should be avoided. At the end of surgery, the mother needs to be fully conscious in order to look after the young.

Induction

- Thiopentone crosses the placenta and affects the neonates. It is fairly long acting and the young may well still be under the influence of this drug when they are delivered, and so less able to suck milk from their mothers

- Propofol is very short acting. In most instances the propofol will have been metabolized by the time the young are delivered. It is the first choice induction agent for Caesarean sections.

Maintenance

- Halothane and isoflurane are both suitable maintenance agents but isoflurane is preferred, as the neonates recover from its effects much more quickly, once they start breathing
- Nitrous oxide will allow lower doses of the other inhalation anaesthetic agent to be used, reducing its respiratory depressant effects on the neonate.

Anaesthetic breathing circuit
Any suitable breathing circuit can be used.

Analgesia

- Opioid analgesics will cross the placenta and are excreted in the milk. They will have a sedative effect on the neonates and so should not be used following Caesarean sections
- Local anaesthetic solutions can be infiltrated into the wound before it is closed. Bupivacaine will provide around 8 hours of analgesia. Do not use local anaesthetic solutions that contain adrenaline, as these will impair wound healing
- Non-steroidal anti-inflammatory drugs are *not* excreted in the milk. Carprofen will produce excellent analgesia but it should be given *after* the neonates have been delivered, so that it does not get into the neonatal circulation.

Special monitoring considerations
The dam must be closely monitored in the immediate postsurgical period to ensure that she is sufficiently conscious to nurse her newborn young.

Tip
The mother should be rotated slightly when in dorsal recumbency so that the weight of the gravid uterus does not press down on her caudal vena cava, reducing venous return to the heart.

Thoracotomies
Risk level depends on indications.

Considerations

- Postsurgical pain is potentially severe following thoracic surgery. It is vital that adequate analgesia is given. Chest pain is not only very unpleasant for the animal; it also impairs respiration, as the patient finds it uncomfortable to breathe
- Thoracic surgery demands facilities for IPPV. Although not an absolute requirement, mechanical ventilators make this a much easier task and allow the anaesthetist to concentrate on caring for the patient. In cats and small dogs, manual IPPV is preferable, but may require further assistance
- Neuromuscular blocking agents greatly facilitate thoracic access, contribute to postsurgical analgesia by reducing soft tissue trauma and are an essential component of balanced anaesthesia. They are less beneficial in cats and small dogs.

3.11 Pure μ agonist opioid doses for thoracotomies

Drug	Cats	Dogs
Morphine	0.1 mg/kg	0.3–0.5 mg/kg
Pethidine	2–5 mg/kg	1–2 mg/kg
Methadone	0.1 mg/kg	0.3–0.5mg/kg

Premedication

- Opioid analgesic should be included in the premedication. Partial μ agonists (such as buprenorphine and butorphanol) should *not* be used as they do not provide sufficient analgesia and reduce the analgesic effects of any pure μ agonists that are given
- Use pure μ agonist opioids at adequate doses (Figure 3.11).

Induction

- Any of the intravenous induction agents can be used
- In patients where the thoracic pathology is affecting gas exchange, preoxygenation with a face mask will be of great benefit.

Maintenance

- Balanced anaesthesia, using a low dose of volatile agent combined with intravenous pure μ agonist opioids and neuromuscular blocking agents, is ideal for thoracic surgery
- Maintenance with volatile agents alone is perfectly acceptable, if not as refined
- Nitrous oxide should not be used in cases of closed pneumothorax. It can safely be used as long as the thorax is open or if chest drains are in place. The analgesic properties of nitrous oxide will reduce the amount of volatile agent required to maintain anaesthesia.

Anaesthetic breathing circuit
Thoracic surgery demands the use of a breathing circuit that can be used for continuous IPPV. Depending on patient size, the T-piece, Bain or circle circuits are all suitable.

Analgesia

- Intercostal nerve block with bupivacaine will provide up to 8 hours of analgesia
- Bupivacaine can also be applied directly to the pleura by introducing it into the thoracic cavity before it is closed. The patient is then positioned in lateral recumbency for a few minutes, with the side of its chest that contains the chest drain placed downwards. The bupivacaine prevents chest pain discomfort
- Pure μ agonist opioids should be used frequently and to effect
- Carprofen can be used to good effect but, in common with other NSAIDs, it can affect blood clotting.

Special monitoring considerations

- Throughout the procedure, blood oxygen saturation should be monitored with a pulse oximeter. The blood oxygen saturation should be maintained above 95%. Any reduction in this figure indicates that ventilation is inadequate

- Particular attention should be paid to the patient's blood oxygen saturation at the end of surgery. Any residual pneumothorax will be reflected in a low blood oxygen saturation
- During the postanaesthetic period, when pulse oximeters become difficult to use due to the patient's movements, the mucous membrane colour should be observed
- Heat loss is rapid during thoracotomies and the patient's temperature should be closely monitored.

Tips

- Try to maintain the patient's body temperature using hot-water bottles or heat pads (it is easier to prevent heat loss than it is to warm up a hypothermic patient)
- When using a 'water trap' chest drain, the water column in the bottle moves with the patient's respiration. This movement can be used as an indication of the degree of lung expansion within the chest. When the lungs are fully inflated, there is very little movement of the water column. If there is a large residual pneumothorax, there will be obvious movement of the water column as the patient breathes in and out.

Diaphragmatic rupture in cats (Risk Level IV)

Considerations

- Diaphragmatic rupture is a common condition in cats that have suffered trauma
- As with all high-risk anaesthesia, wherever possible stabilize the cat before attempting surgery. This will greatly reduce the mortality rate
- Supplement the animal's inspired oxygen whilst it is stabilized
- Cats with a ruptured diaphragm are often quite stable whilst in sternal recumbency, but when placed in lateral or dorsal recumbency the pressure of the intestines on the lungs can cause hypoxia.

Premedication

- If the cat is reasonably calm, sedation should be avoided. It may cause the cat to lie down, adversely affecting its ventilation
- Opioid analgesics should be given prior to the start of surgery. They help to calm a distressed cat, smoothing the induction of anaesthesia.

Induction

- The cat should be preoxygenated using a face mask, if it will tolerate it
- Anaesthesia should be induced using an intravenous induction agent, as this is the least stressful induction technique. Thiopentone, propofol and alphaxalone/alphadalone are all ideal
- Remember: as soon as the abdomen is open the thorax is effectively opened and IPPV should be started (it may even be necessary to start IPPV as soon as the cat's trachea has been intubated, as spontaneous respiration in the recumbent cat may be inadequate).

Maintenance

- Any of the modern volatile anaesthetic maintenance agents can be used in cases of diaphragmatic rupture
- Nitrous oxide should be avoided until the thoracic cavity has been opened to the atmosphere.

Anaesthetic breathing circuit
The T-piece should be used.

Analgesia

- After surgery, respiration will be reduced because the cat finds breathing uncomfortable. Opioid analgesics or carprofen will reduce this pain and so enhance respiration
- A combination of carprofen and a pure μ agonist opioid such as morphine or pethidine, given frequently and to effect, is ideal.

Special monitoring considerations

- The patient's blood oxygen saturation should be monitored using a pulse oximeter. A low blood oxygen saturation indicates poor ventilation. If it occurs once the cat has been allowed to return to spontaneous respiration, it can indicate a large residual pneumothorax
- Anaesthetized cats are normally prone to heat loss but this is more severe in this case, because both the abdominal and thoracic viscera are exposed to cold air. Particular attention should be paid to the patient's temperature.

Tip
A simple oxygen tent can be constructed out of an Elizabethan collar covered in 'clingfilm'. Oxygen is delivered into it using a piece of giving-set tubing. This can be put on the cat to stabilize it whilst preparations are made for the surgery.

Gastric dilation and volvulus syndrome in the dog (Risk Level V)

Considerations

- This surgical emergency occurs when the dog's stomach becomes twisted and dilated, preventing the outflow of stomach contents through either the pyloric or cardiac sphincters. The stomach then rapidly fills with gas. The overexpanded stomach can then put pressure on the caudal vena cava, reducing venous return to the heart
- When these dogs first present, they are hypovolaemic, acidotic and very distressed
- Fluid therapy should be started immediately, using Hartmann's solution
- The stomach should be decompressed, using a stomach tube or percutaneous decompression
- Dysrhythmias, including ventricular premature contractions and ventricular tachycardia, are often seen in these cases. Good preparation of the patient, including well directed fluid therapy and the correction of any electrolyte imbalances prior to anaesthesia, will help to reduce these.

Premedication

- Sedation needs to be sufficient to enable gastric decompression
- In sick dogs, a combination of diazepam (0.2 mg/kg) and pethidine (1 mg/kg) produces safe and effective sedation

- Do not use acepromazine or alpha-2 agonists in cases of gastric dilation and volvulus syndrome.

Induction

- Thiopentone should be avoided because of its tendency to induce cardiac dysrhythmias
- Propofol is the agent of choice but should be administered slowly (there will be a significant delay between intravenous injection and the onset of action of propofol).

Maintenance

- Nitrous oxide should *not* be used, because of its tendency to fill gas-filled spaces
- Isoflurane is the maintenance agent of choice, as halothane is dysrhythmogenic and may make any dysrhythmias worse.

Anaesthetic breathing circuit
Any suitable breathing circuit can be used.

Analgesia

- Morphine can cause an increase in the muscle tone of the pyloric sphincter. For this reason, it should be avoided in these cases
- Pethidine is less likely to slow gastric emptying and is more suitable, provided that it is given frequently enough to be effective.

Special monitoring considerations
Cardiac dysrhythmias are not uncommon during surgical correction of GDVs. An ECG machine will warn the anaesthetist if these dysrythmias become severe enough to warrant treatment with either lignocaine or procainamide.

Patients with liver disease (Risk Level II–V)

Considerations

- These patients are not able to metabolize anaesthetic agents as well as fit animals. This results in an increased duration of action of most anaesthetic drugs
- Short-acting agents should be used, as any increase in the duration of action of these will be less dramatic
- These patients are also less able to metabolize the lactate in Hartmann's solution into bicarbonate. Normal saline or glucose saline should be used as a maintenance fluid instead.

Premedication
Where necessary, diazepam or midazolam, combined with pethidine, produces good sedation in systemically affected patients with liver disease.

Induction
Propofol on its own, or fentanyl and propofol combined, is the preferred induction agent.

Maintenance

- Both halothane and isoflurane are suitable maintenance agents but isoflurane is preferred, because it does not reduce hepatic perfusion as much as halothane

- Although halothane is partly (20%) metabolized by the liver, liver disease should not prolong recovery from halothane anaesthesia, as halothane is eliminated through the lungs and not as a result of liver metabolism
- Nitrous oxide can safely be used in patients with liver disease.

Anaesthetic breathing circuit
Any suitable breathing circuit can be used.

Analgesia

- Non-steroidal anti-inflammatory drugs should be avoided, because they tend to be long acting and potentially more toxic in these cases
- Short-acting pure μ agonist opioids should be used. Pethidine given frequently and to effect is ideal.

Special monitoring considerations

- Normal routine monitoring should be carried out but these patients often recover very slowly from anaesthesia.
- Monitoring should be continued until the patient has recovered fully from the effects of the anaesthetic drugs.

Neonatal anaesthesia (Risk Level II or more)

Considerations

- Puppies and kittens less than 12 weeks of age are considered to be neonates
- They have very poorly developed livers and short-acting drugs should be used
- Venous access can be difficult in these small animals: it may be necessary to induce anaesthesia (using an inhalation anaesthetic agent) before catheterizing a suitable vein
- These patients are very susceptible to heat loss and must be kept warm
- Preanaesthetic starvation should be kept to a minimum. Because of their high metabolic rate, neonates will suffer if starved for long periods.

Premedication
Short-acting sedatives such as diazepam and midazolam, combined with pethidine, can be given if necessary but sedative premedicants should be avoided wherever possible.

Induction
Either intravenous propofol or isoflurane administered via a face mask can be used to induce anaesthesia.

Maintenance

- Isoflurane is preferred, because recovery from anaesthesia is more rapid, allowing the neonate to return sooner to its mother
- Nitrous oxide can safely be used in neonates, provided that precautions are taken to prevent diffusion hypoxaemia from occurring at the end of anaesthesia (the neonate should be allowed to breathe 100% oxygen for 2 minutes after the nitrous oxide has been turned off).

Anaesthetic breathing circuit
The low breathing resistance offered by the T-piece makes it an ideal circuit for use with neonates.

Analgesia

- NSAIDs should be avoided, because of their potential toxicity to neonates. Short-acting pure μ agonist opioids such as pethidine, given frequently to effect, are suitable
- Neonates respond very well to 'tender loving care'. Used in abundance, it will often calm a distressed puppy or kitten.

Special monitoring considerations

- The patient's temperature should be closely monitored, as neonates are prone to hypothermia
- It is easier to maintain the patient's temperature than it is to warm up a hypothermic neonate. Hot-water bottles, heat pads, etc. should be used to maintain the neonate's temperature.

Tip

A good way of reducing heat loss from small patients is to increase the temperature of the operating room. If the temperature in the room is high enough for the patient, the surgeon should be uncomfortably warm.

Urethral obstruction in the cat (Risk Level IV)

Considerations

- Urethral obstruction is a life-threatening condition that prevents the cat from excreting potassium. This leads to a dangerously high blood potassium level (hyperkalaemia), which can cause fatal cardiac dysrhythmias
- Acidosis and hypovolaemia also occur
- Initial treatment is aimed at correcting these metabolic imbalances. The cat should *not* be anaesthetized to relieve the obstruction until the metabolic disturbances have been corrected
- The administration of fluids that do not contain potassium will reduce the hyperkalaemia by simple dilution
- Correction of any acidosis will also reduce the serum potassium ion concentration, because potassium ions (which moved into the extracellular compartment in exchange for hydrogen ions during the acidosis) move back into the intracellular compartment once the animal's pH has been restored to normal
- Calcium can be used to reduce the effects of the potassium on the heart, as calcium is the physiological antagonist of potassium
- Administering glucose saline and insulin combined will help to reduce the extracellular potassium levels still further as extracellular potassium ions are exchanged for intracellular sodium ions when glucose is transported into a cell
- The patient's ECG should be monitored, as cardiac dysrhythmias are common. Hyperkalaemia causes a reduction in amplitude or an absence of the P waves, an increased duration of the QRS complex and spiked T waves on the ECG trace. These classic changes should disappear and the ECG trace return to normal if treatment of the hyperkalaemia is effective
- Whilst the cat is stabilized with fluid therapy, its bladder can be emptied by cystocentesis. This can be carried out without any sedation and allows the surgical correction of the blockage to be postponed until the risk of anaesthesia is minimized.

Premedication

Premedication is not indicated.

Induction

- Diazepam and ketamine, given intravenously to effect, can be sufficient to allow urethral catheterization
- Intravenous propofol is also suitable.

Maintenance

- Catheterization of the bladder is often a very quick procedure and it may not be necessary to use a maintenance agent
- If a maintenance agent is required, isoflurane is less dysrhythmogenic than halothane.

Anaesthetic breathing circuit
The T-piece should be used.

Analgesia
Once the blockage has been removed, this condition is not particularly painful: buprenorphine will produce excellent analgesia.

Special monitoring considerations
The patient's ECG should be closely monitored for evidence of hyperkalaemia-induced cardiac dysrhythmias.

Pyometra in the bitch (Risk Level III–IV)

Considerations

- This is not an emergency. Time spent stabilizing the patient will greatly reduce the risks of anaesthesia
- Correct physiological shock by using intravenous fluids.

Premedication
Do not use acepromazine in patients that are shocked.

Induction
Any of the commonly used intravenous induction agents can be used.

Maintenance
Any of the commonly used volatile anaesthetic maintenance agents are suitable.

Anaesthetic breathing circuit
Any suitable breathing circuit can be used.

Analgesia
Provided that the patient's fluid balance has been restored, any of the common analgesic agents can safely be used.

Special monitoring considerations
Routine monitoring should be carried out.

Tip
The animal should be rolled slightly when she is placed in dorsal recumbency, in order to take the weight of the full uterus off the caudal vena cava.

Geriatric animals (Risk Level II or more)

Considerations

- There is a greater probability that a geriatric patient is suffering from disease. A thorough physical examination should be carried out

- Check for any history of exercise intolerance (which may indicate heart disease) or increased water intake (which can be a sign of kidney or liver disease)
- Check the mouth for any loose teeth that may be dislodged and accidentally inhaled during the induction of anaesthesia
- Water should not be withheld for more than 30 minutes prior to anaesthesia
- Renal insufficiency is common in older cats
- Older dogs are more likely to have developed mitral valve insufficiency: carefully auscultate the chest, listening for any heart murmurs.

Premedication

Unless contraindicated, acepromazine (at a reduced dose) combined with an opioid can be usefully used in geriatric patients. This is especially true for excitable cases.

Induction

- Preoxygenation with a face mask (if it is well tolerated by the patient) will be of great benefit to patients suffering from pulmonary or cardiac disease
- The induction of anaesthesia using an intravenous induction agent is less stressful for the patient than a mask induction
- There is very little difference in the myocardial depressant effects of propofol and thiopentone, but propofol is more rapidly metabolized than thiopentone.

Maintenance

- Any of the common anaesthetic maintenance agents can be used in geriatric patients
- Nitrous oxide can safely be used in geriatric patients unless contraindicated.

Anaesthetic breathing circuit

Any suitable breathing circuit can be used.

Analgesia

Opioid analgesics can safely be used in geriatric patients.

Special monitoring considerations

Geriatric patients are prone to hypothermia and their temperature should be closely monitored and maintained.

Hyperthyroidism in the cat (Risk Level III)

Considerations

- Hyperthyroidism is one of the more common metabolic disorders of older cats. Thyroidectomy is sometimes used to treat this condition
- Hyperthyroid cats should be rendered euthyroid with carbimazole before surgery
- Hyperthyroid cats are thin and therefore susceptible to hypothermia
- They resent being handled and the stress of handling can cause respiratory distress and cardiac dysrhythmias
- They are often suffering from secondary hypertrophic cardiomyopathy; they should be checked for any evidence of congestive heart failure and treated if necessary.

Premedication

- Because of the character of hyperthyroid cats, the premedicant should sedate the cat sufficiently to allow anaesthesia to be induced in a relatively stress-free manner
- Acepromazine in combination with an opioid (such as morphine or pethidine) produces good sedation
- Alpha-2 agonist agents should be avoided, because of their tendency to increase the sensitivity of the myocardium to circulating catecholamines.

Induction

- Ketamine stimulates the sympathetic nervous system and should be avoided in these cases
- Intravenous induction agents are best, and both propofol and alphaxalone/alphadalone are suitable
- Thiopentone should be avoided, as it is dysrhythmogenic.

Maintenance

- Isoflurane is preferred to halothane as it does not sensitize the heart to circulating catecholamines
- Nitrous oxide can be used safely in these cases, as it will reduce the amount of isoflurane required to maintain anaesthesia.

Anaesthetic breathing circuit

The T-piece should be used.

Analgesia

Pure μ agonist opioids can safely be used in these cases.

Special monitoring considerations

- Monitoring should be directed towards the cardiovascular system, because of the tendency of these cats to have underlying heart disease. The ECG traces should be carefully monitored for evidence of cardiac dysrhythmias
- The parathyroid glands are occasionally damaged during this procedure. They form part of the calcium homeostasis mechanism and accidental damage results in a short period of hypocalcaemia. This occurs in the first few days after surgery and lasts for a few days. Cats that have undergone a bilateral thyroidectomy should have daily blood samples for serum calcium assays for 4–7 days to check for evidence of hypocalcaemia. If it occurs, it can be treated with calcium gluconate
- Bilateral recurrent laryngeal nerve damage can occur and this presents as severe respiratory distress when the cat's endotracheal tube is withdrawn. If this occurs, the trachea should immediately be reintubated and a tracheostomy carried out.

Diabetes mellitus (Risk Level III)

Considerations

- All diabetic patients must be stabilized prior to surgery wherever possible
- Facilities for measuring blood glucose levels should be available
- Anaesthesia is best scheduled for first thing in the morning: this means that the patient recovers fully while there are plenty of staff around to observe it

- The patient's normal dietary regime should be upset as little as possible by the surgery – the owners should be asked to bring in the patient's normal food on the morning of surgery, along with its insulin
- Water should not be withheld from these patients, as they are often polydipsic and become dehydrated very quickly
- The owners should be instructed to feed the patient normally the night before the surgery is scheduled. Neither food nor insulin should be given on the morning of surgery.

Premedication

- Sedative premedication should be avoided wherever possible: it is important that these patients are able to eat as soon as possible after they have recovered from anaesthesia
- Opioid analgesics can be used. If sedation is required, acepromazine can be added at a low dose
- Alpha-2 agonist drugs should be avoided, as they affect normal glucose homeostasis
- At the same time as administering the premedication, an intravenous catheter should be placed in each cephalic vein: the first is to administer glucose saline; the second is used to take blood samples during the procedure in order to measure the patient's blood glucose level
- At the same time as the premedication is administered, the patient's blood glucose is measured. The patient is given half its normal insulin dose and an infusion of 5% glucose saline is started at a rate of 5 ml/kg/hour
- The aim throughout the preanaesthetic period, anaesthesia and the recovery period is to keep the patient's blood glucose level between 8 and 16 mmol/l by varying the rate of the glucose saline infusion.

Induction

- Short-acting intravenous anaesthetic agents should be used for anaesthesia induction
- Propofol and thiopentone are both suitable induction agents but propofol is preferred, because it produces a more rapid recovery from anaesthesia.

Maintenance

- Isoflurane is preferred to halothane, because it produces a more rapid recovery from anaesthesia
- Nitrous oxide can be used in patients with diabetes mellitus
- At frequent intervals throughout the anaesthetic, samples of blood should be drawn and the patient's blood glucose level measured. The glucose saline infusion rate is varied in order to maintain the patient's blood glucose level above 8 mmol/l
- It is much more important to make sure that the blood glucose level remains above 6 mmol/l than it is to keep it below 16 mmol/l. Periods of hyperglycaemia are not detrimental to the patient but even a short period of hypoglycaemia can be fatal
- At the end of anaesthesia, the patient is allowed to recover and is offered food at the earliest opportunity
- Once it has eaten its normal morning ration and kept it down for 20 minutes, it can be given the other half of its normal insulin dose. It should be monitored carefully throughout the rest of the day for signs of hypoglycaemia.

Anaesthetic breathing circuit
Any suitable breathing circuit can be used.

Analgesia
Opioid analgesics can safely be given to diabetic patients if required.

Special monitoring considerations
Facilities for blood glucose analysis should be available.

Tip
Simple sticks (similar to urine test sticks) are available that give an accurate indication of blood glucose levels.

Heart disease (Risk Level II or more)

Considerations

- There are many possible causes of heart disease. All affect the heart's ability to pump oxygenated blood around the body and the lungs
- Congestive heart failure occurs when the reduced cardiac output results in the accumulation of fluid in the lungs and body cavities
- Many older patients that present for routine anaesthesia are suffering from some form of heart disease, most commonly mitral valve insufficiency. This condition is often diagnosed on auscultation of a mitral valve murmur, supported by radiographic evidence of heart enlargement
- Younger patients with cardiac conditions are often more difficult to evaluate. Young animals with severe heart murmurs should have the exact cause of their murmur diagnosed before anaesthesia
- Many older animals with congestive heart failure are receiving medication; with the exception of diuretic drugs, these should be given on the morning of surgery
- As a rule of thumb, if a patient is fit enough to walk briskly up and down an average-sized waiting room a couple of times, it should be fit enough to undergo a well managed general anaesthesia.

Premedication

- Acepromazine can cause a profound fall in blood pressure, because of its vasodilatory effects. It should not be used in patients that have severe heart disease
- Some patients can have a loud heart murmur without showing any clinical signs of heart failure. These otherwise lively animals often need some sedative premedication; in these cases it may be necessary to use acepromazine at low doses in combination with an opioid
- Alpha-2 agonist agents should be avoided in patients with heart disease.

Induction
Both thiopentone and propofol produce similar degrees of cardiovascular depression but thiopentone should not be used in patients with dysrhythmias as it will make the dysrhythmia worse.

Maintenance

- Both isoflurane and halothane are suitable maintenance agents
- Halothane should not be used in dogs that have been receiving etamiphylline or theophylline, as this combination may lead to cardiac dysrhythmias.

Anaesthetic breathing circuit
Any suitable breathing circuit can be used.

Analgesia
Opioids, NSAIDs and local anaesthetics are all suitable for use in patients with heart disease.

Special monitoring considerations

- Patients with heart disease are prone to cardiac dysrhythmias under anaesthesia (often because of myocardial hypoxaemia). The patient's ECG should be monitored throughout anaesthesia and any dysrhythmias treated if necessary
- If the myocardial hypoxaemia is thought to be the cause of ventricular premature complexes, intermittent positive pressure ventilation will often help to reduce their frequency or eliminate them completely.

Further reading

Clutton E (1993) Management of perioperative cardiac arrest in companion animals, Part 1. *In Practice* **15**, 267–270

Clutton E (1994) Management of perioperative cardiac arrest in companion animals, Part 2. *In Practice* **16**, 3–6

Clutton E (1995) The right anaesthetic machine for you? *In Practice* **17**, 83–88

Davey A, Moyle JTB and Ward CS (eds) (1997) *Ward's Anaesthetic Equipment*, 3rd edn. WB Saunders, London

Hall LW and Clarke KW (eds) (1991) *Veterinary Anaesthesia*, 9th edn. Baillière Tindall, London

Hall LW and Taylor PM (eds) (1994) *Anaesthesia of the Cat*. Baillière Tindall, London

Seymour C and Gleed R (eds) (1999) *Manual of Small Animal Anaesthesia and Analgesia*. BSAVA, Cheltenham

Short CE (1987) *Principles and Practice of Veterinary Anaesthesia*. Williams and Wilkins, Baltimore

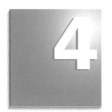

4 Management of a critical care unit

Wendy Adams and Jacqui Niles

This chapter is designed to give information on:

- How and why to set up a critical care unit (CCU)
- Minimum requirements (staff and equipment) for a CCU
- Daily management routines in a CCU
- Specialized equipment found in a CCU and how and when to use it
- Specialized techniques performed in a CCU

Introduction

As the public become increasingly aware of the services that veterinary surgeries can provide, the demand for emergency and critical care facilities is increasing. This awareness has resulted from the recent explosion in media coverage of veterinary work. People now expect the same level of critical care medicine for their pets as they would for themselves and the veterinary profession is obliged to meet these demands.

Veterinary critical care is a rapidly expanding field. This chapter discusses the role that a CCU plays within a veterinary hospital and covers the equipment and techniques that should be provided in such a unit. Good nursing care is the single most important aspect of successful critical care.

When and why to establish a CCU

Public desire for pets to receive a higher level of treatment is an incentive for veterinary practices to improve their facilities and level of care.

Many veterinary patients arrive at veterinary hospitals with critical life-threatening conditions. These result from a wide variety of causes, ranging from trauma to acute respiratory distress, cardiac failure, sudden onset neurological signs or severe metabolic derangement (as seen with Addison's disease, diabetes mellitus, urinary obstruction or renal failure). Other animals, although their condition is not critical, may require intensive nursing and therapy if it is not to become life-threatening. The general hospital ward does not provide an environment suitable to deal with such patients adequately. A CCU, in which high-quality committed and continuous nursing care is given, can provide the optimal environment for these patients. The goals of a CCU are outlined in Figure 4.1.

Animals that benefit from a CCU environment can be broadly classified into three groups:

- Animals requiring nursing care that are stable but require a large amount of nursing time and effort (e.g. patients with spinal disease)
- Animals that are physiologically stable but require intense monitoring or observation. These animals may suffer complications of their disease or postsurgical complications and can be monitored and observed more closely in a CCU; thus problems are likely to be recognized and dealt with more quickly, decreasing morbidity and mortality rates
- Animals that are physiologically unstable and in need of constant veterinary intensive care (e.g. trauma patients). These animals can be monitored constantly in an environment where the necessary equipment, technical expertise and veterinary knowledge are readily available to deal with any change in the patient's status.

How to set up a CCU

Access and reception

A critical care unit may range from a dedicated area within an existing practice to a purpose-built emergency and critical care

4.1 Goals of a critical care unit

- To provide routine treatment and care
- To provide specialized medical and nursing services
- To evaluate continuously the physiological state of the patient by routine monitoring and the use of specialized techniques if necessary
- To provide emergency resuscitative procedures (e.g. for cardiac or respiratory arrest) and treatment in order to save the patient's life.

facility that provides support to a number of practices within the surrounding area.

- Any clinic providing emergency care should be easily accessible by road and the building should be clearly identified by signs
- The reception area of a clinic providing critical care facilities should be designed to help to minimize client anxiety, with information displayed to inform owners about the triage procedure (Figure 4.2) and describing some of the commoner emergencies and first-aid procedures.

Triage is the process of rapid examination and classification of emergency patients based on the severity of their injuries and the urgency with which treatment is required.

Location within the clinic

The CCU should be designed to accommodate the full range of sizes of animals. It should be located centrally within a clinic so that it can easily service patients from all other areas of the building. In most practices the CCU is also the emergency room and it should be possible to move animals to and from the CCU on trolleys or stretchers without obstruction.

4.2 **The triage procedure**

ARRIVAL AT CCU
Obtain only essential information
(i.e. cause of trauma, progression of signs, what first aid has been given).
Obtain permission for treatment

↓

PRIMARY SURVEY
Assess airway, breathing, circulation, level of consciousness

↓

TRIAGE
Classify patient as stable, potentially unstable or unstable

↓

RESUSCITATION OF VITAL FUNCTIONS
Stabilize life-threatening problems

↓

SECONDARY SURVEY
Full physical examination, detailed history, reassessment of original treatment

↓

DEFINITIVE CARE

Facilities within the CCU

- A treatment area should be established with a table, drip stand and facilities for resuscitation kept close by (the resuscitation trolley or 'crash cart' is discussed below)
- Laboratory and radiographic facilities should be available (usually close to but outside the CCU)
- Ideally cages should be arranged so that all patients can be easily seen from any location in the treatment area
- Floors and walls should be durable and easy to clean
- Drainage must be effective, to avoid trapping waste that can encourage the growth of resistant microorganisms
- The area must be well lit and fitted with plentiful electrical outlets so that each cage is within reach of a power point
- Multiple sources of oxygen and suction are necessary (these can be portable or, preferably, wall-mounted)
- Ceiling tracks for intravenous fluids are ideal
- Good ventilation is important
- It is vital that the unit has an emergency generator in the event of power failure
- Storage space for basic equipment (such as animal bedding, heating pads) and specialized equipment (monitors, infusion pumps) is an important consideration, as are adequate facilities for cleaning
- There should be sinks located in the CCU for cleaning hands and equipment.

Figures 4.3 and 4.4 give good examples of CCU design.

Minimum requirements

Staff

The success of a CCU depends to a large extent on the staff that run the facility and their ability to work as a coordinated team. Each member of the critical care team should be responsible for individual jobs within the unit, to ensure proper daily patient care. Emergency medicine is demanding and staff should be experienced enough to be able to cope with the job; they should be able to work under pressure and to communicate well with work colleagues.

The minimum number of staff necessary at any one time is a duty veterinary surgeon and one nurse. Having two nurses is preferable – one is always observing the animals in the CCU whilst the other is available to assist with receiving clients and performing diagnostic and surgical procedures.

The CCU should be staffed 24 hours a day, although at first there may not be critical patients present at all times. As the unit grows it may be possible to introduce two or three shifts of staff within a 24-hour period, with ward rounds at the changeover between shifts to ensure continuity of patient care.

Receptionists

Receptionists are the clients' first point of contact with the practice. They should be able to communicate effectively with stressed and anxious clients and explain the triage procedure to them. Training should be given to ensure that receptionists are able to prioritize emergencies, recognize life-threatening conditions and administer cardiopulmonary resuscitation (CPR). Financial matters should be clearly explained to owners as critical care patients require extensive treatment and monitoring, leading to higher costs than those encountered for routine veterinary services.

4.3 Floor plan of a medium-sized critical care unit

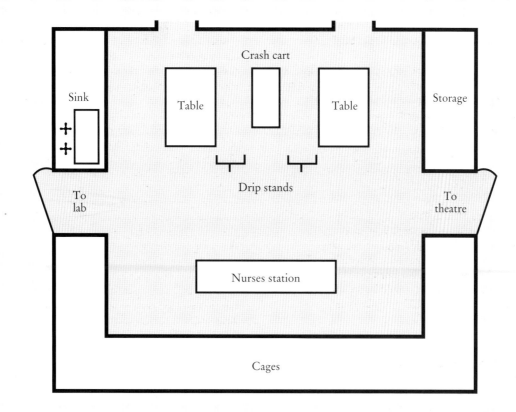

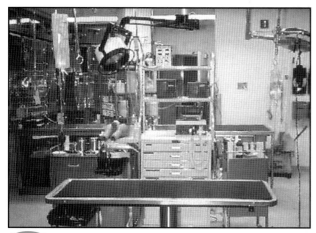

4.4 *A critical care unit.*

Veterinary surgeons

Veterinary surgeons working in a CCU should be competent in the diagnosis and treatment of trauma patients, which comprise the majority of cases seen on an emergency basis. The veterinary surgeon is ultimately responsible for decisions governing patient care and changes in treatment, and should be able to communicate effectively with the rest of the team.

Veterinary nurses

Nurses are vital members of the critical care team. Successful patient care depends on diligent hands-on monitoring and nursing. Critically ill animals are high-risk patients that can exhibit numerous and unpredictable problems. The CCU nurse is usually the first person to recognize changes in the patient's condition and should be able to respond rapidly to such changes in order to manage serious illness and avoid

serious complications. Although increasingly expensive and sophisticated monitoring techniques are available, physical examination of the patient remains the most important means of patient evaluation.

Nursing responsibilities include:

- Direct patient care, such as monitoring of vital signs administration of medication
- Record-keeping
- Attending to patients' physiological and psychological needs.

It should be noted that at present the RCVS considers a large number of the techniques and procedures described in this chapter as acts of veterinary surgery in which a body cavity is entered; therefore they should not be performed by a veterinary nurse.

Equipment requirements of the CCU

Essential equipment and facilities include:

- Basic laboratory facilities to be able to obtain a 'minimum database' following patient admission, including:
  - Packed cell volume (microhaematocrit centrifuge and reader)
  - Total protein (refractometer)
  - Blood glucose (glucometer)
  - Blood urea and urine specific gravity (refractometer)
- Microscope and equipment to be able to perform cytological analysis of fluid and tissue samples obtained (glass slides, pipettes, rapid cytology stain)
- Cardiopulmonary monitoring equipment:
  - Electrocardiogram (ECG) to monitor patients with or predisposed to cardiac abnormalities
  - Equipment to obtain direct or indirect blood pressure measurements

- Resuscitation trolley (see below)
- Blood gas analyser and pulse oximeter
- Intravenous fluid infusion pumps and syringe drivers
- Incubator or thermostatically controlled water bed
- Emergency surgical packs (Figure 4.5)
- Trolley and a stretcher

- Essential drugs (Figure 4.6) and dressings
- Anaesthetic equipment
- Oxygen cage
- Scales
- Clippers
- Vacuum cleaner.

4.5 Emergency surgical packs

Equipment	Basic suture/cut-down pack	Chest drain pack	Tracheotomy pack
Drapes	✓	✓	✓
Towel clips	✓	✓	✓
Scalpel handle and blade	✓	✓	✓
Adson Brown forceps	✓	✓	✓
Mosquito forceps	Curved x 4		x 2
Mayo scissors	✓	✓	✓
Metzenbaum scissors	✓		✓
Needle holders	✓	✓	✓
Swabs	✓	✓	✓
Other		Chest drains, range of sizes Three-way tap Gate clamp	Tracheostomy tubes, range of sizes Gelpi retractors x 2

4.6 Essential drugs

Range of fluids, including:
Lactated Ringer's solution
Dextran
0.9% Saline
Mannitol solution
5% Dextrose
2.5% Dextrose with 0.45% Saline
50% Dextrose

Range of injectable antibiotics, including:
Amoxycillin/clavulanate
Ampicillin
Cephalexin
Enrofloxacin
Gentamicin
Metronidazole
Potentiated sulphonamides

Anaesthetic drugs, including:
Inhalational agents (halothane, isoflurane)
Injectable agents (barbiturates, propofol, alpha-2 agonists, ketamine)
Muscle relaxants and reversal agents

Analgesic agents
Local anaesthetics (bupivacaine, lignocaine)
Morphine
Pethidine
Fentanyl
Buprenorphine
Non-steroidal anti-inflammatory drugs (carprofen)

Additional drugs (appropriate form indicated where necessary)
Adrenaline (1:1000 solution for injection)
Atropine (600 mg/ml solution for injection)
Calcium gluconate and calcium chloride (10% solution for injection)
Chlorpheniramine (solution for injection)
Cimetidine/ranitidine (solution for injection)
Dexamethasone (solution for injection)
Diazepam (for intravenous injection)
Digoxin (solution for injection)
Dobutamine (stock solution for dilution)
Dopamine (stock solution for dilution)
Doxapram (solution for injection and oral drops)
Fludrocortisone (tablets)
Frusemide (for injection)
Heparin (stock solution and heparinized saline, 100 IU/ml)
Insulin (soluble and suspension)
Lactulose
Lignocaine (solution for intravenous injection, without adrenaline)
Methyl prednisolone succinate (for intravenous injection)
Metoclopramide (for injection)
Misoprostol
Naloxone
Nitroglycerin ointment
Nitroprusside (solution for injection)
Omeprazole
Ophthalmic wash and ointments
Oxytocin (solution)
Potassium chloride (stock solution for dilution)
Procainamide (solution for injection)
Propranolol (solution for injection)
Sodium bicarbonate (stock solution for dilution)
Sucralfate
Topical anti-inflammatory and antimicrobial preparations
Water for injection

Ancillary services

These should be readily available for patients admitted to the CCU but are not necessarily part of the facility itself.

- Haematology, biochemistry and electrolyte analysers to obtain a complete blood count, biochemistry and electrolyte profile initially, and then as and when required
- Radiography, including equipment necessary to perform contrast studies and an automatic film processor
- Diagnostic ultrasonography – portable ultrasound machines allow non-invasive and rapid cardiac and abdominal imaging with minimal disturbance to critically ill patients
- Endoscopy equipment suitable for respiratory tract and upper gastrointestinal examinations for animals of all sizes.

Resuscitation trolley ('crash cart')

Equipment and drugs for managing an acute medical crisis should be readily accessible. One of the best ways of achieving this is to have a properly stocked mobile crash trolley ready for use at all times (Figure 4.7).

Equipment for the resuscitation trolley includes:

- Laryngoscope with various blades
- Full size range of endotracheal tubes and syringes to inflate cuffs
- Mouth gags
- Bandages for tying in tubes
- Hypodermic needles (14–22 gauge, 0.5–5 cm in length)
- Spinal needles
- Intraosseous needles
- Syringes (1–50 ml)
- Over-the-needle catheters (14–25 gauge)
- Male urinary catheters suitable for intratracheal injection
- Tape to secure catheters and intravenous lines
- Fresh heparinized saline
- Ready drawn-up doses of adrenaline, atropine and lignocaine
- Drugs (adrenaline, atropine, 10% calcium gluconate, dexamethasone, dobutamine, dopamine, doxapram, lignocaine, naloxone hydrochloride, procainamide, propranolol)
- Drug dose chart
- Fluid bags, fluid giving sets, catheter bungs, three-way taps
- Pressurized fluid infusion cuff
- Ambu bag and line to oxygen source
- Clippers
- Surgical packs (thoracotomy and tracheotomy)
- Chest drains
- Masks, gloves
- Scalpel blades (nos 10, 11 and 15)
- Range of suture materials
- Thermometer
- Stethoscope
- ECG monitor
- Defibrillator.

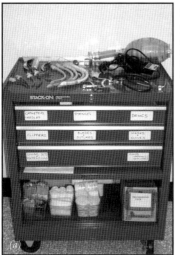

4.7

The crash trolley. (a) Drawers are labelled clearly with contents. (b) Equipment for establishing an airway is laid out on top of the trolley.

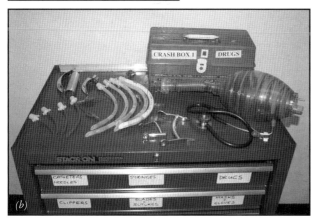

Daily management routines

Daily management routines can be split into three basic areas: patient care, housekeeping and stock-taking. Attention to each area is important to ensure the successful running of a CCU and to ensure the highest standards of patient care.

Patient care

- Morning rounds to update staff on new shifts about each animal's status
- Assessment of cases and updating records accordingly
- Feeding and medicating patients (ongoing throughout the day according to each animal's specific needs)
- Special procedures – catheter care, stoma care, dressing changes, physiotherapy
- Evening rounds.

Housekeeping

- All cages should be cleaned and disinfected thoroughly each day and especially between patients
- Cages should be allowed to stand dry for several hours before they are used again
- All multiple-use equipment (such as oxygen and suction lines, vacuum cleaner, clippers, endotracheal tubes) should be disassembled, cleaned and disinfected or sterilized between uses
- Table tops should be cleaned between each patient
- Work surfaces and floors should be cleaned.

Stock-taking

- The following should be checked and restocked:
  - Drugs and fluids kept in the CCU
  - Equipment (including giving sets, intravenous catheters, Foley catheters, chest drains)
  - Consumables such as bandaging materials, cotton wool

- Surgical packs should be checked and processed
- The crash cart should be checked, tidied and restocked
- Anaesthetic machines and circuits should be checked.

Records

Accurate medical records ensure continuity of care for critical patients. Poor or incomplete record-keeping can lead to compromised patient care.

4.8 SOAP system example

Subjective	Sabre is bright and responsive
Objective	T 38.6°C, P 110 bpm, R 20 pm Body systems evaluation: Cardiovascular: NAD Respiratory: NAD Gastrointestinal: NAD Cutaneous: decubital ulcers 3 cm diameter over lateral surfaces both elbows with minimal exudation (unchanged from yesterday) Musculoskeletal: hindlimb paresis with muscle wastage Neurological: deep pain sensation present (as yesterday). Withdrawal reflexes present but reduced (see neuro exam form) Urogenital: urination when exercised/bladder expressed
Assessment	Neurological status unchanged. Decubital ulcers apparently static and uninfected
Plan	Continue physiotherapy, bladder expression and local wound care. Repeat neurological examination daily. Suggest owners to visit when reporting progress.

T = body temperature; P = pulse; R = respiratory rate;
NAD = No abnormalities detected

The medical records kept may vary, depending on individual preferences of the critical care team, but in all cases they should be simple and complete. An individual unfamiliar with the case should be able to ascertain a particular patient's problem and its current status. Flow sheets are useful to chart various parameters and allow easy assessment of trends in critical patients.

A separate medical record should be maintained for each animal examined. The record should be legible, with the individual patient accurately identified, and should follow the format of a problem-oriented medical record. Problem-oriented medical records have four components:

- Database consisting of the initial information gathered on a patient. From this, problems are identified and should be listed in order of priority
- Problem list, which should be updated and refined throughout the course of hospitalization
- Initial plans (diagnostic and therapeutic), formulated and identified in the record for each problem listed
- Progress notes recorded daily in a standard format with four sections (known as 'SOAP'):
  - Subjective data
  - Objective data
  - Assessment
  - Plans.

A written example of a SOAP is shown in Figure 4.8 and a suggested Daily Progress Record form is shown in Figure 4.9.

Parameters to be monitored at least once daily in the critical patient include:

- Temperature, pulse, respiration
- Capillary refill time
- Total protein, packed cell volume (PCV)
- Urine specific gravity
- Weight and hydration status
- Urine output.

4.9 Daily progress records

Day:		Date:		Clinical Summary:			Page:	
Owner:		Animal:					Case No:	
A.M.	T:	P:	R:	P.M.	T:		P:	R:
Time	Assessment			Time	Assessment			
Plan:				Therapeutics:				
Diagnostic Procedures:				Drug:	Dose:	Route:	Frequency:	

In selected cases the following may also be monitored:

- Serum electrolytes
- Blood glucose
- ECG
- Blood pressure/gases
- Clotting function.

Systems evaluation

The table in Figure 4.10 sets out system parameters that need to be evaluated, abnormalities that might be observed and what the nursing priorities should be.

Respiratory system
Respiratory disorders are common in critically ill patients. It is important to monitor:

- Respiratory rate
- Character of breath sounds
- Breathing patterns
- Mucous membrane colour.

Evaluation of different breathing patterns can aid in localizing the source of respiratory difficulty. For example:

- A slow deep breathing pattern suggests upper airway obstruction
- Rapid shallow respirations are characteristic of a restrictive breathing pattern suggestive of pulmonary parenchymal disease or pleural space disease.

Mucous membrane colour should not be relied on exclusively as an indicator of oxygenation, although the presence of cyanosis (blue or purple membranes) is an immediate indication for blood gas analysis and consideration of supplemental oxygen. The primary nursing aims are to correct hypoxia and decrease the work of breathing.

Circulatory system
There are many causes of circulatory collapse (e.g. shock, heart failure, haemorrhage) and one or more of these may be present in a single patient. Adequate tissue perfusion must be maintained. Methods of evaluating the circulatory system include:

- Monitoring pulse rate and quality
- Monitoring capillary refill time

4.10 Systems evaluation

System	Parameters to be monitored	Common abnormalities	Nursing priorities
Respiratory	Respiratory rate Character of breath sounds Breathing patterns Mucous membrane colour Pulse oximetry (oxygenation)	Hypoxia (underventilation) Respiratory obstruction Pneumonia Pleural effusion (fluid or air)	Maintain oxygenation Decrease work of breathing
Circulatory	Pulse rate and character Blood pressure Tissue perfusion (CRT) Breathing patterns and lung sounds	Shock Circulatory overload Haemorrhage	Detect/stop haemorrhage Maintain circulating volume and tissue perfusion Recognize signs of shock
Gastrointestinal	Appetite Body weight Amount of vomit or diarrhoea Character/consistency of stools	Anorexia Weight loss Vomiting and diarrhoea Ileus Peritonitis	Maintain adequate nutrition Maintain hydration status Prompt diagnosis and management of problems Recognize signs of ileus Recognize signs of peritonitis
Genitourinary	Urine output Urine specific gravity Appearance of urine Frequency of urination Bladder size/consistency	Polyuria Oliguria/anuria Urinary tract infection Urinary tract obstruction	Maintain hydration status and renal function Place/check urethral catheters Check for vaginal and preputial discharges Prevent/treat urine scalding
Neurological	Neurological status Mentation Cranial nerve examination Posturing Heart rate/respiratory pattern Level of consciousness Motor function Deep pain sensation Urinary continence	Dullness Dementia/delirium Stupor Coma Seizures Loss of deep pain sensation	Early detection of changes in neurological status Detect/treat seizures Care of neurosurgical patients Assess motor function and deep pain sensation
Musculoskeletal	Level of mobility Weight-bearing Bandages/dressings	Decubital ulcers Urine scald Muscle atrophy Joint contracture	Patient comfort Physiotherapy Bandage/dressing changes

- Measurement of blood pressure (see later)
- Cardiac auscultation.

Palpation of the peripheral pulses allows a rough estimation of cardiac output. The femoral arterial pulse is the most readily palpable in the dog and cat and the pulse should be characterized with respect to its rate, rhythm and quality. An animal in shock frequently has a weak, rapid, 'thready' pulse that is difficult to palpate. Coupled with pale mucous membranes, this pulse may indicate poor perfusion, low blood volume and low cardiac output.

Gastrointestinal system

Accurate record-keeping is essential to the successful nursing of critical care patients with disorders of the gastrointestinal tract. It is vital to record:

- Changes in appetite
- Character and consistency of stools
- Amount of vomit or diarrhoea
- Changes in body weight.

Of particular concern is the sudden onset of abdominal pain, in association with weakness, collapse and abdominal distension. This can signify an acute abdominal crisis such as peritonitis. Prompt diagnosis and management of the underlying condition is necessary if it is not to prove fatal. (Abdominocentesis and diagnostic peritoneal lavage are considered below.)

Fluid lost in vomit or diarrhoea should be estimated and taken into consideration, along with changes in packed cell volume and total protein, when planning replacement fluid therapy.

Ileus predisposes a patient to ulceration and vomiting and can be secondary to hypokalemia, gastrointestinal disease or malnutrition.

Genitourinary system

Daily examination should include:

- Bladder palpation
- Checking for vaginal or preputial discharge
- Checking for signs of urine scalding around the perineum.

Urine output should be assessed on an ongoing basis. Changes in hydration status or renal function can have a direct effect on fluid requirements. Any changes in an animal's frequency or quantity of urination should be noted down, along with any changes in the physical appearance of the urine and fluctuations in body weight. Changes in urine appearance and specific gravity can be checked easily by obtaining a free-catch urine sample, cystocentesis or catheterization.

Urine output is technically easy to measure and provides useful information about renal perfusion. The rate of urine production in an animal depends on the glomerular filtration rate (GFR) in that animal. Urine production in a normal dog or cat is 1–2 ml/kg bodyweight/hour. Reduced urine production in the critical care patient often occurs in association with decreases in renal perfusion (e.g. hypovolaemic shock), disruption of the integrity of the urinary tract or development of renal dysfunction. An indwelling urinary catheter should be placed (see later) and maintained with a closed collecting system. This procedure is not without risks, since any indwelling catheter will cause mechanical irritation to the urethra and allows bacterial colonization of the urinary tract. Catheters should be removed as soon as possible.

Neurological system

A complete neurological examination should be performed at least twice daily on patients with neurological dysfunction. Serial monitoring is crucial, since deterioration in neurological status often results in irreversible sequelae. Early detection of deterioration may allow successful therapeutic intervention. In addition, the prognosis is often based on clinical progress.

Supportive care for the neurological patient requires monitoring for:

- Changes in mentation, papillary light response and ocular movement
- Posturing
- Changes in heart rate or respiratory pattern
- Signs of hypoxia
- Urinary and faecal continence.

A normal animal should be alert and responsive to external stimuli. Altered levels of consciousness may manifest as:

- Dullness or excessive sleepiness
- Dementia/delirium (resisting restraint, pacing, agitation, over-excitement)
- Stupor (semi-coma, responsive to noxious stimuli)
- Coma (unresponsive to noxious stimuli).

A decreasing level of consciousness on serial examinations suggests a progressive neurological lesion.

Cranial nerve examination should include assessment of pupil size, symmetry and response to light.

- Symmetrical pupils that are normally reactive to light suggest that the third cranial nerves and brainstem are intact
- Miotic pupils generally suggest a better prognosis for an animal than the presence of mydriatic pupils
- Pupils that are bilaterally dilated and non-responsive to light in a comatose patient suggest severe mid-brain disease, which carries a poor prognosis.

Spinal patients exhibiting paresis need to be closely monitored for changes in motor function and deep pain sensation of their limbs. Proper care of these patients is very labour-intensive.

Animals with neurological disorders are prone to a range of complications (Figure 4.11). Recumbent neurosurgical patients are predisposed to urine scald, faecal soiling, limb oedema, muscle wasting, decubital ulcers and pneumonia. Urine scald and faecal soiling result because of altered ability to control elimination and the patient's inability to move out of them.

4.11 Potential complications in animals with neurological disorders

- Seizures post myelography
- Prolonged neurological impairment
- Pain
- Inappetence, fever, depression
- Side effects of recumbency (e.g. urine scald, decubital ulcers)
- Diarrhoea, vomiting, gastrointestinal ulceration
- Untoward corticosteroid effects
- Urinary bladder dysfunction and urinary tract infection
- Surgical wound complications (seroma, infection and dehiscence)

- Absorbent bedding should be provided and should be changed regularly (every 2–4 hours)
- The animal's position should be changed regularly
- As much mobility as the patient's condition permits should be encouraged
- The patient should be frequently cleaned or bathed
- Limb oedema and muscle wasting can be treated with massage and passive range of motion exercises to disperse the oedema and stimulate normal pumping action of muscles.

Prolonged recumbency on pressure points, particularly in heavy patients, may result in decubital ulcers. If a decubital ulcer develops, local wound care and reconstructive surgery may be necessary to resolve the problem.

Recumbent patients may develop pulmonary congestion, due to stasis of blood in the dependent portions of the lungs. Invasion of congested lungs by opportunist bacteria causes pneumonia. Congestion can be treated by facilitating lung expansion and clearance of bronchial secretions. This can be achieved by:

- Encouraging early mobility and barking (in dogs)
- Performing respiratory physiotherapy (See *BSAVA Manual of Veterinary Nursing*, Chapter 4)
- Treating with bronchodilators
- Nebulization (see later).

If bacterial pneumonia is suspected, a transtracheal wash or bronchoalveolar lavage should be performed and antibiotic therapy should be instituted, based on culture and sensitivity results.

Musculoskeletal system

Musculoskeletal disease may be secondary to trauma or surgery (e.g. fracture repair). These patients are often recumbent and require intensive nursing care similar to that for neurosurgical patients. Bandages are often used for protection and support in these cases and require careful observation to ensure that they are fulfilling their intended role and do not become too loose, too tight or soaked with water, urine or faeces. (See Chapter 2 for postoperative care following specific orthopaedic procedures.)

Immobilization of the musculoskeletal system results in stiff atrophied muscles and joint contracture. Regular physiotherapy can help to prevent these complications, improve patient comfort and reduce the length of hospitalization. Patients that can stand and walk should be encouraged to do so; those that can stand but not walk should be encouraged to stand for a few minutes each day, in conjunction with position changes every 4 hours.

Nutrition in the CCU

Each animal's nutritional needs should be considered from the moment it enters the CCU.

Anorexic critical patients rapidly develop a negative energy and protein balance, which will result in compromised host defences and muscle strength, visceral organ atrophy and dysfunction and, eventually, gastrointestinal barrier breakdown, pneumonia, sepsis and death. Anorexic patients must be tempted to eat with highly palatable foods. If food is uneaten after an hour it should be removed and replaced with fresh food. If animals are recumbent they must be fed carefully to prevent aspiration of food.

If the nutritional and caloric requirements of the animal are not being met, alternative methods of nutritional support should be instituted before the patient's condition deteriorates further. Absolute indications for enteral nutritional support are given in Figure 4.12.

4.12 Absolute indications for enteral nutritional support

- Recent weight loss of more than 10%
- Inappetence for more than 5 days
- Anticipated anorexia or inability to eat for more than 5 days
- Increased nutrient loss (e.g. open peritoneal drainage, burns)
- Increased nutritional needs (e.g. sepsis, multiple trauma)
- Low serum albumin
- Hepatic lipidosis in cats
- History of chronic disease

Note: Nutritional support may be indicated earlier if any of these conditions occur concurrently.

Feeding methods include naso-oesophageal or oesophagostomy tube feeding, gastrostomy or jejunostomy tube feeding or total parenteral intravenous hyperalimentation. Each of these methods has its advantages and disadvantages but enteral nutrition has more advantages than parenteral nutrition (Figure 4.13). In general enteral feeding tubes placed more proximally are more physiological and less prone to cause gastrointestinal disturbance than those placed distally.

Whatever method of supplemental feeding is used, clear and concise nursing instructions are vital to ensure that the correct type and amount of diet is fed by the correct route. For further information on assisted feeding, see Chapter 4 in *BSAVA Manual of Veterinary Nursing*.

Tube feeding – general points

- The animal's daily nutritional requirement should be determined and split into four to six feeds daily
- On the first day, the patient should be given 30% of its nutritional requirements
- This should be increased by 30% each day until the full daily requirement is provided
- Food should be fed at room temperature
- Tubes should be flushed with water prior to and after feeding to prevent clogging.

With gastrostomy and jejunostomy tubes, care should be taken to ensure that food does not run down the outside of the tube and contaminate the abdominal wound.

Tablet medication can be crushed and administered via the tube but solutions or suspensions are preferable.

Tip
If the tube becomes clogged, flushing with a few millilitres of a carbonated drink may relieve the blockage.

Naso-oesophageal tubes

These are one of the most commonly used feeding tubes. They are easy to place, inexpensive and generally well tolerated.

Tube type	Advantages	Comments
Pharyngostomy	(Offers no significant advantages over other methods of enteral feeding)	Incorrect placement may lead to aspiration pneumonia and damage to the larynx or hyoid apparatus
Naso-oesophageal	Easily placed without sedation, so useful in unstable patients Inexpensive	Limited to liquid diets and prone to blockage Most useful for short-term feeding (< 14 days)
Oesophagostomy	Very easy to place under sedation and well tolerated by cats and dogs	Useful for intermediate-term feeding and tubes are larger diameter than naso-oesophageal tubes
Gastrostomy	Large-diameter tubes placed either surgically, by endoscopy or percutaneously Patient tolerance is excellent	Ideal for long-term feeding (> 14 days); special low-profile tubes are available for prolonged feeding
Jejunostomy	Better than intravenous nutrition	May be of use in selected patients but patients require intensive care and are prone to develop diarrhoea

They can be placed in a conscious animal and are thus useful in patients that are a poor anaesthetic risk.

Soft flexible silicone or polyurethane tubes are preferable to plastic and polyvinyl chloride tubes, which are not as pliable. The placement technique is described in Figure 4.14.

Complications

Complications are usually minimal. They include rhinitis, oesophagitis, vomiting, tube removal/migration and aspiration.

4.14 Placement of a naso-oesophageal tube

1. Place one to two drops of topical ophthalmic anaesthetic solution into one of the patient's nostrils.
2. Measure the length of the tube from the tip of the nose to the level of the ninth rib, to ensure that it terminates just short of the lower oesophageal sphincter.
3. Use the largest tube diameter that fits comfortably into the nares (3.5–5 F in small cats, 6 F in larger cats and small dogs).
4. Lubricate the end of the tube.
5. Push the nares upwards slightly to facilitate passage of the tube into the ventromedial meatus (Figure 4.15).
6. Never force the tube. If resistance is met, withdraw the tube and reinsert it.
7. Swallowing should be detected as the tube passes into the oesophagus.
8. Check tube placement:
   – Infuse 5–10 ml air
   – Auscultate the caudal thorax, listening for air bubbling in the stomach
   – Alternatively, gentle aspiration with a 10 ml syringe will produce immediate suction if the tube is in the oesophagus, due to collapse of the oesophagus over the end of the tube. (This does not occur with tracheobronchial intubation.)
   – If in doubt, evaluate the position of the tube radiographically.
9. Secure the tube with permanent adhesive (cyanoacrylate glue) or butterfly tapes and fine nylon sutures.
10. Divide the daily intake into small frequent meals.

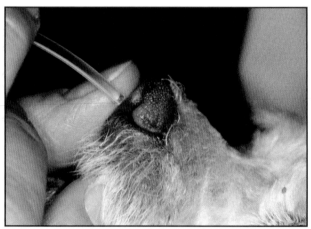

4.15 Pushing the nares dorsally facilitates the passage of a naso-oesophageal tube into the ventromedial meatus.

Gastrostomy tubes

One of the preferred methods of assisted nutrition in animals that are unable or unwilling to eat is the placement of a gastrostomy tube. These can be placed surgically or percutaneously, either 'blind' or with the use of an endoscope (percutaneous endoscopic gastrostomy – PEG). A general anaesthetic is required for either method of placement. Mushroom-tipped tubes can be placed endoscopically or at surgery. Foley catheters can also be used, but only with surgical placement.

The tubes are well tolerated by patients, allow feeding directly into the patient's stomach and can be left *in situ* for weeks to months without complication. The large diameter of these tubes means that obstruction of the tube is less of a problem than with naso-oesophageal or pharyngostomy tubes.

The technique for placement of a PEG tube is described in Figure 4.16 and illustrated in Figure 4.17.

In addition to mushroom-tipped catheters supplied singly, kits including all the necessary equipment (except the endoscope) are available, but are more expensive.

Gastrostomy tube care

Gastrostomy tubes are relatively easy to maintain. The stoma may discharge a little for the first few days and should be cleaned regularly (once or twice daily) and a sterile dressing applied. A conforming bandage or stockinette 'vest' should be used to support and protect the tube.

4.16 Placement of a PEG tube

1. Following a 12-hour fast, the patient is anaesthetized and placed in right lateral recumbency.
2. An area approximately 12 cm x 12 cm is clipped just behind the last rib on the left.
3. The endoscope is passed into the stomach and air is insufflated.
4. The tip of the scope is placed close to the stomach wall in the fundic region so that the light is visible through the abdominal wall.
5. A small skin incision is made where the light can be seen and an intravenous catheter is placed through this incision into the gastric lumen.
6. Nylon suture is fed down the catheter into the stomach, visualized by the endoscopist and grasped with biopsy forceps so that it can be pulled up through the oesophagus and out of the mouth whilst the other end is held by an assistant.
7. The connecting end of a 20 F mushroom-tipped catheter is removed with scissors and a further 2 cm length is removed.
8. A stab incision is made in this 2 cm length and the cut end of the catheter is passed through the incision to create an internal flange next to the mushroom tip.
9. The proximal end of the catheter is cut to form a V-shape.
10. The suture is threaded through a plastic cone (such as a pipette tip).
11. The suture is stitched to the proximal end of the catheter and the pipette tip is pushed on to the tube to form a pointed end; then it is pulled back down the oesophagus, into the stomach and out through the abdominal wall.
12. The mushroom and internal flange are retained in the stomach, which is pulled firmly against the abdominal wall, and the catheter is held in place using a Chinese finger-trap suture (see Figure 4.21).
13. The catheter is stoppered, the area is dressed and the tube is supported by a light bandage.

4.17 PEG tube placement

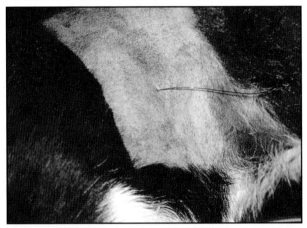

The patient has been placed in right lateral recumbency and an area just caudal to the last rib has been clipped and prepared aseptically. A nylon suture has been passed through an intravenous catheter, into the lumen of the stomach, and the catheter has been removed.

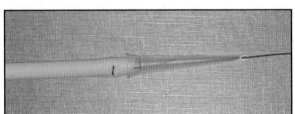

The proximal end of the mushroom-tipped catheter. The suture that has been passed through the abdominal wall is grasped with endoscopic forceps and withdrawn back through the mouth. The suture is passed through a plastic pipette tip before being sutured to the end of the catheter.

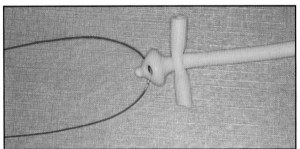

The distal end of a mushroom-tipped catheter following removal of the connecting end. A further 2 cm has been removed and used to create a flange next to the mushroom tip – this helps to prevent displacement of the catheter from the gastric lumen. The suture loop aids in retrieval of the catheter should the suture on the proximal end break.

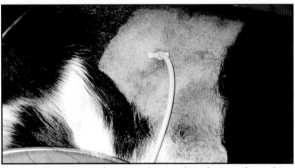

Using gentle traction on the proximal suture, the catheter is advanced into the stomach and out through the abdominal wall. A further 2 cm length of tube can be used to create an external flange or alternatively a Chinese finger-trap suture (Figure 4.21) can be used to anchor the tube in place. Courtesy of J. Williams

Patients generally do not interfere with the tube but if this is a problem an Elizabethan collar should be used. Feeding can be initiated 24 hours after placement and a variety of canine and feline diets are available.

Gastrostomy tubes should remain *in situ* for a minimum of 5–7 days to ensure that adequate adhesions form between the stomach and the abdominal wall. Earlier or premature removal may result in leakage of gastric contents into the abdomen, leading to peritonitis.

Tubes can be removed by cutting the skin sutures, deflating the bulb (if a Foley catheter was used) and applying gentle traction. Mushroom-tipped catheters can be removed by traction, which will collapse the tip and allow withdrawal, or they can be cut against the skin and the tip left to migrate through the intestine or retrieved endoscopically. The hole left in the abdominal wall generally heals quickly and will seal within 72 hours.

Total parenteral nutrition (TPN)

TPN refers to the delivery of every nutrient via the intravenous route and is applicable to those animals that are temporarily unable or have limited capacity to assimilate nutrients from the gastrointestinal tract. This form of nutrition requires specialized training and equipment. Since the special solutions for intravenous feeding are best delivered continuously, 24-hour patient monitoring is required.

Management of a critical care unit | **95**

Delivering nutrients via the intravenous route bypasses normal gastrointestinal physiology and hence complications (sepsis and various electrolyte disturbances) are more frequent and severe than with enteral nutritional support. For further information, see chapter on nutritional support of the critical patient in *BSAVA Manual of Canine and Feline Emergency and Critical Care*.

Infections in the CCU

Infections acquired by patients during the course of their hospitalization are known as nosocomial infections.

Critically ill animals have an increased susceptibility to infection related to the stress of their disease, a catabolic metabolic state and the invasive diagnostic and monitoring techniques employed. Diseases such as diabetes mellitus, hyperadrenocorticism, neoplasia, uraemia, burns and trauma compromise the immune system and predispose to the development of nosocomial infections. Also treatments received by critical patients can contribute to further immunosuppresssion (chemotherapy, corticosteroids).

The most common sites of nosocomial infections are the lower urinary tract, respiratory tract, surgical wounds and indwelling catheter and tube sites. Bacteria are the most common agents involved and tend to come from the endogenous flora of the patient or exogenously from the hospital microflora. Those commonly implicated tend to be environmentally resistant and have an increased antibiotic resistance.

Nosocomial infections are transmitted by contact exposure, contaminated objects (fomites) and airborne spread. Direct transmission by contact between patients or members of staff is the most prevalent method of infection. An increased number of staff having contact with the animal and an increased length of hospitalization are the most important risk factors. Strategies to decrease the chances of nosocomial infection are listed in Figure 4.18.

4.18 Strategies to decrease the chances of nosocomial infection

- Strict aseptic technique when placing catheters, tubes and drains
- Cover tubes, drains and catheters with sterile dressings
- Minimize the use of indwelling tubes – only use them if necessary and for the shortest period possible
- Wash hands between each patient and before handling medications and intravenous lines between patients
- Change intravenous fluid lines every 24–48 hours
- Use disposable gloves when handling patients, and change them between patients
- Appropriate antibiotic use to minimize development of resistant bacterial strains
- Keep the duration of hospitalization as short as possible
- Thorough cleaning of equipment between uses (e.g. clipper blades)
- Place soiled bedding and bandages in appropriate containers
- Careful monitoring for evidence of infection, and record-keeping of the same
- Establish and follow a strict cleaning and disinfection protocol for the facility and equipment.

Specialized techniques

Care of indwelling vascular catheters

The major risk from intravenous and intra-arterial catheters is local infection or bacterial dissemination in the blood stream; skin bacteria surrounding the catheter site are the most common pathogens. The incidence of catheter-related infections can be greatly decreased by giving careful attention to basic nursing procedures.

- Catheters should be inserted with strict aseptic technique
- Prolonged indwelling catheters should be placed in large-bore veins (e.g. jugular vein)
- The catheter should be fixed to the skin at the puncture site to minimize movement of the catheter
- There should be strict adherence to aseptic technique during injection and sampling procedure
- All three-way tap ports should be fitted with injection caps to maintain a closed system
- The catheter should be flushed at least twice daily with heparinized saline solution
- Justification for continued use of the catheter should be reassessed daily
- The catheter should be removed if there are any signs of phlebitis, thrombosis, patient discomfort, systemic fever or catheter malfunction
- Peripheral catheters should be changed every 48 hours
- Extension sets (e.g. T-piece extensions) should be used to minimize handling of the catheter itself.

Urinary catheters

Indications for urethral catheters in the CCU

- Collection of urine samples for analysis
- Measurement of urine output
- Measurement of postmicturition residual urine volume
- Relief of urethral obstruction to urine flow
- Relief of urine retention.

Equipment

Catheters are made from a variety of different materials and are available in a range of diameters and lengths. The catheter selected should be no larger in diameter than is necessary for its intended purpose and it should be flexible and pliable to minimize injury to the urinary tract.

The French (F) scale is commonly used to measure the diameter of urinary catheters. Each French unit is equivalent to 0.33 mm; for example, a 9 F catheter has an external diameter of 3 mm.

- The simplest catheters have a single lumen and one or more openings (eyes) at the proximal end
- Canine urinary catheters made from plastic or rubber are flexible and may be used to catheterize male or female dogs
- The edges around the eyes of polypropylene catheters are often rough. These catheters are relatively inflexible and can cause trauma to the urethral mucosa
- Foley catheters are available and inflation of the balloon when the tip of the catheter is within the bladder prevents migration of the catheter
- For cats, disposable polypropylene tom cat catheters are available from commercial manufactures
- Most catheters are intended for once-only use and should not be re-used.

A proper catheterization technique is essential (see Chapter 4 in *BSAVA Manual of Veterinary Nursing*). The three basic types of catheterization are single diagnostic, repeated intermittent and indwelling.

There is a risk of inducing an infection whenever a urethral catheter is used. This risk is greater with indwelling than with intermittent catheterization and greater with repeated intermittent than with single short-term catheterization. Development of infection is an almost inevitable consequence of indwelling catheterization and the major factors influencing this include:

- The initial catheterization technique
- Care of the catheter
- Duration of catheterization
- Urine drainage system
- Condition of the lower urinary tract.

The risk of urinary tract infection increases in proportion to the duration of catheterization. Systemic antibiotics administered prophylactically are of little or no value and may in fact predispose to the development of a resistant bacterial infection.

Indications for indwelling urethral catheters

- Close monitoring of urine output in critically ill patients
- During the immediate period following relief of urethral obstruction if:
  - There is lack of a relatively normal urine stream
  - There is persistence of intraluminal material or extraluminal compression
  - There is loss of detrusor contractility and over-distension of the bladder that causes ineffective micturition despite urethral patency.

Long-term management of indwelling catheters

- The duration of catheterization should be kept to the minimum necessary
- Prophylactic antibiotics should not be used
- Urine output should be monitored and recorded regularly
- The catheter should be checked at least twice daily to ensure that it is still in place. If necessary, water-soluble iodine-based contrast material can be injected into the catheter and its position confirmed by radiography
- A closed urine collection system should be maintained (Figure 4.19)
- An Elizabethan collar should be used to prevent premature removal
- On removal of the catheter, a urine sample should be obtained for bacteriological culture and sensitivity testing. Antibiotic therapy based on the results obtained should be instituted
- Flushing with antiseptic solutions is of no proven value.

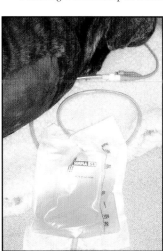

4.19

Long-term management of urinary catheters includes maintaining a sterile closed urine collection system. This allows collection and measurement of urine and helps to prevent urine scalding in the recumbent patient.

Cystostomy tubes

Indications

- Temporary bypass of the urethra in cases of obstruction due to inflammation, neoplasia, reflex dyssynergia
- (Rarely) permanent bypass of the urethra as a palliative treatment for urethral neoplasia.

Technique

Cystostomy tubes are placed via a caudal laparotomy incision (Figure 4.20).

4.20 Placement of a cystostomy tube

1. At laparotomy, a purse-string suture is placed through the serosa and muscular layers of the bladder.
2. A stab incision is made into the bladder within the purse-string.
3. A Foley catheter is introduced through the skin into the bladder lumen.
4. The purse-string suture is tied and omentum incorporated around the catheter.
5. The bladder is secured to the abdominal wall.
6. The catheter is secured to the skin using a Chinese finger-trap suture (Figure 4.21).

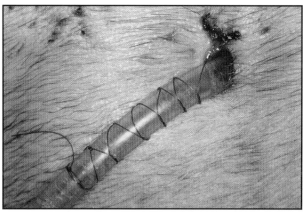

4.21 *A Chinese finger-trap suture, used to secure indwelling tubes (e.g. gastrostomy, cystostomy and chest drains). Courtesy of J Williams*

Cystostomy tube care

- The catheter should be connected to a closed collecting system
- Antiseptic ointment should be applied around the stoma and should be covered with a protective dressing
- An Elizabethan collar should be used to prevent premature removal by the patient
- Catheters must be left in place for a minimum of 5 days to allow adhesions to form between the bladder and abdominal wall
- After tube removal the stoma should be left to granulate
- Urine may leak for 1–2 days. Placing antibiotic ointment around the stoma can help to prevent urine scalding of the skin.

Abdominocentesis

If fluid is present in the abdomen, abdominocentesis is a simple and rapid method of obtaining a sample for analysis. The technique is described in Figure 4.22.

How to perform abdominocentesis

1. Clip and prepare the abdomen aseptically.
2. Have the animal standing if possible.
3. Wear sterile gloves.
4. Introduce a large-bore (14–18 gauge) intravenous catheter attached to a three-way tap.
5. Perform a four-quadrant tap to increase the chances of recovering fluid.
6. Fluid obtained should be analysed to determine if it is an exudate or transudate. Cytology should be performed and a sample sent for bacterial culture.
7. If abdominocentesis is negative, diagnostic peritoneal lavage (DPL) is used.

Diagnostic peritoneal lavage

The technique is described in Figure 4.23.

4.23 **Peritoneal lavage**

Equipment

- Peritoneal lavage catheter, peritoneal dialysis catheter or large intravenous catheter with added side holes
- Scalpel blade
- Warmed lactated Ringer's or 0.9% sodium chloride
- Intravenous fluid giving set.

Technique

1. Empty the bladder manually or via catheterization prior to performing this procedure.
2. Place the animal in left lateral recumbency to avoid hitting the spleen.
3. Locally infiltrate the skin with lignocaine 1–2 cm caudal to the umbilicus in the abdominal midline.
4. Make a small incision in the skin with a scalpel blade.
5. Under sterile conditions a large-bore multifenestrated drain is directed caudally and dorsally into the abdominal cavity until the fenestrated component is entirely within the abdomen.
6. Fluid may flow freely. If it does not, gently roll the animal from side to side.
7. If fluid is still absent, administer 22 ml/kg of warmed 0.9% sodium chloride or lactated Ringer's solution via the drain.
8. Then roll the animal gently from side to side to distribute the fluid within the abdomen.
9. Allow fluid to drain out via the giving set and analyse as stated above.

Complications

- Subcutaneous haematoma or leakage of lavage fluid
- Visceral perforation – especially if organomegaly is present.

Open peritoneal drainage

This technique is used to manage patients with peritonitis after laparotomy has been performed and the cause of the peritonitis has been corrected. The laparotomy wound is allowed to remain open by means of a loose simple continuous suture of nylon or polypropylene (Figure 4.24a). The incision is covered with sterile, non-adherent dressings and then layers of absorbent material, followed by an outer protective layer. The bandage should be large enough to extend beyond the cranial and caudal aspects of the incision and constructed so that it will not slip.

These patients require intensive nursing care. The bandage should be changed aseptically at least twice daily, if not more frequently, depending on the quantity of fluid drainage (Figure 4.24 b,c). Intra-abdominal adhesions may need to be broken down gently with a sterile gloved hand during bandage changes. If necessary, samples of fluid can be obtained for cytology and culture. The bandage should be weighed before and after placement to estimate fluid loss – this information can be used to help to calculate fluid requirements and to monitor the trend in abdominal fluid production.

Once drainage has declined (usually within 4–6 days) the abdominal incision is closed.

4.24

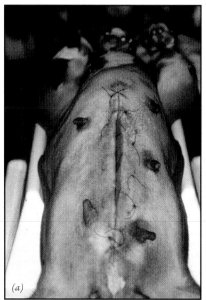

(a)

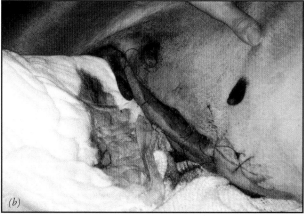

(b)

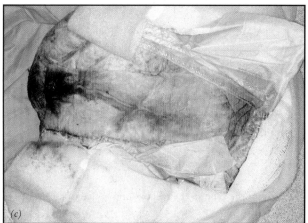

(c)

(a) Suturing a laparotomy wound with loose sutures of polypropylene allows continued drainage from the abdomen in cases of peritonitis. (b,c) The abdomen should be covered with sterile absorbent dressings that should be changed at least twice daily, if not more frequently, depending on the quantity of fluid produced.
Courtesy of J. Williams

Complications

- Loss of fluid and protein from the peritoneal cavity – can be a serious problem in these patients; it is vital that they receive supportive intravenous fluid therapy to prevent dehydration
- Severe hypoproteinaemia – will develop if the animal is not eating adequately; these animals may require hyperalimentation
- Electrolyte loss, especially potassium – occurs concurrently; electrolytes should be monitored and intravenous fluids may need to be supplemented
- Evisceration – the abdomen must be securely bandaged and the animal prevented from traumatizing the bandage by use of an Elizabethan collar; exercise should be kept to a minimum
- Ascending and nosocomial infection – the bandage should be kept as clean as possible. Urethral catheterization may be necessary in male dogs.

Tracheotomy

Indications

- To relieve airway obstruction causing marked hypoxia not amenable to conservative management or definitive treatment
- To provide ventilatory support during upper airway surgery
- To improve access for extensive oral or pharyngeal surgery
- After airway surgery when severe swelling and postoperative obstruction are anticipated (e.g. after surgery for brachycephalic obstructive syndrome).

Contraindications

- **Absence of satisfactory tube management**
- Tracheal abnormalities such as tracheal collapse or hypoplasia.

Equipment

- Tracheotomy surgical kit (see Figure 4.5).

Technique

This is described in Figure 4.25.

4.25 How to perform a tracheotomy

1. Tracheotomy can be performed under sedation with local anaesthesia but it is preferable to induce general anaesthesia and intubate patient if possible.
2. Position in dorsal recumbency with the head and neck extended over a sandbag (Figure 4.26a).
3. Clip and prepare the surgical site (ventral midline of neck from the larynx caudally).
4. Make a midline incision through the skin and subcutaneous tissue, extending approximately 3 cm caudally from the caudal border of the cricoid cartilage of the larynx.
5. Identify the paired sternohyoideus muscles and separate in the midline.
6. In the region or the third or fourth tracheal rings, make a hemicircumferential incision through the annular ligament.
7. Choose correct diameter tube and insert correctly so as to cause minimal mucosal damage.
8. Place stay sutures around the tracheal rings proximally and distally to allow manipulation of the trachea, to facilitate tube replacement (Figure 4.26b).
9. Suture the tube to the skin, in preference to tape ties (which can come undone).

4.26 Tracheotomy technique

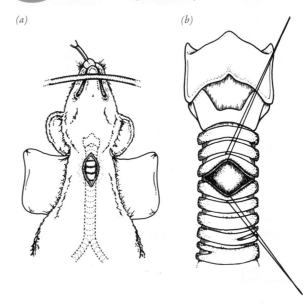

(a)   *(b)*

(a) Dog positioned in dorsal recumbency with head and neck extended over a sandbag. (b) Circumferential incision into the trachea and placement of stay sutures around the tracheal rings on each side of the incision.

An alternative technique is the use of a needle tracheotomy kit (available commercially).

Tracheostomy tube care

 A patient with a tracheostomy tube requires careful constant monitoring. It is essential to clean the tube regularly.

- Ideally, tubes should have an inner sleeve that can be removed to facilitate cleaning
- The inner cannula should initially be removed and cleaned every 20–30 minutes; later it can be done every few hours
- The tube should be cleaned every 3–4 hours for the first 2 days
- The frequency of cleaning can be decreased the longer the tube remains *in situ* (every 6–8 hours for the next 3–4 days, decreasing to every 12–24 hours thereafter)
- Suction equipment should be kept available and ready for use, especially during the first few days after tracheotomy when tracheobronchial secretions increase secondary irritation
- Suction tubing should be of suitable diameter to remove any mucus or debris but without blocking the diameter of the trachea; a soft urethral catheter is suitable
- Preoxygenation should be performed prior to suctioning
- The tip of the tube should be inserted into the trachea to the level of the carina without suction. Suction is only applied during withdrawal of the tube
- The tube should be withdrawn slowly with a gentle twisting motion
- Tracheal suction should be performed for 15 seconds or less, since it is possible to precipitate hypoxia and cardiac arrest by prolonged suction

- Humidification of inspired air is essential, to prevent tracheitis and crust formation within the tube
- Inspired air should be humidified by flushing the tube with sterile saline (0.25–5 ml, depending on size of patient) every 4–6 hours or by nebulizing water into the cage
- The wound should be cleaned frequently (at least twice daily) and antibiotic ointment should be applied.

Removal of the tracheostomy tube

- The tube should be removed once the airway is patent (timing can be difficult in some cases)
- The size of the tube can be reduced to allow air to bypass the tube and pass into the upper respiratory tract
- The tube can then be occluded to determine if an adequate airway is present
- The patient should be observed closely for the first 12 hours following tube removal. The tube may have to be replaced if the patient becomes dyspnoeic
- The incision is usually left to heal by second intention, as this minimizes the chances of subcutaneous emphysema.

Complications

Complications associated with temporary tracheotomy are shown in Figure 4.27.

 4.27 **Complications associated with temporary tracheotomy**

Complication	Cause
Surgical injury to cervical structures (e.g. recurrent laryngeal nerve, oesophagus)	Usually due to dissecting too lateral or too deep to the trachea
Dislodgement of the tube	Tube too short Inadequate observation
Occlusion of the tube	Occurs if cleaning and suctioning are not performed frequently enough
Bronchopneumonia	Inadequate suctioning and humidification
Tracheitis	Can be caused by a tube that is too large or too long or if humidification is inadequate
Tracheal necrosis	Usually only a problem if cuffed tubes are used
Cervical cellulitis	Inadequate wound care
Subcutaneous emphysema	Skin sutured too tightly around tube Primary wound closure following tube removal
Tracheocutaneous fistula	Tube left *in situ* too long

(Modified from: Aron DN and Crowe DT (1985) Upper Airway Obstruction – General Principles and Selected Conditions in the Dog and Cat. Veterinary Clinics of North America (Small Animal), WB Saunders, Philadelphia.)

Thoracocentesis

Thoracocentesis is the removal of air or fluid from the pleural space for diagnostic and therapeutic purposes (see Chapter 6).

A large gauge chest tube should be placed if an animal is suffering from a large or continuous accumulation of fluid or air in the pleural space, since multiple thoracocenteses are associated with an increased risk of trauma to the thoracic organs and a higher mortality rate. In an emergency situation, thoracocentesis can be performed rapidly to allow patient stabilization (e.g. tension pneumothorax) prior to placement of a chest tube.

Equipment

Preferably the equipment (Figure 4.28) should include:

- A 14–18 gauge, 2–3-inch over-the-needle catheter
- Three-way tap
- Large syringe (20–50 ml)
- Intravenous extension tubing.

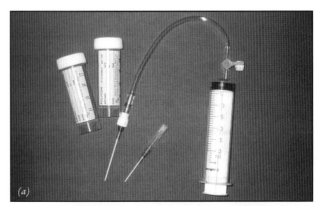

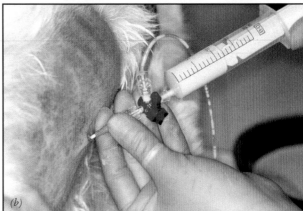

4.28 *Equipment for thoracocentesis. (a) A three-way tap and extension tubing minimizes movement as the syringe is manipulated. Samples of fluid should be collected for cytology and bacteriology. (b) Addition of an extension tube to the side-arm of the three-way tap allows drainage of fluid with reduced risk of contamination or aerosol formation.*

In an acute emergency a needle can be used instead of a catheter but this carries a higher risk of lung laceration. In the cat, a scalp vein set is a useful alternative.

This is described in Figure 4.29.

Percutaneous placement of thoracostomy tubes

Indication

- Accumulation of air or pleural fluid sufficient to require repeated drainage.

Equipment

- Sterile thoracotomy pack (see Figure 4.5) containing tubes with a range of diameters.

Technique

This is described in Figure 4.30 and illustrated in Figure 4.31.

Care of the chest drain is discussed in Chapter 2.

4.29 Performing thoracocentesis

1. Perform aseptically, although this may not always be possible in an emergency.
2. Fluid is most effectively collected in the ventral third of the fourth to seventh intercostal space, with the animal standing or sternally recumbent.
3. Air is collected from the dorsal thorax if the patient is standing, or from the mid thorax if the patient is laterally recumbent.
4. Local anaesthetic is usually not needed.
5. Advance the catheter or needle into the pleural space at an angle of 45 degrees, with the bevel toward the patient.
6. Stop advancement immediately on entering the pleural space.
7. Place a three-way tap and extension tube between the syringe and catheter. This allows the catheter to be held steady whilst the syringe is manipulated and allows more than a single aspiration.

4.30 Placement of a thoracostomy tube

1. Use the largest diameter tube that can comfortably fit between two ribs:
   - For cats, 14–18 F
   - For medium-sized dogs, 20–28 F
   - For large dogs, 28–36 F.
2. Location and number of tubes is determined by the location and volume of air/fluid, based on clinical examination and thoracic radiographs.
3. Clip and prepare a large area of the thorax on the required side (Figure 4.31a).
4. Local anaesthetic can be used if necessary (Figure 4.31b).
5. Make a small skin incision in the dorsal third of the lateral thoracic wall around the 10th–12th intercostal space (Figure 4.31c).
6. A subcutaneous tunnel is bluntly dissected forwards in a cranioventral direction over two to three intercostal spaces (Figure 4.31d).
7. Using the stylet, the drain is introduced through the seventh or eighth intercostal space with a controlled thrust directed towards the opposite shoulder.
8. Avoid the intercostal artery, vein and nerve which lie on the caudal border of each rib.
9. The tube is fed into the pleural space, clamped and sutured to the skin using a Chinese finger-trap suture (Figure 4.31e).
10. Antiseptic ointment applied around the entry site helps to prevent leakage of air.
11. Cover with a protective dressing and loosely bandage to the chest (Figure 4.31f).
12. Confirm position with a radiograph.

Tube removal

Tubes are removed when they are no longer productive. After it has been *in situ* for several days, the tube itself can induce an effusion of 2–4 ml/kg/24 hours and this effusion will not resolve until the tube is removed.

Technique

1. Cut the sutures holding the tube in place.
2. Hold a gauze swab with antibiotic ointment over the stoma and tube.
3. Remove the tube rapidly and press the swab over the stoma (the ointment helps to seal the stoma).
4. Bandage the swab in place for 24 hours.

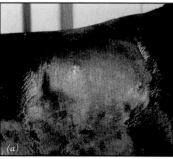
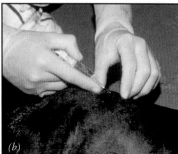

4.31 *Thoracostomy tube placement. (a) A large area of the thorax is clipped and aseptically prepared. (b) Local anaesthetic can be infiltrated into the skin. (c) A stab incision is made through the skin in the dorsal third of the lateral thoracic wall, using a scalpel blade. (d) The thoracostomy tube has been placed through the skin incision (11th intercostal space) and tunnelled subcutaneously prior to introducing the drain into the pleural cavity with a controlled thrust (8th intercostal space). (e) The tube is secured in place with a Chinese finger-trap suture and clamped, and a three-way tap is placed on the end of the tube. (f) The tube is covered with a protective dressing, and a stockinette 'vest' is used to hold the tube against the chest.*

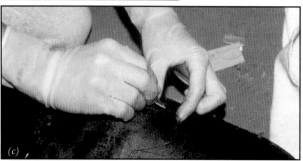
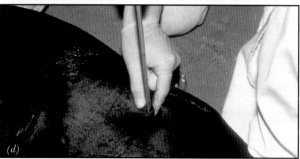
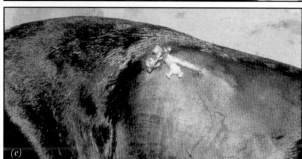
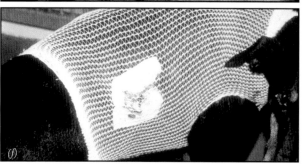

Respiratory monitoring and therapy

Assessment of the patient

To minimize stress to the dyspnoeic patient, physical examination should be carried out as quietly and calmly as possible. Any stress may seriously compromise the patient's chances of survival. It is best to take time over the examination, and even to perform different parts of the examination in stages, allowing the animal to rest in between. Cats are particularly prone to stress when handled, and simply restraining a cat may precipitate respiratory failure.

Much information can be gained about the patient's respiratory function simply by watching it quietly for a few minutes.

Respiratory rate and effort

Attention should be paid to the respiratory rate (normally 15–30 breaths per minute, depending upon species and age) and to the effort exerted by the patient to achieve this. During normal respiration very little chest movement is visible, because most of the respiratory movement is driven by the diaphragm, which displaces the abdominal contents backwards. Changes in the degree of abdominal movement or significant movement of the chest wall are indicative of respiratory compromise and are often seen concurrently with an increase in respiratory rate.

Paradoxical respiration may also be seen as the patient's condition worsens. In paradoxical respiration, abdominal effort at inspiration and expiration is increased to such an extent that the thoracic wall is drawn inwards on inspiration and forced outwards at expiration. This is the reverse of normal respiration – hence paradoxical.

Postural changes

Dyspnoeic animals often choose a posture that helps their breathing (orthopnoea). Typically, they will prefer to sit or stand rather than lie down. Often the elbows are abducted and the neck is extended. Such animals may also exhibit mouth breathing.

In general, dogs prefer to stand rather than sit, whilst cats will crouch in sternal recumbency. Lateral recumbency in conjunction with mouth breathing is a very bad sign in both species.

Respiratory pattern

In certain cases the pattern of breathing can be useful in determining the origin of the dyspnoea.

- In general, upper airway obstruction produces a prolonged inspiratory time, often with an associated stertor or stridor, and a short expiratory time
- In lower respiratory tract (small airway) disease, this pattern is reversed, with a longer expiratory phase than normal.

Auscultation

A quiet environment is essential for auscultation of any patient. Auscultation of the dyspnoeic patient can be difficult.

- It is important to cover the whole of the lung field on each side of the chest
- Lung sounds should be symmetrical on both sides of the chest

- Attention should be paid to any areas of dullness, which may indicate filling of the pleural space (e.g. air, tumour, fluid, abdominal viscera)
- Increased lung sounds are usually associated with lower respiratory tract disease; however, noises from the upper airway can be amplified and referred to the chest.

Percussion

When an area of dullness is suspected, it can be confirmed by gently percussing the thoracic wall over the lung fields whilst auscultating the chest. This will make the area of dullness clearer, and may help to determine the nature of pleural filling.

Mucous membranes

Mucous membrane colour can be useful as a guide to respiratory function. Normal mucous membranes are pale pink to pink in colour, with a capillary refill time of 1–2 seconds. Cyanotic (blue or purple) mucous membranes indicate dangerously low arterial oxygen levels, and oxygen supplementation should be started immediately.

Pulse oximetry

Oxygen delivery to the tissues can be more accurately measured with a pulse oximeter (Figure 4.32). The pulse oximeter probe passes light through the tissues of an extremity and detects the amount of light absorbed by the haemoglobin in those tissues at two different wavelengths. The wavelengths used correspond to the wavelengths of light absorbed best by oxygenated and deoxygenated haemoglobin. The pulse oximeter then compares the amount of absorbed light at each wavelength and uses this to calculate the proportion of haemoglobin that is fully saturated. Most pulse oximeters display oxygen saturation (SpO_2, expressed in %) and pulse rate.

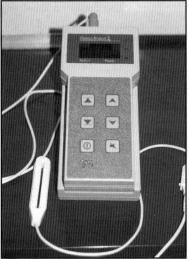

4.32

A pulse oximeter can be used to measure tissue oxygenation.

In the normal animal, oxygen saturation should be close to 99% (certainly > 97%). As a general rule, oxygen supplementation should be considered if SpO_2 falls below 93%, and is essential if it is less than 90%.

In the past, pulse oximeter probes have been adapted for veterinary use from human medical equipment, and many of these probes are unsuitable for use in very small patients. However, probes that have been specifically designed for veterinary use are now available and these have eliminated some of the problems previously encountered.

Probes should be positioned on hairless unpigmented skin or on mucous membranes – for example, on the pinna of the ear, on a nipple, on the vulva, or on the tongue (unconscious or anaesthetized animals).

Limitations of pulse oximetry
Poor perfusion is the most common reason for getting poor or variable readings. There are two main reasons for this:

- Hypovolaemia and tissue hypoperfusion (the pulse oximeter used in the authors' clinic fails to give a reading when the patient's mean arterial pressure falls below 40 mmHg)
- Gradual tissue compression by the probe, resulting in a localized reduction of perfusion.

Other reasons for variable readings include:

- Pigmented skin
- Very thin tissue, such as the pinnae of cats
- Carbon monoxide (CO) poisoning. CO binds to haemoglobin with a much greater affinity than oxygen, but the pulse oximeter cannot distinguish between HbCO and HbO_2
- Movement artefacts (e.g. shivering).

Capnometry
The capnometer (Figure 4.33) is a device that is used to monitor the carbon dioxide (CO_2) levels in the airway. Some capnometers incorporate a recording device and produce a permanent record of the changes in airway CO_2. This type of recording is known as capnography. The CO_2 level is expressed as either tension (mmHg) or concentration (%).

In normal animals, the CO_2 level at the end of expiration (end tidal CO_2, sometimes expressed as $P_{ET}CO_2$) should be 35–40 mmHg. Deviations from the normal value indicate hypoventilation (increased CO_2) or hyperventilation (decreased CO_2). Values of 50 mmHg or greater are associated with significant respiratory acidosis.

From a practical point of view, use of capnometry in the CCU can be somewhat limited. It is of most value in patients undergoing artificial ventilation via either a tracheostomy or an endotracheal tube. In some models of capnometer, the sampling device can be substituted for a hypodermic needle, and this can be passed percutaneously into the proximal trachea.

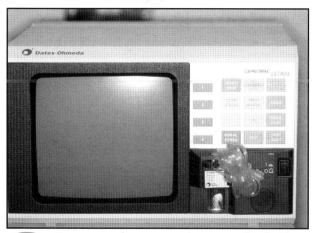

4.33 Capnometer used to measure respiratory gas carbon dioxide content.

Blood gases
Arterial blood gas analysis is the best way of assessing and monitoring respiratory function. Ideally a catheter should be placed in an artery if multiple sampling is anticipated. In the long run this minimizes distress to the patient, compared with repeated arteriopuncture, although in practice placement of arterial catheters can be difficult, particularly in a conscious patient.

Oxygen supplementation
It is often necessary to increase the proportion of oxygen delivered to the critical patient. This may be necessary as a short-term emergency treatment for an animal in acute respiratory distress, or in the longer term for an animal with chronic respiratory disease or anaemia.

It is important to remember that oxygen, as well as being essential to life, is a poison at high concentrations. As a general rule, toxicity is only a problem if very high levels (> 60%) are maintained for longer than 12 hours. For longer-term oxygen therapy, the proportion of inspired oxygen should be reduced to 40% or lower.

It is also essential to humidify the inspired gas whenever oxygen therapy is to be continued for more than a few hours.

Indications for oxygen therapy
- Cyanosis
- Hypoxaemia (SpO_2 < 90%)
- Anaemia (Hb < 5 g/l or PCV < 10%).

There are several ways of delivering an oxygen-enriched atmosphere to the patient, as follows.

Mask
Oxygen can be given via a face mask in animals that will tolerate one; however, many animals object to this and the stress caused can make matters worse. With a snugly fitting mask and high flow rates, high levels of inspired oxygen can be achieved. It is important not to have the mask fitted so tightly that the animal rebreathes carbon dioxide.

'Flow-by' oxygen
This is another very simple method, where the oxygen supply is simply held close to the patient's nose. This is much better tolerated than a mask.

Oxygen cage or tent
The simplest oxygen tent can be made by fitting the animal with an Elizabethan collar covered with cling-film, and supplying oxygen into this at around 5–10 l/min. This is poorly tolerated by some patients, particularly cats. Purpose-built oxygen cages (Figure 4.34), or those improvised from a standard cage using polythene sheeting to cover the mesh front, provide a very convenient way of supplementing oxygen.

The main disadvantage of the oxygen cage is the isolation of the animal and difficulty in examining it, but reduced handling of the patient can be greatly to its benefit. Another problem with enclosed oxygen cages is the risk of hyperthermia, particularly if the patient is panting or pyrexic.

Intranasal oxygen
This is useful for longer-term oxygen supplementation, where the levels of oxygen required are lower. Nasal oxygen can be supplied via a urinary catheter or nasogastric feeding tube inserted into one nostril to the level of the medial canthus of the eye. It is then secured in place with sutures

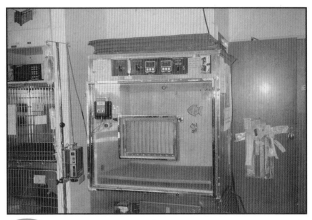

4.34 *Oxygen cage.*

or cyanoacrylate adhesive. This is suitable for most dogs and cats, the chief exceptions being brachycephalic breeds of both species. Alternatively, nasal prongs designed for humans can be used in dogs. Oxygen supplied in this way at 2–3 l/min will increase the inspired oxygen concentration to around 35%.

Transtracheal
Oxygen may be supplied directly into the trachea via an intravenous catheter (14–18 G) placed percutaneously into the trachea. This is preferable to nasal oxygen delivery in brachycephalic animals and those that are mouth-breathing.

Tracheotomy
Standard anaesthetic circuits can be connected directly to a tracheostomy tube to supply 100% oxygen. For longer-term supplementation, oxygen can be supplied via a suitable catheter positioned in the tracheostomy tube.

Endotracheal intubation
This is included for completeness, but it is not a suitable route for oxygen therapy for more than a few hours at most. It is only possible in the unconscious or anaesthetized patient.

Humidification
Humidity refers to the amount of water vapour present in the atmosphere, and is temperature dependent. Normally, atmospheric air in the UK is 30–40% saturated with water vapour. In addition, this is further humidified and warmed in the upper respiratory tract at inspiration, and so by the time it reaches the alveoli the inspired air is close to 100% saturated and at body temperature.

Medical gases are dry, and the nasal turbinate system is bypassed by many of the delivery systems for supplemental oxygen. There are a number of detrimental consequences of a cold, dry source of inspired gas:

- Hypothermia, especially smaller patients. The patient uses energy to heat and humidify the inspired gas
- Increased water loss from the respiratory tract
- Drying of the lower airway. This may result in inflammation, decreased mucociliary activity and excessive mucus production, predisposing to pneumonia.

Humidification of the gas source is therefore necessary for all patients requiring long-term oxygen supplementation. It is *essential* in patients undergoing artificial ventilation.

Types of humidifier

Ambient temperature water vapour supply
Basically, this is a bottle or jar of sterile water through which the gas supply can be bubbled. The system is simple to set up, and to improvise if necessary (an old Boyle's bottle, found on some older anaesthetic machines, serves this purpose very well indeed). Similar saturation levels to room air are reached. It is adequate for humidifying air for animals receiving oxygen supplementation by most routes, but not adequate for animals undergoing intermittent positive pressure ventilation (IPPV) via a tracheostomy or endotracheal tube.

Heated water vapour supply
This is similar to the ambient temperature humidifier but with a thermostatically controlled heater. The water and gas supply are warmed. The system can produce an inspired gas close to 100% humidity and body temperature. The thermostat prevents thermal damage to the airway.

Nebulizer
This device produces fine droplets of water, rather than water vapour. They may be incorporated in the inspiratory limb of the breathing system, or used independently to humidify the atmosphere in an oxygen cage. They are very efficient humidifiers and do not require heat to produce 100% saturation of the inspired gas. Indeed, they should be used with caution as it easy to achieve over-humidification of the airway. Nebulizers can also be used for the administration of drugs, such as bronchodilators.

Heat and moisture exchanger
The HME, or 'artificial nose', is a small disposable device that attaches between the endotracheal or tracheostomy tube and the breathing system. It behaves rather like the nasal turbinates, trapping warm water vapour from the expired air and using this to warm and humidify the inspired gas. The increase in functional dead-space and resistance is not normally a problem for most dogs or patients undergoing IPPV, but can present problems in small dogs and cats.

Artificial ventilation
In the severely compromised patient, or in aggressive or intractable animals, it may be necessary to induce anaesthesia and to intubate the trachea in order to secure an airway and to control ventilation. This is normally reserved for the most severely affected patients, those that do not respond to oxygen therapy by other routes, or those that will not tolerate them.

There are several techniques for controlling ventilation in the critical patient, including:

- Intermittent positive pressure ventilation (IPPV)
- Positive end expiratory pressure (PEEP)
- Continuous positive airway pressure (CPAP).

IPPV via an anaesthetic breathing system is the simplest and most commonly used method in the critical patient. It may be manual ('bag squeezing'), or controlled mechanically by a ventilator.

PEEP and CPAP are advanced techniques used in the medium- to long-term management of patients with respiratory disease, and should only be employed under expert supervision.

Manual IPPV via an anaesthetic circuit

1. Close off the expiratory valve in the circuit (in an Ayre's T-piece with the Jackson–Rees modification, close the open end of the reservoir bag).
2. Squeeze the reservoir bag gently to produce filling of the lungs. Monitor chest movements as the bag is squeezed to ensure adequate but not excessive ventilation.
3. Release the bag and the expiratory valve.
4. Ventilate the animal at a rate similar to its own physiological rate (10–30 per minute for a dog, 20–30 for a cat), with an inspiratory:expiratory ratio of 1:2 or 1:3.
5. If possible, monitor the efficiency of ventilation by pulse oximetry or blood gas analysis.

Mechanical IPPV

Mechanical IPPV is also carried out using an anaesthetic breathing system. Most (but not all) ventilators replace the reservoir bag in the anaesthetic circuit. If mechanical ventilation is to be used, it is important that the operation of the particular ventilator used is well understood, since there is a wide range of different types available, working in a number of ways (see Chapter 3).

Long-term ventilation

Artificial ventilation of the veterinary critical patient for more than a few hours is rarely undertaken, although it is commonplace in human critical care medicine. Most animal patients will not tolerate artificial ventilation without heavy sedation or general anaesthesia.

Considerations for long-term ventilation include the following.

- A secure airway is mandatory, either by endotracheal intubation or tracheostomy tube (cuffed if possible)
- Poorly tolerated by the conscious patient
- Heavy sedation (e.g. propofol infusion, 0.2–0.4 mg/kg/min) or general anaesthesia usually required
- Nursing care for recumbent animals should be applied (fluid and nutritional support, regularly turning to prevent pressure sores, regular emptying of bladder)
- Inspired gas should not be 100% oxygen
- Inspired gas should be humidified
- Continuous monitoring is essential.

Nebulization

Nebulization is the formation of microdroplets (3–7 microlitres) of fluid for inhalation. Droplets of this size will be inhaled to the smallest airways and can be used to hydrate and mobilize bronchial secretions or to carry drugs (e.g. antibiotics or corticosteroids) into the airways. In practical terms, a commercially available ultrasonic or oxygen-driven nebulizer is used to vaporize sterile saline or water in which drugs may be dissolved. Usually the animal is placed into a closed cage or a basket covered by plastic film and nebulization carried out three or four times daily. Following nebulization, the animal is encouraged to cough and the thoracic wall percussed ('coupage') to loosen and aid the expulsion of secretions.

Cardiovascular monitoring and therapy

The cardiovascular system can be monitored in a variety of ways, including palpation of peripheral pulses, assessment of the mucous membranes (colour and capillary refill time) and auscultation of the heart. More detailed information can be acquired by means of monitoring blood pressure, both indirectly and by direct means.

Auscultation

Auscultation permits evaluation of heart rate and rhythm, and may reveal the presence (or absence) of murmurs. Certain conditions may make this difficult; for example, a pericardial effusion will muffle the heart sounds (a helpful finding in itself). Similarly, conditions such as a space-occupying mass or pleural effusion may move the heart, so that the normal heart sounds cannot be heard clearly where one might expect.

In most normal unstressed dogs, the heart rate is between 60 and 180 beats per minute (bpm), and the rhythm should be regular. In cats, a resting heart rate of 110 to 180 bpm is considered normal. Many normal dogs will have sinus arrhythmia, where the heartbeat varies *regularly*, and this variation can be correlated to the animal's respiratory pattern. This occurs because changes in intrapleural pressure during respiration produce reflex changes in the heart rate (at least three reflexes are involved in this – it is very complicated). Sinus arrhythmia is a normal finding in healthy dogs.

Peripheral pulses

Palpation of the peripheral pulses can be extremely useful in patient assessment. Not only can one assess cardiac rate and rhythm, but a great deal can be learnt about the cardiovascular system as a whole.

The most useful sites for assessment of the pulse are the dorsal metatarsal artery (found on the dorsomedial aspect of the metatarsus) and the femoral artery (medial aspect of the thigh, superficial to the femur). The metatarsal pulse is lost before the femoral in animals with a compromised cardiovascular system, and this makes it a useful, if a little crude, means of assessing blood pressure. Another useful site can be the carpal pulse, found just medial of midline on the palmar aspect of the metacarpus, distal to the carpal pad.

Palpation of the peripheral pulses can be difficult, particularly in cats and very small dogs, and practice is required to become proficient in the technique. It is advisable to practise on normal patients whenever the opportunity arises.

Normal pulses should be at the same rate and rhythm as the heartbeat, and should not vary in strength from beat to beat. Variations in pulse strength may indicate a deficit in circulating volume. Variations in rate or rhythm may be indicative of an arrhythmia and should be followed up with electrocardiography.

Electrocardiography

Continuous monitoring of the electrocardiogram (ECG) can be useful in the critical patient, and is advisable in cases that exhibit dysrrhythmia. Most ECG leads come equipped with crocodile clips but adhesive patches are better tolerated, particularly for long-term monitoring. Any abnormalities in the ECG, such as dysrhythmia or abnormal wave forms, should be noted. Placement of leads and the interpretation of the ECG is covered in Chapter 1.

Mucous membranes

The buccal mucous membranes are usually the best and easiest from which to assess the membrane colour and capillary refill time (CRT). The gum just above the incisors or canine teeth is the best site for assessing CRT. In animals with a pigmented oral mucosa the conjunctiva may be useful, although some changes may be masked by concurrent ocular disease. In female patients the vulva may also be used.

In the normal animal, the oral mucosa should be pink and the colour should return rapidly (in 1–1.5 seconds) after firm pressure is applied to the gums.

- A prolonged CRT is indicative of reduced peripheral blood flow, most commonly seen in hypovolaemia and heart failure.
- A rapid CRT is commonly seen in excited animals, and those with fever or the so-called systemic inflammatory response syndrome (SIRS).

The mucosa should feel moist, not dry or 'tacky'. Abnormalities in membrane colour and their respective causes are:

- Pink – normal
- Pale, white, grey or 'muddy' – poor perfusion, hypovolaemia or anaemia
- Red or congested – excitement, pyrexia, SIRS, endotoxaemia, sepsis, severe pancreatitis or neoplasia
- Cyanotic (blue or purple) – severe life-threatening hypoxaemia
- Icteritic (yellow or jaundiced) – obstructed biliary flow, destruction of erythrocytes or liver disease.

Arterial blood pressure

Systemic arterial blood pressure can be measured directly by arterial puncture or catheterization, or indirectly using a variety of techniques. Percutaneous placement of an arterial catheter can be successfully employed in small animal patients. However, indirect methods are often better tolerated in the conscious patient.

Invasive (direct) methods of measurement

Direct measurement of arterial blood pressure is accomplished by the catheterization of an artery using a standard intravenous catheter. In small patients, a number of arteries may be used for catheterization, including the dorsal pedal artery, the femoral artery and the palmar metacarpal artery. The catheter can then be attached to a device to measure the pressures within the vessel. Commonly used measuring devices include the aneroid manometer and the pressure transducer.

Transducers and recorders allow beat-to-beat measurement of arterial blood pressure and assessment of the arterial pressure waveform. Arterial catheters also provide convenient access ports for the sampling of arterial blood gases. Periodic flushing with heparinized saline is required to maintain the patency of arterial catheters.

Aneroid manometer

A standard aneroid manometer can be adapted to fit to the arterial catheter by using a length of non-compliant tubing and a three-way tap. The manometer should be centred on the level of the heart (point of the shoulder or sternal manubrium). The mean arterial pressure is estimated by noting the upper deflection as the needle swings on the dial of the manometer.

Pressure transducer

Electronic pressure transducers are more sophisticated (and expensive) methods for measuring blood pressure. Changes in arterial blood pressure are transmitted through a column of fluid within non-compliant tubing to the transducer, where they cause distortion of a metal diaphragm. This distortion changes the electrical conductivity through the transducer, which is then displayed on an oscilloscope screen. To avoid any extraneous influences on pressure, the transducer should be centred at the level of the heart and then set to zero.

Non-invasive (indirect) methods of measurement

Indirect methods are used to monitor blood pressure in human patients and can also be employed in small animals. They are generally well tolerated, but suffer the disadvantage that they are relatively insensitive during periods of hypotension.

Conventional sphygmomanometry

Arterial blood pressure can be estimated by auscultation of the characteristic Korotkoff sounds. These are produced by blood flow through an artery as pressure is released from an occluding cuff which is linked to a manometer. This method can be used to assess trends in systolic blood pressure.

Doppler ultrasonography

A number of devices for measurement of arterial blood pressure rely on Doppler ultrasound. Doppler techniques can estimate both systolic and diastolic arterial blood pressures but the diastolic estimate is less reliable. Blood flow is detected by transmitting, receiving and amplifying the changes (Doppler shift) in an emitted frequency as blood flows through the vessel, and the effect of applying a pressure cuff above the vessel.

Oscillometric devices

Oscillometric devices measure the magnitude of arterial pulsations produced in an air-filled cuff. The main advantage of oscillometric devices is their ease of use. They do not require constant attention, being fully automated. The disadvantages include expense and inaccuracy, particularly with movement, dysrhythmia, hypotension or bradycardia (heart rate below 25 bpm).

Electronic sphygmomanometry

This method indirectly estimates arterial blood pressure by detecting vibrations in the arterial wall in the sub-audible range. Electronic sphygmomanometry requires training of the operator and may be unreliable in hypotensive animals.

Central venous pressure

Central venous pressure (CVP) is an estimate of the right ventricular filling pressure and will vary with the body weight of the patient. It is a balance between blood volume, venomotor tone and cardiac function, and is influenced by drugs and by positioning of the patient. It is usually measured via a jugular catheter, long enough to extend at least into the thoracic inlet. As for direct arterial blood pressure measurements, this is then attached to a measuring device.

CVP can be measured (in cm H_2O) using a fluid-filled manometer system or via an electronic pressure transducer with zero set at the level of the right atrium. Single measurements of CVP are of little value; trends are more important.

- Marked changes may reflect changes in blood circulating volume, venous tone and systemic vascular resistance, venous return and right ventricular systolic and diastolic function
- Plasma volume contraction and venous pooling will reduce CVP
- Exercise, right heart failure, pericardial disease and overinfusion of fluids to cause volume overload will all raise CVP.

Fluid therapy

Fluid therapy is one of the key components of managing the critical care patient. The main aims of fluid therapy are to correct any volume deficits, electrolyte and acid–base disturbances, and then to maintain these parameters at normal levels. For convenience, fluid therapy may therefore be considered in two phases, which can be termed acute and chronic.

- Acute fluid therapy involves the correction of any imbalances
- Chronic fluid therapy can be thought of as maintenance therapy once the patient has been stabilized.

Basic physiology

Body water

Total body water represents 55–75% of body weight in the normal animal, depending upon age, sex and body fat (60% can be considered as average for an adult animal). It is distributed between extracellular and intracellular compartments.

- Extracellular water represents about 25% of body weight
- Intracellular water represents about 40% of body weight.

Extracellular water is further distributed between the circulatory system (intravascular water) and the space between cells in the tissues (interstitial water).

- Intravascular water is equivalent to the plasma water and does not include the water within the red cells
- Intravascular water represents about 5% of body weight
- Blood volume (about 8–10% body weight) is equal to intravascular water plus red cell volume
- Interstitial water constitutes about 20% of body weight.

Electrolytes

The main electrolytes (ions) in the body are sodium, potassium and chloride. They are collectively responsible for maintaining normal cellular function, and the concentrations of these ions are normally controlled by the body's homeostatic mechanisms to within very tight boundaries. During many disease processes, these balances may be disrupted and, furthermore, the homeostatic mechanisms may be impaired.

Extracellular fluid (intravascular and interstitial) contains large amount of sodium and chloride ions, whereas the main intracellular ion is potassium. In addition to these ions,

calcium is very important for the maintenance of normal cellular function – in particular, excitable tissues such as nerves, muscle and the heart.

Assessment of fluid requirements

Fluid therapy in the critical patient should be directed at the specific requirements of the patient – that is, the volume deficits, acid–base disturbances and electrolyte imbalances. This should be accompanied by monitoring of the patient to assess the efficacy of therapy, and its changing needs. Fluid requirements can be split into two components: maintenance and replacement.

Maintenance

An animal's maintenance requirement is defined as the amount of water and electrolytes required to replace those lost through normal physiological processes, i.e. through respiration, perspiration and excretion via the alimentary and urinary tracts. In the normal animal, the maintenance requirement for water is 50 ml/kg body weight/day, or 2 ml/kg/h.

In addition to supplying water, the maintenance fluid should replace electrolytes. Normal fluid losses are hypotonic to the extracellular fluid but contain more potassium. The ideal maintenance solution therefore is 4% dextrose with 0.18% sodium chloride, supplemented with 20–30 mEq potassium per litre.

In the diseased animal, maintenance requirements are often greater than this because the ongoing losses are larger than normal. A good example is the patient that is panting heavily, thereby losing more water than normal by evaporation from the respiratory tract. The patient's maintenance requirements must be provided *in addition* to any fluid replacement therapy.

Replacement

In order to implement a fluid replacement plan, one must first determine the nature of fluid loss. Many conditions produce characteristic types of fluid loss, and it is worth remembering the more commonly occurring of these. Once the nature of fluid loss has been established, the general rule is to replace like with like. The principal types of fluid loss are summarized in Figure 4.35, along with conditions in which each type of loss commonly occurs.

Types of fluid

Crystalloids

Crystalloid fluids contain salts and/or glucose. They may be hypotonic, isotonic or hypertonic. They can also be classified according to their use and suitability for different purposes, such as volume replacement or maintenance (Figure 4.36).

4.35 Types of fluid loss

Nature of loss	Common conditions	Comments	Diagnostic aid
Primary water loss	Fever Panting Diabetes insipidus	Water is lost from all body compartments	Elevated serum sodium, PCV and TP
Extracellular fluid loss	Vomiting Diarrhoea	Most common Water and electrolytes lost	Elevated PCV and TP
Protein-containing loss	Burns Some effusions	Relatively uncommon	Elevated PCV TP normal or low
Whole blood	Wounds Fractures Haemorrhage into body cavity	May not be obvious Watch for signs of shock	PCV normal acutely

4.36 Types of intravenous fluids

- Volume restoration
  - Hypertonic saline
  - Normal saline
  - Hartmann's
- Maintenance
  - 5% Dextrose
  - 0.18% Saline in 4% dextrose
- Colloids
  - Gelatin-based
  - Dextrans
  - Hetastarch

Colloids

These contain large molecules to increase the colloid pressure in the solution (and within the circulation), in addition to electrolytes. They are used for replacement of plasma losses, rather than for replacement of fluid loss generally (Figure 4.36).

Whole blood and blood products

The RCVS considers only the collection and use of blood from a donor animal for the treatment of another specific patient to be ethical; collection and storage for future use is not considered to be an act of veterinary surgery. For this reason, fresh whole blood is used almost exclusively in the UK. However, in theory, blood may be processed and separated and blood products or components used in therapy. In some countries, such products (Figure 4.37) are available commercially.

Choice of fluid

In order to decide which type of fluid is needed, it is necessary to decide the nature of the patient's deficits, and then the general principle is to 'replace like with like' (Figure 4.38).

Routes

Intravenous

Intravenous access is central to the management of critical patients, and is best achieved by placement of an indwelling catheter for the administration of fluids and pharmaceuticals. In addition to this, centrally placed catheters may be used to monitor central venous pressure. Currently, the RCVS considers catheter placement to be an act of veterinary surgery in which a body cavity is entered, and therefore it should not be performed by a veterinary nurse. Figure 4.39 shows the types of intravenous catheters that may be used in different circumstances.

Catheters may be placed either peripherally (typically in the cephalic or saphenous veins) or centrally (in the jugular or femoral vein). A description of catheter placement is given below. The importance of strict asepsis as core to catheter management cannot be overemphasized.

Intraosseous

For very small patients, such as neonates, venous access can be difficult to establish. In such patients, a needle can be inserted into the medullary cavity of a long bone, usually the femur, for the administration of fluids. As in the case of intravenous catheters, the skin should be prepared aseptically prior to placement of the needle. An intraosseous needle (Figure 4.40) or a 20 G spinal needle is ideal for the procedure.

4.37 Blood and blood products

Product	Indication	Notes
Fresh whole blood	Specifically indicated for replacement of red cells, platelets and clotting factors	Most commonly used platelets and clotting factors deactivated within a few hours
Stored whole blood	Volume and red cell replacement	Platelets and clotting factors lost
Platelet-rich plasma	Volume and platelet replacement (uncontrolled bleeding problems)	Difficult to produce without specialized equipment
Plasma	Volume or albumin replacement	Can be produced by careful centrifugation of whole blood
Cryoprecipitate	Replacment of clotting factors or antibody donation	Only produced with specialized equipment

4.38 Selection of intravenous fluids for use in the CCU

Fluid	Indication	Notes
Ringers' solution Hartmann's solution	Volume replacement	Use for maintenance may lead to sodium overload
0.9% saline	Volume replacement	Use for maintenance may lead to sodium overload and potassium deficiency
4% glucose with 0.19% saline 5% glucose	Water replacement/maintenance treatment of hypoglycaemia	Potassium supplementation required for medium/long term use
Mixtures of the above	Water replacement/maintenance	Potassium supplementation required for medium/long term use Preferred by some clinicians
Amino acids solutions Lipid emulsions Concentrated glucose solutions	Parenteral nutrition	Careful formulation and administration required

4.39 Types of intravascular catheters used in the CCU

Indication	Types	Notes
Short-term IVFT	Peripheral over-the-needle or over-the-needle intravenous catheters	Not usually recommended for use beyond 48 hours Not suitable for hyperosmotic fluids
Long-term IVFT Parental nutrition Central venous pressure monitoring	Central venous catheter (usually in jugular vein); Seldinger type, through-the-needle, sheathed needle	Suitable for long term use if placed aseptically Require careful maintenance
Cardiac output monitoring	Swan–Ganz catheter	Placed in jugular vein Highly specialized technique
Concurrent treatment and monitoring	Multilumen central venous catheter	Used to allow concurrent CVP measurement, fluid therapy or nutrition and blood sampling
Direct blood pressure measurement	Peripheral over-the-needle or over-the-needle intravenous catheters	Rarely used except in the short term

IVFT = intravenous fluid therapy

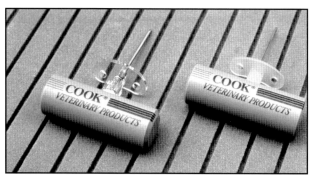

4.40 *Intraosseous needles.*
Courtesy of Cook Veterinary Products.

Intraperitoneal

In some circumstances, it may be necessary to administer fluids directly into the peritoneal cavity, from which they are absorbed into the circulation via the peritoneum. A bolus dose of fluid (usually an isotonic crystalloid solution) is administered from a needle. This method can be particularly useful where the temperament of the patient makes management of an intravenous catheter difficult. The intraperitoneal route is not considered to be suitable for acute volume replacement.

Subcutaneous

This is included for completeness, but is not considered to be an appropriate route for effective fluid administration.

Intra-arterial

Intra-arterial catheters are generally used for monitoring purposes rather than for the administration of fluids or medication. Typically they are used for direct arterial blood pressure monitoring and for obtaining blood samples for blood gas analysis.

Placement of a peripheral catheter

Equipment

- An assistant
- Clippers
- Skin scrub (e.g. chlorhexidine solution)
- Surgical spirit
- Scalpel blade (No. 11) (optional)
- Sterile gloves
- Over-the-needle catheter of appropriate gauge (cats 24–22; dogs 22–18)
- Injection bung, three-way tap or T-piece extension
- Tape or cyanoacrylate adhesive
- Heparinized saline (this can be made cheaply by adding 100 IU heparin to 100 ml 0.9% saline aseptically).

Technique

This is described in Figure 4.41.

4.41 Placement of a peripheral catheter

1. Clip an area over the vein.
2. Prepare the skin aseptically as for surgery. This is important and is the key to good catheter management.
3. Clean hands and put on sterile gloves.
4. Make a stab (facilitating) incision over the vein (optional).
5. Ask an assistant to raise the vein.
6. Insert the catheter into the vein, bevel up, until a 'flash back' of blood is observed.
7. Advance the catheter and stylet a few millimetres along the vein.
8. Run the catheter off the stylet, keeping the stylet still.
9. Place the bung or three-way tap over the end of the catheter and flush with a little (1–2 ml) heparinized saline.
10. Secure the catheter with tape, sutures or superglue.
11. In some patients (for example, those in circulatory collapse) it may be necessary to cut down surgically to expose the vein prior to catheterization.

Sites for catheter placement

The most commonly used site for catheter placement is the cephalic vein, but it is not always the most appropriate or accessible site in CCU patients. Alternative sites include the lateral and medial saphenous veins, the jugular vein, and even the auricular vein if no other site is available.

Catheter management

Strict asepsis is the key to effective catheter management. If care is taken to avoid contamination following aseptic placement, a normal short-stay over-the-needle catheter can be left without replacement for 3–4 days. The catheter site should be monitored for signs of sepsis or phlebitis, such as redness, swelling, heat and pain. If any of these signs are detected, replacement of the catheter, preferably at a different site, should be considered.

The catheter should also be monitored every 4–6 hours for patency and evidence of phlebitis or fluid extravasation. If not in continuous use, the catheter should be covered with a light dressing, and flushed with 0.5–1 ml sterile heparinized saline every 4–6 hours to maintain patency and prevent clotting.

Blood transfusions

The indications for blood transfusion fall into three groups:

- Restoration of oxygen-carrying capacity of the blood
- Restoration of blood volume
- Provision of clotting factors.

Collection of blood for transfusion

- Blood for transfusion should be taken from a jugular vein
- The donor animal may require sedation or, in rare cases, general anaesthesia
- The donor should be a healthy and tractable young adult in good physical condition, at least 30 kg in weight for a dog (4 kg for a cat)
- Blood should be collected into either a commercial blood collection bag or a syringe pre-treated with anticoagulant.

Anticoagulants

The best anticoagulants are citrate based. Heparin can be used (2 IU/1 ml blood) in an emergency, but blood collected using heparin must be used within 48 hours.

Commercial blood collection bags contain either acid citrate dextrose (ACD) or citrate phosphate dextrose (CPD) as the anticoagulant. CPD is the better of these, since it is more effective than ACD in preserving red cell viability.

Collection from dogs

Blood can be collected from donor dogs directly into commercial blood bags. As a rule of thumb, approximately 1% of body weight (e.g. 300 ml from a 30 kg dog) can be collected at each donation.

Collection from cats

Blood can be collected from cats into syringes which contain CPD (0.14 ml CPD/1 ml blood), up to a maximum of 25–30 ml per cat. Donor cats should be screened for viruses such as FIV and FeLV.

Storage of blood

Storage of blood and blood products is not approved by the RCVS. However, where it is permitted, blood collected using CPD as the anticoagulant can be stored for up to 28 days at 1–6°C (e.g. in a domestic refrigerator). The storage time is less for ACD.

Blood-typing

Chapter 6 gives details about blood-typing and cross-matching.

Transfusion reactions

The term 'transfusion reactions' is usually applied to any immune-mediated adverse reactions to a blood transfusion. They may be classified broadly into immediate and delayed reactions. Immediate transfusion reactions may be further divided into haemolytic and non-haemolytic:

- Non-haemolytic or hypersensitivity reactions are mediated by the same type of immune response as asthma or hay fever. The response is mediated by immunoglobulin E, and the clinical signs are produced by histamine release
- Haemolytic transfusion reactions are caused by interactions between recipient antibodies and the donor red cells. They may also occur when the donor has been sensitized (e.g. has previously had a blood transfusion itself) and donor antibodies react with recipient red cells. These should be eliminated by cross-matching.

Immediate transfusion reactions are unlikely during a first transfusion in both dogs and cats but there is one important exception to this. Cats from blood group B carry anti-A antibodies, and therefore cannot receive blood from a group A donor.

Signs of transfusion reactions include tachycardia, hypotension, urticaria, muscle tremors, panting and pyrexia.

Delayed transfusion reactions may occur for up to 2 weeks post transfusion, and occur when the recipient mounts an immune response to the donor's red cells. These reactions can be eliminated by blood typing prior to transfusion.

Other adverse transfusion reactions

Not all problems encountered during transfusion are mediated by the immune system. The most common of these are:

- Septicaemia, caused by poor attention to cleanliness when taking blood from the donor, or from placing the intravenous catheter in the recipient; also caused by inadequate storage and handling conditions
- Transmission of infections or parasites from the donor
- Volume overload
- Citrate toxicity. This is rare because citrate is rapidly metabolized in the liver, but toxicity can occur in patients with severe hepatic disease.

Blood administration

A blood giving set should always be used. This includes a filter to remove any microthrombi and debris from the blood. The giving set should be flushed through with sterile saline prior to use.

 Never use Hartmann's solution (lactated Ringers') for this, since it contains calcium and may trigger the clotting cascade.

The blood may be administered intravenously, or via the intraosseous route, from which 95% is absorbed within 5 minutes. The peritoneal route may be used; however, blood should be administered slowly and recovery of red cells is poor.

Blood should be warmed to 37°C before administration. This reduces viscosity and prevents hypothermia in the recipient. It is important not to overheat the blood (> 40°C), as this will cause auto-agglutination and protein breakdown.

Amount of blood

The amount to be administered depends on why the blood is being given.

- If it is administered to treat acute haemorrhage, then the volume lost by the patient should be estimated and this volume should be given rapidly

- If the transfusion is to correct a low PCV, then the volume required can be estimated using the following formula:

Volume needed = [(desired PCV – recipient PCV)/PCV of donor] x recipient blood volume

Total blood volume in litres can be estimated as approximately 8% of body weight (kg).

As a rule of thumb, giving 2 l blood/kg body weight will raise the recipient's PCV by 1%, assuming the donor's PCV to be 40%.

Rate of administration
This depends on the reason for the transfusion.

- To treat acute and massive haemorrhage, the blood should be given as rapidly as possible
- In all other cases:
  - The blood should be given slowly at first (0.2–0.5 ml/kg for the first 30 min)
  - The patient should be monitored for signs of acute transfusion reaction
  - After the first 30 min, the administration rate should not exceed 10 ml/kg/h (5 ml/kg in cats). Transfusion can be continued at this rate until the desired PCV is reached
  - The patient should be monitored for signs of volume overload and transfusion reactions.

Autotransfusion
This may be considered when an animal is bleeding uncontrollably into a body cavity but fresh blood is not available, or there is no time to cross-match. The blood should be drawn into a large (20–50 ml) syringe containing anticoagulant, through as large gauge a needle or venous catheter as is available. The blood must be administered through a filter.

Electrolyte imbalances
Imbalances of electrolytes (particularly potassium, sodium, calcium and chloride ions) are common in patients admitted to the CCU. In many animals, these are secondary to dehydration or shock and correction of volume depletion will enable homeostasis to be restored. In certain instances, when a primary electrolyte abnormality is present or when the disorder is severe enough to be immediately life-threatening, direct treatment is indicated. Electrolyte abnormalities, their causes and treatment are addressed in Figure 4.42.

Analgesia and pain management

The relief of pain is a very important aspect of veterinary critical care. Veterinary professionals have an ethical duty to minimize pain and anxiety in animals. The subject of analgesia is covered in detail in Chapter 3. However, because of its importance, an overview in the context of the critical patient is given here.

Assessment of pain
This can be extremely difficult in the critical patient. Often the disease process itself produces depression, and overt signs of discomfort such as vocalization can be uncommon. Signs of pain exhibited by the patient will depend upon its species, breed and personality as well as the nature of its condition. Often the only guide is a change in behaviour, which may range from a change in posture to aggression and self-mutilation. It is also useful to consider the disease process when assessing pain – for example, the type of surgery that has been performed, or the nature of injuries sustained (Figure 4.43).

Analgesia
Measures to alleviate pain should be undertaken as soon as possible. In patients undergoing surgery, appropriate analgesia should be administered preoperatively, since this will block sensitization of the central nervous system to painful stimuli. In other critical patients, pain should be assessed and treated appropriately.

It is important to bear in mind that many systemic analgesic drugs may have depressant effects on the cardiovascular, respiratory and central nervous systems. These effects may be harmful to the patient – either directly, or indirectly by masking changes in the patient's condition. Analgesia in the CCU should aim to alleviate pain as much as possible without compromising the patient.

4.42 Electrolyte imbalances

Abnormality	Common causes	Signs	Treatment
Hypernatraemia	Primary water loss CNS disease	Depressed mentation Seizures	Water replacement
Hyponatraemia	Water intoxication Protracted vomiting and diarrhoea	Lethargy Coma	Sodium chloride infusion
Hyperkalaemia	Hypoadrenocorticism Renal failure Urinary obstruction Diabetic ketoacidosis	Weakness Cardiac dysrhythmias/arrest	Treatment of primary disease Volume replacement in extreme cases Intravenous glucose/insulin therapy
Hypokalaemia	Failure of food intake Idiopathic in oriental cats	Weakness Ventroflexion of the neck	Cautious intravenous potassium supplementation
Hypercalcaemia	Paraneoplastic disease Hypoadrenocorticism Renal failure	Polydipsia/polyuria Weakness Leads to renal failure	Diuresis with IVFT Frusemide
Hypocalcaemia	Lactation	Seizures	Cautious intravenous calcium

IVFT = intravenous fluid therapy

4.43 Pain levels associated with surgery or trauma to different regions

Severity of pain	Site of surgery/injury
Severe	Thorax
	Cranial abdomen
	Ophthalmic surgery, injuries involving the orbit and eye
	Nasal cavity
	Perineum
	Aural surgery (e.g. TECA/LBO)
	Spinal column
Moderate	Caudal abdomen
	Long bone fractures
	Major joints
Mild	Superficial skin
	Extremities

Options

For clarity, the strategies that can be used to control pain and anxiety have been divided into two groups: those that require the administration of medication and those that do not.

Non-drug-dependent

- Immobilization (for example, of a fractured limb)
- Application of hot or cold compresses
- Distraction (by holding, stroking or talking to the patient). This may be particularly useful in the recovery period following general anaesthesia, or whilst waiting for medication to take effect.

Drugs

- Opiates (covered in detail in Chapter 3) have an important role in critical care medicine. The use of transcutaneous fentanyl is discussed below
- NSAIDs (non-steroidal anti-inflammatory drugs) may not always be appropriate for the critical patient because of their effects on renal function and the gastrointestinal tract. However, newer drugs such as carprofen and meloxicam have a role in pain management in the CCU. NSAIDs are absolutely contraindicated for patients undergoing corticosteroid therapy
- Sedation or tranquillization may be required to augment the effects of systemic analgesics
- Local analgesic techniques.

Fentanyl patches

Transdermal therapeutic system technology is a relatively recent advance in therapeutics. It provides a method of steady-state long-term administration of medication without the need for venous access.

The fentanyl patch (Durogesic, Janssen Pharmaceuticals) (Figure 4.44) was developed for human use in the management of chronic pain, and is particularly well suited to patients

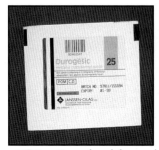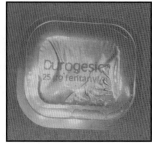

4.44
Fentanyl patch for transdermal analgesic delivery. (a) In foil packaging. (b) Ready for application.

4.45 Fentanyl patch requirements for patients of various sizes

Weight of patient (kg)	Size of patch required
< 10	25
10–20	50
20–30	75
> 30	100

unable to tolerate oral medication or those in which the use of NSAIDs is contraindicated. This makes the fentanyl patch ideal for providing analgesia to veterinary critical care patients.

The patch is available in a range of doses (25–100 mg) suitable for animal use (Figure 4.45). In dogs, application of the patch provides analgesia that reaches a steady state within 24 hours and lasts for 3 days. In cats, steady state is reached within 2–6 hours and lasts for 4 days.

For very small patients, part of the patch should be covered or folded to prevent contact with the skin. Patches should never be cut, since this will affect the release of the fentanyl.

Further reading

Aron DN and Crowe DT (1985) *Upper Airway Obstruction – General Principles and Selected Conditions in the Dog and Cat*. Veterinary Clinics of North America (Small Animal), WB Saunders, Philadelphia

King L and Hammond R (eds) (1999) *BSAVA Manual of Canine and Feline Emergency and Critical Care*. BSAVA, Cheltenham

Kirby R and Crowe DT (eds) (1994) *Emergency Medicine*. Veterinary Clinics of North America (Small Animal Practice), WB Saunders, Philadelphia

Murtaugh RJ (ed.) (1995) Critical care. In: Bonagura JD (ed.) *Kirk's Current Veterinary Therapy XII*. WB Saunders, Philadelphia, pp. 95–199

Murtaugh RJ and Kaplan PM (eds) (1992) *Veterinary Emergency and Critical Care*. Mosby, St Louis, Missouri

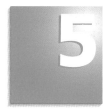

5 Advanced imaging

Deborah J Smith

This chapter is designed to give information on:

- Applications and techniques of radiographic contrast studies. The veterinary nurse can perform many of these. Some of the more advanced techniques, such as myelography and arthrography, will be performed by a veterinary surgeon but the veterinary nurse has an important role in preparing and positioning the patient properly. An understanding of the procedures is invaluable when it comes to explaining to owners the potential benefits, complications and alternatives
- Basic principles and applications of ultrasonography
- Basic principles and applications of advanced techniques such as image intensification and nuclear medicine
- New imaging modalities that have become available to the veterinary profession in recent years – in particular, computed tomography and magnetic resonance imaging
- Capabilities and limitations of various techniques

Radiographic contrast studies

On plain radiographs, where structures of the same radiographic density contact each other, there is nothing to provide contrast and the structures are therefore indistinguishable. For example, the soft tissue density of the urinary bladder wall contains urine, which is also of soft tissue density. No information can be gained from a plain radiograph about the thickness of the wall or condition of the mucosal surface. If soft tissue densities (e.g. blood clots or radiolucent cystic calculi) are present in the urine, they will not be visible on a plain radiograph.

If the urine is removed and replaced by something of different radiographic density, this provides contrast with the surrounding tissues and enables the mucosal surface, bladder wall thickness and luminal contents to be assessed. The following types of study may be performed:

- *Negative contrast* – the urine is replaced by something of reduced radiographic density (e.g. air)
- *Positive contrast* – uses something of increased density (e.g. an iodine-containing solution)
- *Double contrast* – negative and positive contrast agents are used in combination (Figure 5.1).

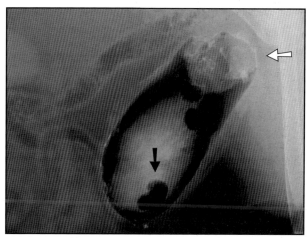

5.1 *Double contrast cystogram demonstrating bladder neck tumour (white arrow) and blood clots within positive contrast pool (black arrow).*

In some situations, the need for contrast studies has diminished due to the use of newer investigative techniques, such as ultrasonography and endoscopy. Ultrasonography has the advantage of being non-invasive and not requiring general anaesthesia. However, in many cases the techniques are complementary and can help to build a more complete picture of a patient's condition.

Types of contrast media

General requirements for contrast media are that they should be non-toxic and non-irritant and should provide optimum contrast to the surrounding tissues. The main types of contrast media are:

- *Barium sulphate* – ideal for most alimentary tract studies; it is inert and insoluble and provides excellent mucosal detail
- *Conventional water-soluble iodine-based media* – used for a wide range of studies. A significant incidence of side effects is associated with these agents, many of which (e.g. palpitations, nausea and hot flushes, experienced by human patients) are rarely a problem in veterinary use as patients are usually anaesthetized. However, it is important to appreciate their potential to produce severe side effects, including profound hypotension and damage to brain, heart and kidneys when used intravascularly, and local irritation if injected perivascularly
- *Non-ionic low osmolar iodine-based media* – much safer in all respects than the above and can be used for vascular studies in compromised patients. They are also suitable for myelography, which conventional media are not, but they are considerably more expensive than conventional media
- *Negative contrast agents* – the most commonly used and readily available is air. Oxygen, carbon dioxide and nitrous oxide can all be used but are less convenient and have to be taken from pressurized cylinders.

Barium and iodine have high atomic numbers and therefore absorb a large number of photons from the primary beam, resulting in a white area on the radiograph. Gases have a lower physical density than surrounding soft tissues and do not attenuate the beam very much, resulting in a black area on the film.

Patient preparation

Proper preparation is essential. The following points should be considered:

- The hair coat should be clean and dry. Dirt or water on the coat produces artefacts on radiographs, as will any positive contrast agent on the animal, X-ray table or cassette
- For alimentary and urinary tract studies, the gastrointestinal (GI) tract should be empty of ingesta and faeces
  - Starve patient for 12–24 h before study
  - For upper GI studies, withhold water for 4 h (provided it is not clinically contraindicated to do so)
  - For upper GI studies, allow adequate opportunity for patient to evacuate bowels before any sedative is given. For large bowel and urinary tract studies, administer suitable enema before sedation (e.g. low volume lubricant type for small dogs and cats or a phosphate enema for larger dogs – avoid soapy water enemas because of gas bubbles produced within the colon)
- Use appropriate sedation or general anaesthesia
  - For alimentary studies: no general anaesthesia. Sedation acceptable if required (e.g. acepromazine/opiate combination) but will have some effect on motility and more care is required to avoid inhalation of contrast agent if administered orally
  - For urinary tract studies: general anaesthesia preferable in most cases.

Plain films

These must always be taken before commencing a contrast study:

- To ensure that the patient is properly prepared for the examination
- To avoid masking a diagnosis
- To check that exposure factors are appropriate
- To help to estimate the quantity of contrast agent required
- To provide a means for comparison with contrast films.

Alimentary tract studies

A suspension of barium sulphate is used for most studies. Many texts recommend using a water-soluble iodine-based agent when perforation of the tract is suspected. This is because barium is inert and there is a risk of granuloma formation in the thoracic or abdominal cavities if it were to leak from the tract. However, this response is less important than the inflammatory response likely to result from leakage of ingesta from the tract. Also, most perforations will require surgical intervention, thus providing the opportunity for flushing of the cavity at that time.

A major disadvantage of using a conventional iodine-based agent is its hypertonicity. A patient with alimentary tract perforation is likely to be dehydrated and may well have severe electrolyte disturbances; the osmotic pull of a hypertonic agent could further compromise such a patient, as well as reducing the quality of the study by diluting the contrast. The non-ionic low osmolar media are suitable for this purpose but their expense is prohibitive except in the smallest patients.

Gastrointestinal tract studies are best started early in the day so that contrast can be followed as far through the tract as required.

Oesophagus

Barium swallow
The technique is described in Figure 5.2.

5.2 How to perform a barium swallow

1. Starve the patient before the study, in case a lack of findings from the swallow leads on to a GI study
2. Use mild sedation if necessary
3. Obtain plain films including the entire oesophagus (from pharynx to stomach). Large patients may require separate cervical and thoracic films
4. Administer barium
   - Use 100% w/v liquid barium suspension. Quantity: 5–50 ml (depending on size of patient)
   - Using a syringe or plastic bottle with some sort of nozzle, insert nozzle behind the canine tooth and direct across the mouth. Give the liquid slowly, allowing the patient time to swallow, to avoid aspiration
   - Hold a towel beneath the chin to catch any barium that dribbles from the animal's mouth.
   (If megaoesophagus or a partial stricture is suspected, liquid barium alone may not delineate the lesion and a mixture of liquid barium and meat may be needed. Most patients with such lesions tend to be very hungry and will eat the mixture voluntarily. The meat produces filling defects within the barium, therefore a follow-through study of the remainder of the alimentary tract cannot be performed immediately afterwards if the barium swallow is normal)
5. Obtain a lateral radiograph of the thorax and neck immediately after administration of contrast agent. A second view is often not required, but if indicated (e.g. in evaluation of oesophageal displacement) more contrast agent will normally need to be given.

Stomach

The technique chosen depends on the information required:

- *Pneumogastrography* (air alone) – to assess gastric position or evaluate an extramural mass
- *Positive contrast gastrography* – best for evaluation of gastric emptying time and good for assessing gastric position, size and shape
- *Double contrast gastrography* – best for delineating foreign bodies and assessing stomach wall lesions (which may be masked by large volumes of positive contrast material).

Gastrography

Gastrography may require moderate to heavy sedation to allow stomach tubing; this will have a significant effect on motility and gastric emptying. General anaesthesia may be used but will have an even more profound effect and is normally to be avoided. The technique is described in Figure 5.3.

5.3 How to perform gastrography

1. Obtain lateral ± ventrodorsal (VD) views centred on the cranial abdomen (over the last rib)
2. Pass a stomach tube. Barium can be given orally but stomach tubing is best – a large volume of liquid can be deposited in the stomach in a short time and radiographs obtained before gastric emptying commences. A stomach tube is definitely needed if air is to be given for a negative or double contrast study.
3. Inject barium suspension (100% w/v) and/or air slowly from a syringe at the end of the stomach tube. If any resistance to injection is encountered, or the animal shows discomfort, the tube may have doubled back on itself at the cardia and should be withdrawn slightly and repositioned. Volumes required:
   - Positive contrast: 3–10 ml liquid barium/kg (low end of range for large patients; high end for small patients)
   - Negative contrast: approximately 5 ml air/kg (total 50–300 ml, depending on size)
   - Double contrast: 5–30 ml liquid barium (depending on size) followed by 50–300 ml air (depending on size); then rotate animal gently to distribute barium
   (When injecting air, palpate abdomen for moderate gastric distension to know when sufficient has been introduced, or stop if any resistance to injection is felt)
4. Withdraw stomach tube
5. Obtain immediate and follow-through films as directed. Views required will depend on the purpose of the study. An immediate lateral may suffice to show stomach position, whereas four views at right angles to each other are needed for complete evaluation. Take left lateral recumbent and VD views first, as contrast moves more readily into the duodenum under gravity when in right lateral and DV positions.

Gastric emptying often begins almost immediately and should certainly commence within 30 min of barium administration. If liquid barium alone is used, emptying will normally be complete by 2–3 h (often less in the cat or immature dog). In nervous or heavily sedated animals, emptying times can be greatly increased. Once most of the barium has moved into the small bowel, take a further radiograph to include the stomach. Foreign bodies and wall lesions (e.g. ulcers, or tumours breaching the mucosa) may have been masked by the large volume of barium in the full stomach and are often most easily identified by the adherence of barium after the stomach has emptied.

As with all GI studies, an unusual appearance may be due to peristaltic movements of the tract. The presence of a suspicious lesion should be confirmed by demonstrating a matching appearance on at least two films.

Small intestine

Small intestinal contrast studies often involve following through barium given to examine the stomach when a diagnosis has not been reached. They are of most value in assessing obstructive lesions and determining the position of the small intestine if it is not apparent on plain films. They are often unhelpful in evaluating mucosal disease and rarely add any information in the investigation of chronic inflammatory bowel disorders. Complete obstructions often have diagnostic plain film findings, in which case a barium series is of little benefit to the patient, surgeon or owner as it delays time to surgery and increases cost for the owner. However, plain film findings can be equivocal in cases of partial small bowel obstruction, and a contrast study may be useful to confirm or rule out a suspected lesion.

Small intestinal contrast study

The technique is described in Figure 5.4. Precise timing of follow-through films cannot be given, as transit times are very variable. It is possible to miss significant lesions by taking films at random. Some radiologists prefer to follow a standard protocol; others prefer to decide after examining each film what subsequent ones will be required. If a lesion is suspected but not confirmed on a particular film, another one should be taken immediately and centred over the region in question to check if the appearance is persistent. Small intestinal transit time is around 30 min to 2 h; emptying takes up to 5 h. The study should continue until all contrast has reached the large intestine (which may take until the next day). A rough guideline to timing of radiographs is:

- Dog: 5 min, 1 h, 3 h, 5 h
- Cat: 5 min, 30 min, 1 h, 2 h.

5.4 How to perform small intestine contrast radiography

1. Obtain lateral and VD plain abdomen radiographs
2. Pass stomach tube
3. Introduce liquid barium via the tube. If the study is for small intestine alone, dilute the barium suspension to 25% w/v with water – this reduces its transit time through the small intestine (which can be rather slow if more concentrated). Dose rate: 3–12 ml/kg body weight (low end of range for large patients; high end for small patients)
4. Withdraw stomach tube
5. Obtain lateral and VD abdomen radiographs. VD views are often most useful for the intestines - there is less superimposition than on a lateral, but sometimes both are necessary.

Large intestine

Follow-through radiographs after upper GI studies serve to demonstrate the large intestine's position but a barium enema is necessary to outline the lumen and wall properly. Many large-bowel lesions can be adequately evaluated by proctoscopy and contrast studies are rarely required. As with the stomach, negative, positive and double contrast techniques can be used.

Barium enema
This technique is described in Figure 5.5.

5.5 How to perform a barium enema

1. Ensure colon and rectum are empty by administering enema and allowing patient adequate opportunity to defecate before any sedation is given
2. General anaesthesia is preferable, but administration of air to demonstrate the position of the distal large intestine may be possible under sedation
3. Obtain lateral and VD plain films
4. Place a Foley catheter in the terminal rectum and inflate bulb. If necessary place a purse-string suture in the anus and tighten around the catheter, to ensure no leakage of contrast from rectum and to allow proper filling of large intestine
5. Administer barium
   - Dilute liquid suspension to 25% w/v with warm (body temperature) water
   - Use a 50 ml syringe, or allow the bowel to fill under gravity from a reservoir (e.g. a drip bag or plastic bottle) connected via a tube to the catheter
   - Use 2–10 ml suspension/kg to fill the large intestine. (The barium should not progress proximally beyond the terminal ileum, so take initial radiograph after instilling a volume at the lower end of the dose scale and use this to evaluate the need for more contrast to fill the entire colon and caecum)
   - Inject slowly and stop if any resistance to contrast flow is felt
6. For a double contrast study, drain as much barium as possible from the large intestine (elevate front end of animal and lower hindquarters to achieve this). Then introduce air via catheter using enema pump or 50 ml syringe. (For pneumocolonography, to demonstrate the position of the large intestine, introduce a small volume of air directly into the rectum through an enema pump i.e. without the Foley catheter)
7. Obtain lateral and VD views – include entire large bowel (collimate beam to last rib cranially and perineum caudally)
8. When removing catheter from rectum after completion of the study, do so over a drain to prevent bowel contents leaking out over the table.

Urinary tract studies

Water-soluble iodine-based agents are used for positive contrast studies of the urinary tract. Conventional ionic media are suitable on most occasions, but one of the low osmolar non-ionic media may be considered for intravenous use in a severely compromised patient.

Kidneys and ureters

Contrast studies are used to demonstrate changes in kidney shape and structure and to demonstrate the size and position of the ureters.

Intravenous urography (IVU) (intravenous pyelography, excretory urography)
The technique is described in Figure 5.6.

Slight variations in the protocol may be required depending on the findings on initial radiographs, and it may be necessary to follow the contrast through for longer, at the radiologist's discretion.

5.6 How to perform intravenous urography

1. Ensure colon and rectum are empty by administering enema and allowing patient adequate opportunity to defecate before any sedation is given
2. General anaesthesia is normally used. IVU can be performed in conscious patients, but general anaesthesia is preferred as timing of exposures is important and the contrast agent may cause unpleasant side effects (conventional media)
3. Place intravenous catheter in a peripheral vein
4. Obtain lateral and VD plain abdomen radiographs
5. Empty the urinary bladder. If determining the position of the distal ureters is important (e.g. incontinence investigations) introduce a small volume of air (10–100 ml)
6. Place animal in dorsal recumbency. Centre X-ray beam in midline at level of last rib and collimate beam to include as much of the caudal abdomen as possible
7. Inject contrast rapidly via the catheter. Use a water soluble iodine-based agent containing 300–400 mg iodine/ml. Dose rate: 1–2 ml/kg body weight. To reduce viscosity and allow rapid injection, warm the agent to blood temperature first
8. Take VD radiographs 30 s and 5 min after completion of injection
9. Take lateral views 10 min after injection to include kidneys and bladder
10. If information about distal ureters is required, take VD and lateral views at 15 min; centre on the bladder.

Bladder
Cystography may be performed on its own, or together with urethrography. It can demonstrate bladder position, wall lesions, calculi and rupture. Negative (pneumocystography), positive or double contrast techniques may be employed – a pneumocystogram will demonstrate the bladder's position, whereas a double contrast study gives superior detail of the mucosal surface. A positive contrast study is best for demonstrating bladder rupture, with leakage of contrast into the peritoneal cavity. Air can cause a fatal air embolus and should not be used if trauma is suspected.

Cystography
The technique is described in Figure 5.7.

If there is any evidence of reflux of contrast from bladder into ureters and renal pelvices on the radiograph, a course of systemic antibiotics should be given to prevent pyelonephritis.

Vagina and urethra
Retrograde vagino-urethrography is used to investigate urinary incontinence and evaluate lesions of the vagina or urethra. Positive contrast agent from the urethra flows into the bladder, so the study may be followed by a double contrast cystogram if required.

Retrograde vagino-urethrography
The technique is described in Figure 5.8.

The contrast should flow retrogradely to fill the urethra once the vagina has filled. The volume of contrast required to do this varies; if there is insufficient on the first radiograph, a top-up injection is made and a repeat radiograph taken. If the bitch is in oestrus the vagina can dilate markedly and the cervix will be open, allowing contrast to flow into the uterus. Much greater volumes of contrast are required and it is best to avoid performing the study during oestrus if possible.

5.7 How to perform cystography

1. Prepare as for IVU except in emergency cases
2. General anaesthesia normally used (may be avoided if rupture suspected)
3. Obtain plain lateral radiographs centred on caudal abdomen
4. Catheterize and empty bladder. Leave catheter in position and attach three-way tap and syringe
5. Introduce contrast material:
   - *Pneumocystogram* – use 30–500 ml air, depending on size of animal. Inflate bladder until moderately distended, gently palpating abdomen to assess degree of filling
   - *Double contrast study* – use 5–10 ml of water-soluble iodine-based agent, then rotate animal to coat bladder mucosa before introducing air as above
   - *Positive contrast* (only likely to be used on its own for suspected bladder rupture) – use 5–10 ml of water-soluble iodine-based agent
6. Close the three-way tap after introducing contrast material and withdraw catheter into urethra
7. Take lateral radiograph centred on bladder. A single lateral view is usually sufficient but occasionally VD or oblique views may be requested
8. Empty bladder once study is completed.

5.8 How to perform retrograde vagino-urethrography

1. Prepare as for IVU
2. General anaesthesia required
3. Obtain plain lateral film centred on caudal abdomen; collimate to include perineum
4. (Empty bladder if going on to perform double contrast cystogram)
5. Attach three-way tap and syringe containing contrast medium to a dog catheter and fill the catheter with contrast (to prevent introduction of artefactual air bubbles into the vagina). Insert catheter about 2 cm into vestibule, then seal vulval lips around catheter using a bowel clamp. (Alternatively, use a Foley catheter with the tip removed and the bulb inflated in the vestibule)
6. Introduce contrast agent. Use approximately 1 ml water-soluble iodine-based agent/kg (300–400 mg iodine/ml solution diluted 1:1 with sterile water or saline). Inject slowly and stop if any resistance to injection is felt
7. Obtain a lateral radiograph. Oblique views may sometimes be necessary if looking for ectopic ureters.

Retrograde urethrography in the male dog or cat

The technique is described in Figure 5.9.

Myelography

This technique is quite commonly used in general veterinary practice. It involves the injection of a contrast agent into the subarachnoid space to delineate the spinal cord. Such a study may demonstrate a lesion causing spinal cord compression or obstructing the flow of cerebrospinal fluid (CSF) and allows a distinction to be made between lesions that are outside the meninges (extradural), those between the meninges within the subarachnoid space (intradural) and lesions actually within the spinal cord (intramedullary) (Figures 5.10 and 5.11). The technique for myelography is described in Figure 5.12

5.9 How to perform retrograde urethrography in the male

1. Prepare as for IVU
2. General anaesthesia preferred
3. Obtain plain lateral film of caudal abdomen; collimate to include bladder, perineum and prepuce in the dog
4. Pre-fill a urinary catheter with contrast material to prevent the introduction of artefactual air bubbles into the urethra
5. Place the urinary catheter approximately 2 cm into the urethra in the cat and to the level of the distal os penis in the dog. In the dog, place a bowel clamp over the end of the prepuce (take care to avoid the penis), to prevent leakage of contrast on to the X-ray table and cassette. Alternatively, in the dog, place a 6 FG or 8 FG Foley catheter into the penile urethra and inflate the bulb; this avoids the need to clamp or hold the prepuce.
6. Wear protective clothing. Unless using a Foley, manually occlude the urethral opening around the catheter to prevent leakage. (In male cats, an Allis tissue forceps can be used to occlude the prepuce)
7. Inject contrast agent rapidly. The exact volume is not critical (5–30 ml generally required in the dog). Use a water-soluble iodine-based agent (300–400 mg iodine/ml, diluted 1:1 with sterile water or saline)
8. On completion of injection, stand back from the patient and simultaneously call for the exposure to be made of a lateral radiograph centred and collimated as above.

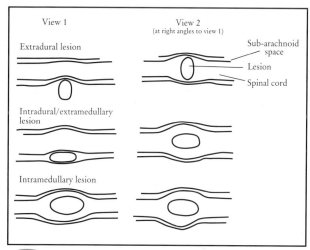

5.10 *Differentiation of lesions by myelography.*

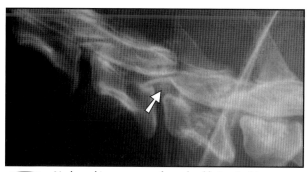

5.11 *Myelographic appearance of extradural lesion, in this case a C5-6 intervertebral disc protrusion (arrow).*

5.12 Technique for myelography

1. General anaesthesia is essential. It is probably best to avoid acepromazine for premedication because of the risk of seizures. A suitable alternative would be an opiate (e.g. pethidine at 1–3 mg/kg i.m.) approximately 30 min prior to induction

2. Plain lateral and VD films are obtained covering all areas of the spine in which the lesion may be located (as determined by the neurological examination)

3. The injection site is prepared by clipping the hair from an area approximately 8 cm x 8 cm and preparing the skin as for surgery. Strict asepsis is essential to avoid the risk of introducing infection. The injection sites are:
   - Cisternal puncture – in the midline, halfway between the palpable landmarks of the external occipital protuberance and the wings of the atlas (Figure 5.13)

     Lumbar puncture – in the midline, just cranial to the dorsal spinous process of the more caudal of the two vertebrae between which the injection is to be made (Figure 5.14)

4. Introduction of the needle and injection of contrast agent will be performed by a veterinary surgeon. The role of the nurse is to assist in correct positioning of the animal to facilitate this:
   - Cisternal puncture
     - Place animal in lateral recumbency with the spine along the edge of the X-ray table
     - The table may be tilted slightly to elevate the head and prevent contrast flowing cranially
     - Flex the neck and hold the nose at right angles to the spine and parallel to the tabletop. This can cause kinking of the endotracheal tube and may occlude the airway (Figure 5.15), especially in small patients, and so it is important to check the rebreathing bag for movement at this time
     - A hypodermic needle with short bevel or a spinal needle is used. The size depends on the size of the patient. A 20–23 G needle between 25 and 65 mm in length will be used and is introduced into the subarachnoid space
     - CSF will flow from the needle hub without suction and can be collected into a sterile vial for analysis if required
     - Injection of contrast agent is made slowly over a couple of minutes. Approximately 0.3 ml/kg body weight is used, up to a maximum of 10 ml. Injection is stopped immediately if any resistance is perceived. As soon as injection is complete the needle is removed, the head elevated and the table tilted for a few minutes to assist the caudal flow of contrast

   - Lumbar puncture
     - The needle may be introduced with the animal either in lateral recumbency with the spine and hips flexed or in sternal recumbency with the hindlimbs drawn forwards beside the body
     - A spinal needle with short bevel and stilette is used and may need to be up to 90 mm in length
     - Once the needle is placed, the stilette is removed. Backflow of CSF confirms correct positioning but there is often none from the lumbar site, even though the bevel is in the subarachnoid space
     - If lateral recumbency is used, a radiograph can be taken to check needle placement. A small test injection of contrast (0.5 ml) can be made to ensure that the needle tip is within the subarachnoid space rather than the epidural space
     - If sternal recumbency is used, the animal cannot be safely moved into lateral recumbency with the needle still in place. A horizontal beam projection with the cassette 'propped' vertically at the patient's side may be used, if appropriate safety precautions are used
     - The volume of contrast agent required is as for cisternal puncture and the injection is made slowly over a few minutes. A lateral radiograph can be taken before the needle is removed to check how far cranially the contrast has reached and further contrast can be injected if required. The needle is then removed.

5. Obtain lateral and VD radiographs. Several views may be needed, sometimes including oblique or 'dynamic' views, for which the spine is positioned in a fully flexed or extended position. It may be necessary to tilt the animal further to promote caudal (for cisternal puncture) or cranial (for lumbar puncture) flow of contrast agent before obtaining repeat films. (For radiographs of the caudal cervical spine in deep-chested dogs, DV positioning produces better contrast than VD, due to pooling of the agent when in sternal recumbency)

6. When the study is complete, it is advisable to administer a benzodiazepine (diazepam or midazolam, i.m. or i.v.) to lessen the risk of seizures during recovery. This is not necessary if the animal is going on to surgery, as the contrast will have been at least partially cleared from the CSF by the time anaesthesia is complete.

Myelography involves risk to the patient and should only be performed if the outcome will influence case management and be of benefit to the animal. If surgical intervention is an option, myelography is required to localize a lesion precisely and to assess whether or not it is amenable to surgery. In some cases, myelographic findings may lead to a decision to perform euthanasia on humane grounds. If a case is to be referred to a specialist centre for possible surgery, it is best to leave the myelography to them, as they will almost certainly prefer to perform their own study, and radiography and surgery can be carried out under the same general anaesthetic. Myelography is best performed only when automatic processing is available, since the ability to produce reliable images rapidly is crucial.

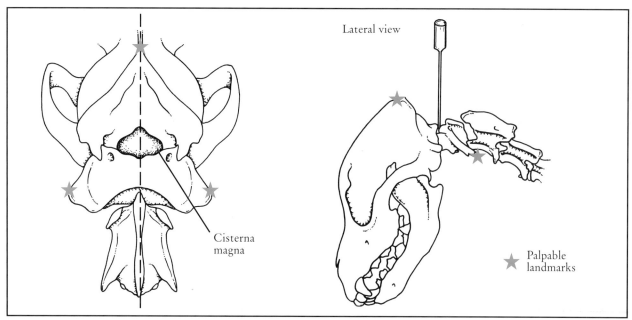

Site for cisternal puncture.

Lateral view

Cisterna magna

Palpable landmarks

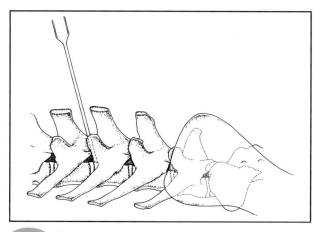

5.14 *Site for lumbar puncture.*

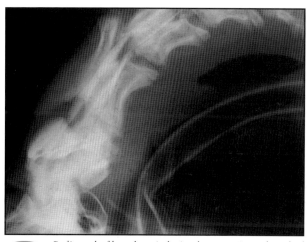

5.15 *Radiograph of lateral cervical spine demonstrating endotracheal tube occlusion caused by neck flexion.*

Potential complications associated with myelography include:

- Seizures on recovery from anaesthesia
- Spinal cord damage if the needle is placed incorrectly
- A worsening of the neurological signs for which the patient initially presented (usually transient but can be permanent)
- Septic meningitis.

A water-soluble iodine-based contrast agent is used for the study and *must* be one of the non-ionic low osmolar types. The conventional ionic iodine-based media are contraindicated. Iopamidol, iohexol and iotrolan are all suitable and a concentration of 200–300 mg iodine/ml is normally used. The injection can be made into either the cisterna magna (at the base of the skull) or the lumbar spinal canal – usually at L3–4 or L4–5.

It is technically easier to make the injection into the cisterna magna and also to be sure of correct needle placement, as cerebrospinal fluid (CSF) flows more readily from this site. However, contrast flow from a cisternal injection is under gravity and pressure must not be exerted to force contrast past an obstructive lesion because of the risk that it will flow forwards into the ventricles of the brain, which would increase the risk of seizures. Also, flow from a cisternal injection may not reach as far as the lumbar region, which is unsatisfactory if the lesion is at this site.

A lumbar injection often produces a superior study as the contrast agent can be introduced under a small amount of pressure to force it past an obstruction. Occasionally, both sites will be used in the same patient – for example, to delineate cranial and caudal aspects of a lesion in the thoracolumbar spine.

A complete neurological examination to localize the suspected lesion as accurately as possible is essential before commencing myelography.

Arthrography

This technique (Figure 5.16) is used to evaluate peripheral joints. It is not a routine procedure and tends to be performed mainly by orthopaedic specialists. The main clinical application of arthrography is in examination of the shoulder joint of the dog, where it is most frequently used to assess changes within the bicipital tendon sheath and osteochondrosis lesions. Its use in the dog's stifle is described but probably has little advantage over manual manipulation and plain radiographs. Negative, positive or double contrast studies may be performed but a positive contrast arthrogram is preferred. Negative and double contrast studies may be marred by air bubbles, which can form as the air mixes with synovial fluid or contrast agent.

5.16 Technique for shoulder arthrography

1. General anaesthesia is preferred
2. Obtain plain lateral and caudocranial views
3. Turn the dog over so that the leg to be studied is uppermost. Clip the hair over the cranial aspect of the shoulder. Prepare the skin as for surgery
4. The needle is introduced into the joint and the synovial fluid aspirated by the veterinary surgeon. A 20 G needle (25–50 mm, depending on the size of the patient) is used, preferably with a short bevel to reduce any risk of damaging the articular cartilage. The site for needle insertion is approximately halfway between the greater tubercle of the humerus and the acromion process of the scapula, with the needle directed medially, caudally and slightly downwards (Figure 5.17).
5. 1–6 ml of contrast agent is injected. A water-soluble iodine-based agent is used and can be diluted 1:1 with sterile saline. A low osmolar agent may provoke less tissue irritation than a conventional one. To assess the subchondral bone and the presence of any cartilage flaps, only a small volume (1 ml) should be used, even in a large dog. To fill the joint, including the bicipital tendon sheath, more will be required (4–6 ml)
6. The needle is withdrawn and the joint manipulated gently to distribute the contrast agent. Then turn the dog back on to the affected side
7. Obtain lateral and caudocranial views immediately. (The contrast agent is absorbed within about 15 min of injection.)

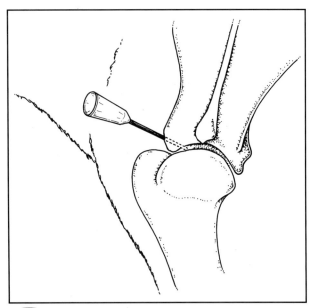

5.17 *Site for needle insertion in shoulder arthrography.*

Angiography

All of the angiographic studies described involve the use of a water-soluble iodine-based contrast agent injected into a portion of the vascular system. Ionic media can be used but the non-ionic agents are preferred, particularly in animals with metabolic disturbances. The contrast may be injected into a blood vessel to demonstrate its course and/or patency, or into a heart chamber, usually to demonstrate a congenital defect. Many angiographic procedures require specialized equipment and facilities and are infrequently performed. If available, image intensification is preferred for these studies, so that the passage of contrast can be followed through the vasculature, rather than relying on spot images which may miss significant lesions. Ultrasonography offers a non-invasive and much safer alternative for the evaluation of many lesions that would previously have required an angiogram to diagnose.

Portal venography

This is used to outline the hepatic portal system to diagnose and identify the position of portosystemic shunts. The commonest technique is operative mesenteric portovenography, in which a laparotomy is performed so that a jejunal mesenteric vein can be catheterized. Contrast medium is injected and a lateral radiograph of the abdomen and caudal thorax taken immediately upon completion of injection. This requires the surgeon to be wearing a protective lead apron underneath the operating gown.

Selective angiocardiography

A selective angiocardiogram involves the injection of contrast agent into a selected cardiac chamber. A specially designed long flexible catheter is inserted into a peripheral artery or vein and fluoroscopy is used to guide the catheter tip into the desired position. The injection must be made very quickly, so that the contrast medium travels as a bolus through the cardiac chambers, and a special pump can be used to achieve this. A rapid film changer is required, to make a series of exposures at very short time intervals during the course of and immediately after injection. The technique can therefore only be performed in specialized centres with these facilities and has anyway been largely superseded by echocardiography. In the veterinary field, its main use is in the diagnosis of congenital cardiac defects.

Non-selective angiocardiography

This is a much simpler procedure, which can be used in general practice and demonstrates the passage of contrast medium through the heart, great vessels and lungs. Contrast agent (at a dose rate of 1 ml/kg) is injected as a rapid bolus through a large-bore catheter placed in a cephalic or jugular vein (warming the contrast to body temperature prior to injection will aid rapid injection by reducing viscosity). Results are best in small patients because of the volume of agent involved. Several exposures can be taken close together on completion of injection, either by using a vertical stack of lead-backed cassettes that can be removed in sequence, or by using a series of cassettes taped together side by side so that they can be pulled in sequence through a tunnel beneath the animal.

This technique can be useful to outline an atrial thrombus in cats with cardiomyopathy, or to distinguish between hypertrophic and dilated forms, if ultrasonography is unavailable. A single lateral exposure made 6–10 s after injection may suffice for this purpose. A second exposure centred on the abdomen made approximately 15 s after injection can be used to demonstrate a saddle embolus, if present.

Study	Contrast agent	Structure(s) outlined	Indications
Sialography	Water-soluble iodine-based	Salivary glands and ducts	Obstruction, dilations and defects of ducts; tumours of gland
Dacrocystorhinography	Water-soluble iodine-based	Nasolacrimal ducts	Obstructions, defects
Epidurography	Low osmolar iodine-based	Epidural space in lumbosacral canal	Lesions associated with cauda equina syndrome
Sinography and fistulography	Water-soluble iodine-based or oily if available	Sinus tracts	To show extent and possibly cause (e.g. foreign body)
Pneumopericardiography	Air	Pericardial cavity	Intrapericardial masses (largely superseded by ultrasonography but may occasionally be used if ultrasonography fails to find a suspected mass)
Pneumoperitoneography	Air	Abdominal contents	(Obsolete – superseded by ultrasonography)
Bronchography	Special, oily, non-irritant	Airways	Obstruction, distortion and deviation (obsolete – superseded by endoscopy)
Cholecystography	Cholecystopaque (i.v.) (water-soluble, binds protein excreted through bile)	Gall bladder	For example, to assess function after feeding small fatty meal to stimulate emptying (obsolete – superseded by ultrasonography)

Peripheral angiography

This may be used to demonstrate an anomaly in a peripheral artery or vein and may be selective or non-selective. Contrast medium is injected into a vessel proximal to the site of the suspected lesion and a rapid series of radiographs is obtained immediately.

Other contrast studies

Other contrast studies (Figure 5.18) are rarely performed because in most cases the indications are few. As with other techniques, some have been largely replaced by other imaging techniques.

Ultrasonography

Ultrasonography is a complementary technique to radiography, each having its advantages and disadvantages. In many situations, both will be used to gain the maximum amount of information about a particular lesion. In radiography, someone who understands the physical principles involved but who may not have any interpretation skills can obtain good images. By contrast, ultrasonography is a dynamic technique, for which operators needs to appreciate what they are seeing in order to obtain the maximum amount of information.

Advantages of ultrasonography

- Most patients can safely be manually restrained for ultrasonography. Sedation or general anaesthesia are required only for the most fractious or aggressive animals, or if an ultrasound-guided biopsy is to be performed. Many examinations can therefore be performed on an outpatient basis
- In contrast to radiography, ultrasonography poses no health risk to personnel performing the examination or restraining the animal and at diagnostic levels there is no conclusive evidence that ultrasonography poses any risk to the patient

- Ultrasonography is excellent at differentiating between fluid and soft tissues (which have the same radiographic density), giving ultrasonography the advantage over radiography in situations where fluid is in contact with soft tissues. It can therefore be used to examine the structure and contents of fluid-containing organs (e.g. heart, uterus, urinary bladder). To do this radiographically requires the use of invasive contrast studies. Another example is a patient with a fluid-filled abdomen: on a radiograph, contrast is lost and little information is available about the viscera, whereas free fluid in the abdomen actually enhances an ultrasonographic examination by separating the viscera (Figure 5.19)
- Radiographs demonstrate the size, shape and position of body organs but do not give any information about the parenchyma. Ultrasonography does give this information and so is particularly useful for examining the internal architecture of organs such as the spleen, liver (Figure 5.19) and kidney
- Ultrasonography is a dynamic technique and can be used to gain information about organ movement. It is particularly useful in the assessment of cardiac function. On more expensive machines with the capability to perform Doppler ultrasonography, information can be obtained about the direction and speed of blood flow. This is again of particular value in cardiac assessment, especially when evaluating congenital abnormalities.

Disadvantages of ultrasonography

- Ultrasonography is of no use for imaging bones or lung, and large volumes of bowel gas can produce artefacts when imaging parts of the abdomen
- Many imaging artefacts may be produced when performing ultrasonography that can reduce the quality of the images obtained

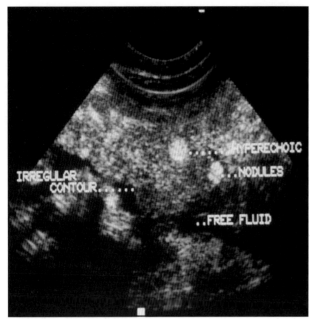

5.19 *Ultrasound image of liver showing hyperechoic parenchymal nodules and free abdominal fluid.*
Courtesy of E. Munro.

- Several controls on an ultrasound machine adjust the image electronically. Misuse of these can cause a significant loss of information and deterioration in image quality
- Misinterpretation of artefacts and lesions and over-diagnosis by those new to the technique are common. Hands-on practice is the only way to gain the experience necessary to become a competent ultrasonographer.

Basic principles

An ultrasound machine works by sending sound waves into the body. These sound waves are reflected back from the body tissues, to a greater or lesser extent depending on their composition. The returning waves (echoes) are picked up by the machine, which then converts them electronically into an image of the tissues based on the strength of the returning waves and the time taken for them to travel back to the machine.

Properties of ultrasound

- Sound waves are longitudinal waves, produced by vibration of an object. The vibrations superimpose a backwards and forwards motion on the particles of the medium through which the sound is transmitted
- The motion of particles in a sound wave is along the direction of wave travel
- Sound waves require a medium for their transmission and are therefore unable to travel in a vacuum
- The frequency of a sound wave is equal to that of the vibrating source
- Ultrasound frequencies are higher than the upper limit audible to the human ear (approximately 20 kHz). Diagnostic ultrasonography utilizes frequencies in the range 2 to 10 MHz
- The speed of sound varies depending on the material in which the wave is travelling. Rigid materials transmit sound much more rapidly than gases (Figure 5.20).

5.20 **Speed of sound in various materials**

Material	Speed (m/sec)
Air	330
Water	1480
Bone	2700–4100
Body tissues	1540 (average speed)

Acoustic impedance

The characteristic acoustic impedance of a body tissue is a measure of how readily that tissue transmits sound, which depends on the density of the medium and the velocity of sound in it. Air has very low characteristic acoustic impedance; water, fat and soft tissues have mid-range values (similar but slightly different to each other); and bone has a high value. Sound is reflected back when it meets an interface between two tissues of differing acoustic impedance and this forms the basis for diagnostic ultrasonography. The proportion of energy reflected depends on the size of the difference in acoustic impedance between the two tissues:

- Where there is a big difference, a large proportion of sound is reflected back, leaving very little to continue into the deeper tissues, e.g. soft tissue–air interfaces (99.9% of the incident sound energy is reflected back) and bone–muscle interfaces (approximately 30% reflected)
- Where there is only a small difference in acoustic impedance values (e.g. at soft tissue–water or fat–muscle interfaces) only up to 1% of the incident sound energy is reflected, allowing most to continue into the deeper tissues
- If acoustic impedances are identical (e.g. within fluids), no sound is reflected.

In real-time (B-mode; see below) imaging, reflection of a large proportion of the sound produces a white (hyperechoic) area and a lack of reflections produces a black (anechoic) area (Figure 5.21).

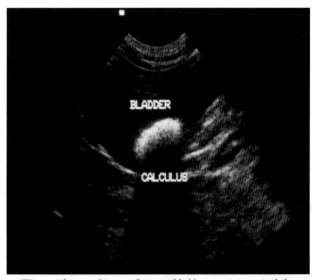

5.21 *Ultrasound image of urinary bladder containing a single large calculus. Urine appears black and the highly attenuating mineral calculus produces a very strong reflection, thus appearing bright white. Note also the strong acoustic shadow thrown by the calculus.*
Courtesy of E. Munro.

Attenuation

The intensity of a sound wave passing into the body tissues is gradually reduced (attenuated) by a combination of factors including reflection, scatter and absorption. Absorption involves the conversion of ultrasound energy into heat and accounts for around 90% of attenuation in soft tissues. The amount of absorption is directly proportional to the frequency of the sound waves: the higher the ultrasound frequency, the greater is the absorption in the tissues and the shorter the distance into the body that the wave can travel. Due to attenuation, echoes from deep structures are weaker than ones from identical interfaces that are more superficial. The electronics of the ultrasound machine take this into account and compensate for the loss of intensity when producing a visual display of the structures imaged.

The transducer

The transducer produces sound waves and receives returning echoes. A single transducer produces ultrasound waves of a specific frequency, so different transducers need to be used for different situations. High frequency transducers (7.5–10 MHz) provide the best image resolution and therefore the ability to distinguish fine detail. However, they only allow examination of superficial structures, as high frequency waves are unable to penetrate far into the tissues. They may be used for scanning eyes or horses' tendons. To allow adequate tissue penetration to scan the chests and abdomens of large dogs, a lower frequency transducer (3.5–5 MHz) is required.

Some machines have a selection of transducers of differing frequencies.

The piezo-electric effect

The sound waves are produced and received by a piezo-electric crystal, which is usually a synthetic ceramic. When a voltage is applied across the surface of the crystal, its shape deforms and a sound wave is produced. The wave frequency depends on the crystal thickness. The voltage is applied across the crystal intermittently, producing short pulses of sound. During the period between pulses, the crystal is able to receive returning echoes from the last pulse emitted. The returning echoes mechanically deform the crystal and the change in crystal shape is recognized and converted back into electrical signals, which are analysed by the machine electronics and converted to a visual display on the screen.

Near and far fields

The diameter of the beam of sound waves emitted by the transducer is approximately the same as the diameter of the crystal, and the beam continues almost parallel for a certain distance (the near field). Beyond this, the sound waves tend to spread out (the far field; Figure 5.22). Once this happens, resolution is lost, and so the aim is for objects of interest to be within the near field.

The length of the near field and the angle of beam divergence in the far field depend on the frequency of sound emitted and the diameter of the crystal. A high frequency transducer, or one with a large diameter, has a longer near field and less beam divergence in the far field than one with a lower frequency or smaller diameter.

Focusing

Transducers can be designed so that beam width is reduced at a particular tissue depth. Known as beam focusing, this produces stronger echoes and improved resolution from that depth (the focal zone) but it restricts the tissue depth over

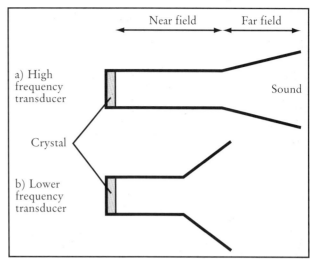

5.22 *(a) Near and far fields for a high frequency transducer. (b) A lower frequency transducer of the same diameter has a shorter near field and increased far field divergence.*

which the beam can usefully be used. It is important that the structures under examination lie within the focal zone. The greater the degree of focusing, the shorter and closer to the skin surface the focal zone will be and the greater the divergence of the far field.

Between the transducer and the focal zone is a zone that cannot be used for scanning. To image structures close to the skin surface that fall within this zone, a stand-off is needed to increase the distance between the transducer and the skin and bring those structures into the focal zone. A stand-off may be built into the transducer or may be a separate water-filled bag or gel block, which does not reflect or absorb the sound beam. Beyond the focal zone the sound beam diverges rapidly and resolution is lost.

Beam focusing can be achieved by:

- Using a crystal with a concave surface (Figure 5.23)
- Using a plastic converging lens fixed to the surface of the crystal
- Electronic focusing using an annular array: the crystal face is divided into a series of concentric rings to which the voltage is applied in sequence, starting with the outermost ring.

The latter method has the advantage that by changing the time delay between energizing successive rings, the depth of focus can be varied. The depth of the focal zone can therefore be altered without changing the transducer, giving improved resolution over a greater depth of tissue.

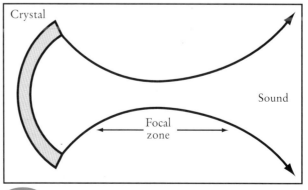

5.23 *Ultrasound beam focusing.*

Types of transducer

Mechanical sector scanners

Probably the most commonly used transducers in small animal veterinary work, these consist of either a single circular crystal that oscillates backwards and forwards (Figure 5.24a), or of three to five crystals mounted on a rotating wheel (Figure 5.24b). The crystal may be divided into an annular array to allow electronic focusing. These configurations produce a fan-shaped field of view, the size of which can be varied. The sound beams are diverging in the fan shape and so there is some loss of resolution, which is more pronounced the wider the field of view.

The ultrasonic beam sweeps across an area of the body, each sweep producing one image frame. By altering the rate of crystal oscillation or rotation the frame rate can be varied. These scanners only require a small skin contact area, making them easy to use, particularly in small patients. The moving parts make these transducers prone to wear and tear.

Phased array sector scanners

These consist of an array of about 60 tiny piezo-electric elements, which do not move. Electronic delays are applied to the individual elements both in transmission and receipt of signals, to allow the beam to be electronically 'steered' (Figure 5.25) to produce a fan-shaped field and also to focus the beam. They have no moving parts and are more compact than mechanical scanners, but they are much more expensive.

Linear and curved array scanners

These consist of 100 or more crystals arranged in a line, which are activated in small groups in sequence (Figure 5.26). They produce a large, rectangular field of view and can be electronically focused. They are relatively bulky, therefore requiring a larger skin contact area than sector scanners and are more awkward to manipulate. Their use is more common in large animals, particularly for tendon and reproductive examinations, where the large contact area is not a problem.

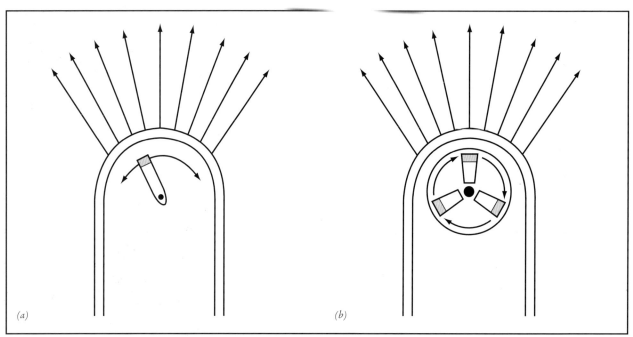

5.24 *Mechanical sector scanners: (a) single oscillating crystal; (b) multiple rotating crystals.*

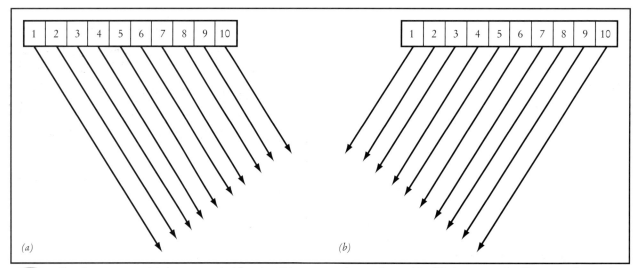

5.25 *Phased array scanner: (a) elements energized from 1 to 10 in sequence – beam swings to right; (b) elements energized in reverse – beam swings to left.*

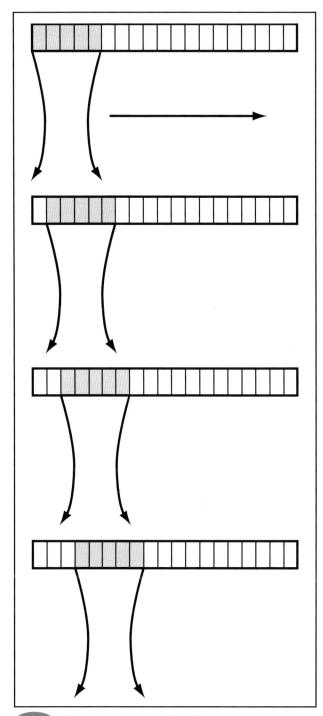

5.26 *Linear array scanner with beam focusing.*

Image display

A-mode (amplitude mode)

This is the simplest form of ultrasound imaging and only shows the position of tissue interfaces. A single pulsed beam of ultrasound is used and the image is displayed by a spot of light on a screen. The light spot moves at a constant speed across the screen, tracing out a horizontal line. When an echo is received back from a tissue interface a small voltage is generated in the transducer crystal, resulting in a vertical trace on the screen. The height of the vertical trace is proportional to the strength of the returning echo, whilst its location along the horizontal axis indicates the depth of the tissue interface. By repeating the pulse approximately 1000 times per second a sustained image is produced.

Early applications of this form of ultrasonography were in large animal reproduction but the information gained is very limited and it is now rarely used.

B-mode (brightness mode)

This involves sending pulsed beams of ultrasound back and forth across a two-dimensional section of the patient to produce an image of a slice through the patient (Figure 5.27a). The returning echoes are displayed as small bright dots on a screen, corresponding to each of the interfaces encountered by each sound beam. Only interfaces approximately at right angles to

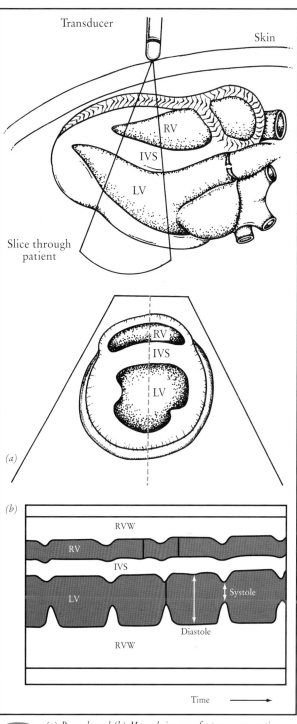

5.27 *(a) B-mode and (b) M-mode images of a transverse section through the heart. Selection of position of M-mode beam is taken from B-mode image (blue line). RV, right ventricle; RVW, right ventricular free wall; IVS, interventricular septum; LV, left ventricle; LVW, left ventricular free wall.*

the sound beams are imaged. The position of each dot on the screen represents the position in the body of the interface producing the echo. A computer is used to make the brightness of each dot in the image representative of the strength of the returning echo. This allows tissue differentiation and is known as grey scale imaging.

Black areas in the image represent an absence of echoes and may be described as *anechoic* or *echolucent*. Fluids (e.g. urine, blood, ascitic fluid) are anechoic. Grey (*hypoechoic*) areas represent intermediate reflection of sound. Most soft tissues are hypoechoic, appearing as various shades of grey depending on their composition and the number of internal interfaces within them. White areas represent strongly reflecting interfaces (e.g. bone or gas), described as *hyperechoic* or *echogenic*.

Real-time imaging involves scanning the image rapidly in a succession of frames, so that tissue motion can be demonstrated or an entire organ examined in a short time. The image can be frozen on the display screen at any time, so that permanent copies can be taken or measurements (e.g. of organ or tumour size) can be made.

M-mode (time–motion)

Most B-mode machines have transducers that can also be used to produce M-mode images when required. M-mode uses a single ultrasound beam from a stationary transducer (as in A-mode). The returning echoes are displayed as dots in a vertical line on the screen, the position and brightness of the dots representing the depth of the reflecting interface and strength of the echo, respectively (Figure 5.27b). The line of dots is continuously updated with time as the screen scrolls horizontally. As the transducer is stationary, this therefore displays movements of

structures along the path of the beam of ultrasound with time. The B-mode image is used to select the path through which this single beam of ultrasound will be directed.

The main application of this display mode is in cardiology, where it can be used to assess cardiac function (myocardial contraction in particular). The direction of the beam is chosen to intersect the moving surfaces of the heart as nearly as possible at right angles. The M-mode display can be frozen on the screen for measurements to be made. Contractions of the heart muscle can be evaluated by measuring the distance moved by the ventricular walls between end systole and end diastole.

Doppler ultrasonography

If sound waves are reflected back from a moving interface, there is a change in the frequency of the reflected wave compared with that of the incident wave. This is known as *Doppler shift*. If the interface is moving towards the sound source (Figure 5.28a), there is an increase in frequency; if it is moving away (Figure 5.28b), the frequency decreases. The faster the interface is moving, the greater the shift in frequency.

This effect is used in ultrasound imaging to determine the direction and speed of blood flow in the circulation, where the moving interfaces are the surfaces of red blood cells. Maximum Doppler shift occurs when motion is in line with the direction of the sound wave. The effect is reduced if the sound wave is at an angle to the direction of movement and is absent if motion is at right angles to the transducer. (Compare this with normal scanning, where the strongest echoes are from interfaces at right angles to the sound beams). The angle of incidence of the sound beam therefore needs to be taken into account when calculating speed of movement.

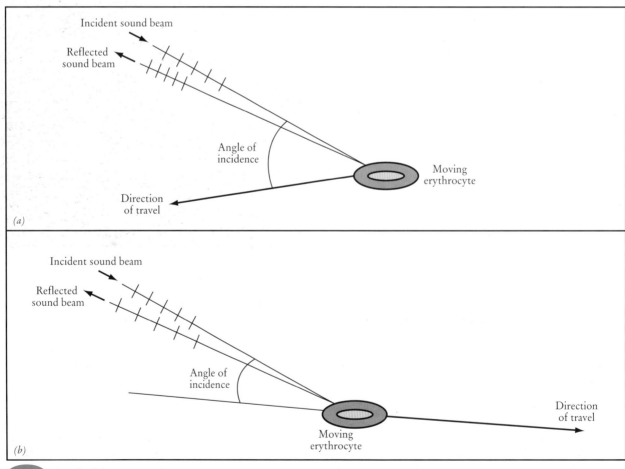

5.28 *Doppler shift.*

Continuous wave Doppler

This uses two transducers: one emits a continuous ultrasound beam, while the other receives reflected echoes. Pulsatile blood flow, such as occurs within the circulation, involves a wide range of velocities, producing a spectrum of Doppler frequencies. These frequencies are analysed by computer and can be displayed on a screen as velocity of movement against time. Alternatively they may be played through a loudspeaker, allowing the signal to be heard as a rushing sound: the higher the pitch, the greater is the velocity of blood flow; the harsher the sound, the greater is the turbulence.

This method can measure a wide range of velocities but does not allow location of the moving object.

Pulsed Doppler

The short pulses of ultrasound used for normal imaging cannot be used to obtain accurate flow information but a compromise, using longer pulses, can be used to provide some information of both position and flow.

Duplex scanning combines B-mode and Doppler imaging. The simplest scanners combine a sector scanner with a single pulsed Doppler transducer together in the scanning head. The B-mode image is used to choose the path for the Doppler beam. The pulsed Doppler transducer both emits and receives the Doppler signal, the depth of the moving interface being located by the time taken for the reflected echo to return.

A velocity–time spectrum corresponding to the range of frequencies in the Doppler signal is displayed, together with the cross-sectional B-mode image on the same screen.

Real-time colour flow imaging

Instead of having to select a path for the Doppler beam, this method displays velocity information across the whole of the cross-sectional image. This is displayed as colour superimposed on the grey scale B-mode image of stationary tissues. Flow towards the transducer is normally displayed in red, flow away from the transducer in blue and turbulence in green or yellow. The depth of each colour varies according to flow velocity.

This is a very useful technique, particularly in the assessment of congenital cardiac defects but also in other areas. Machines with this capability are very expensive and are likely to remain available only within specialist centres for the foreseeable future.

Imaging artefacts

If not recognized, image artefacts may lead to misinterpretation and misdiagnosis. Commonly encountered artefacts include the following.

Reverberation

Where there is a strongly reflecting interface close to the body surface, the reflected echoes reaching the transducer may be reflected back from it into the body tissues. When these echoes reach the same interface, they are again reflected back and the same thing can happen several times. This produces multiple images of the reflecting interface parallel to and deep to the original. This is most often seen at soft tissue–gas or fluid–gas interfaces.

Double reflection (mirror image artefact)

This also occurs at strongly reflecting interfaces and is due to multiple reverberations between the reflecting interface and other body tissues. It is sometimes seen at the interface between the lung and the diaphragm, when a mirror image of the liver appears beyond the diaphragm (Figure 5.29).

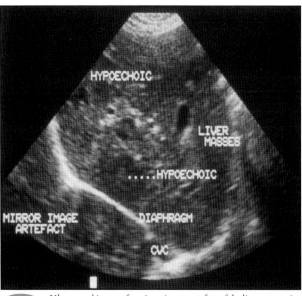

5.29 *Ultrasound image of a mirror image artefact of the liver, appearing on the far side of the diaphragm. Courtesy of E. Munro.*

Acoustic shadowing

A strongly attenuating structure (e.g. gas in the bowel or lung, bone, or urinary tract calculi) produces a bright image from the surface but there is a dark area or shadow cast beneath this because of the reduction in beam intensity beyond the interface (Figures 5.21 and 5.30).

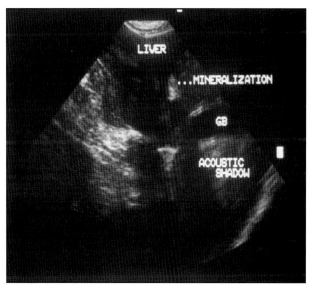

5.30 *Ultrasound image of an acoustic shadow thrown by an area of mineralization within the hepatic parenchyma. Courtesy of E. Munro.*

Acoustic enhancement

Fluid-filled structures (e.g. urinary bladder) do not attenuate the sound beam and so reflections from structures beyond the fluid appear particularly bright (Figure 5.31). Time gain compensation makes acoustic shadowing and enhancement worse.

Recording the image

The methods commonly used are:

- *Polaroid camera.* The camera is swung round to fit over the front of the screen and a photograph is then taken of a frozen image on the screen. Image quality is relatively poor on such prints

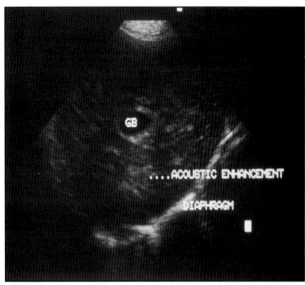

5.31 *Ultrasound image of acoustic enhancement, producing stronger echoes from the region deep to the fluid-filled gall bladder. Courtesy of E. Munro.*

- *Video printer*. This is linked to the ultrasound machine via a cable and produces good quality prints of a frozen image quickly. Such printers are more expensive than Polaroid cameras but individual prints are cheaper
- *Multiformat camera*. This produces images on X-ray film, which can then be processed routinely. Image quality is excellent. As with the video printer, individual images are relatively cheap to produce but the camera itself is more expensive
- *Video recorder*. This can be linked to the screen, allowing recording and replay of the full examination if required. This can be especially useful when performing cardiac examinations and allows measurements to be taken at leisure, without the animal becoming restless.

Machine controls

The controls listed are those that may be found on B-mode machines. On some machines they will not all be present.

- *On/off switch*
- *Power*. Governs the amount of sound emitted and therefore overall image brightness. If too high or too low then detail is lost. The power used should be the lowest possible that still allows good tissue differentiation
- *Time gain compensation* (sometimes called *depth gain compensation*). Due to attenuation, reflections from an interface deep within the body are weaker than those from an identical interface near the surface. Time gain compensation allows echoes from identical interfaces to appear the same irrespective of their depth within the body. Gain should be adjusted so that image density is even throughout the depth of the scanning field
- *Pre- and post-processing controls*. Can be used to enhance certain details in the image either before it is displayed or after it has been frozen on the screen. It is very easy to produce artefacts and to lose information with these controls
- *B-mode/M-mode selection*
- *Freeze-frame*
- *Cursors*. Can be placed at two points on a frozen image and the distance between them measured. This can be especially useful when making comparisons on follow-up examinations

- *Zoom*. Allows magnification of a part of the image
- *Field of view angle*. Allows selection of a wide or narrow field of view. A wide field allows more structures to be seen together and their relationships examined but either frame rate or resolution is compromised
- *Frame rate*. A slow rate provides better resolution, whereas a fast one gives the best image of moving structures.

Patient preparation

- For gastrointestinal tract scans, it is best to withhold food for several hours prior to the examination. Barium within the tract reduces image quality so if ultrasonography may be required it is best to plan this either prior to a barium study or on the following day
- Scans of the urinary bladder, uterus or prostate gland are facilitated by the presence of urine in the bladder and so it is helpful if the animal is not given the opportunity to urinate for an hour or two before the examination. Air in the bladder is detrimental to image quality: if a pneumocystogram is to be performed it should be done after ultrasonography
- Sedation or general anaesthesia is rarely necessary when performing ultrasound examinations. They may occasionally be used, for particularly anxious or aggressive animals, or sometimes when ultrasound-guided biopsies are to be performed and inappropriate patient movement could pose a risk. For echocardiography, chemical restraint is best avoided as it can influence heart rate and contractility
- To produce the best image possible, an appropriate site (*acoustic window*) on the skin needs to be chosen to place the transducer. Bone and gas are very poor materials through which to image: because they reflect a large proportion of the sound beam, a very white (hyperechoic) area is produced on the screen with virtually no deeper structures imaged due to attenuation of the beam. The acoustic window used is therefore an area – usually as close as possible to the organ under examination – that avoids any bony or gas-containing structures on the path between the skin and the organ
- The hair coat must be clipped from the scanning area and the skin cleaned (with methylated spirit) if necessary. Good contact between skin and transducer is very important, as any air trapped between the two reflects sound back, preventing it reaching the tissues
- A coupling gel or oil is applied between the transducer and the skin, avoiding any bubbles of air, and the transducer is pressed against the patient to scan
- When positioning the patient for the examination, remember that a comfortable animal is more likely to be cooperative. For example, if placing the animal in dorsal recumbency a foam-padded trough or blanket beneath it will be more comfortable than a plastic cradle or hard tabletop. An animal with an abdomen full of fluid may find breathing easier when on its side than on its back, or may prefer to stand. Unlike radiography, for most ultrasonographic examinations the exact position of the animal is not critical and usually a position can be found that suits both patient and ultrasonographer.

Basic scanning technique

The technique is described in Figure 5.32.

5.32 Basic scanning technique

1. Prepare the patient as described in the text.
2. Position the animal in a consistent orientation on the scanning table (this will make learning and consistent orientation of images easier).
3. If right-handed, it is usually easiest to hold the transducer in the right hand and use the left hand to make control panel adjustments.
4. Dim the room lighting to reduce reflections from the screen and enhance visualization of the image.
5. Choose the highest frequency transducer possible for the patient and area under examination. This provides the best resolution but also limits depth of penetration of the sound beam.
6. Set the power setting as low as possible but so that the most distal structure in the field can be seen.
7. Use the time gain compensation control to obtain an image of uniform brightness.
8. Do not press the transducer too hard against the patient as this may cause discomfort. Simply use sufficient pressure to maintain good contact between the skin and the transducer.
9. Scan slowly and thoroughly to ensure complete examination of each structure, scanning organs in at least two planes to allow a three-dimensional impression to be built up from the cross-sectional images.

Ultrasound-guided biopsies

Ultrasonography can be used to guide placement of hypodermic or biopsy needles to obtain tissue from lesions for cytology or histopathology, respectively. Advantages over blind needle placement are that important structures can be avoided and there is a much better chance of obtaining a diagnostic sample from the correct site. In some cases, the technique will obviate the need for invasive surgery.

It is important to ensure that the needle is introduced in the same plane as the beam of sound waves from the transducer, so that it can be visualized in the image. Special biopsy guns are available to attach to the transducer to facilitate this.

When an ultrasound-guided biopsy or fine needle aspirate is to be performed, the skin must be aseptically prepared, sterile gel used and the transducer covered with a sterile sleeve (e.g. a surgical glove), remembering to use gel within the sleeve and avoiding any air bubble entrapment.

Sites for scanning and applications of ultrasonography

Figure 5.33 gives a general guide to sites of skin preparation for imaging various organs, together with an indication of some instances in which ultrasonography is useful. It is not intended to provide an exhaustive list of lesions that can be detected with ultrasonography, nor does the inclusion of a

5.33 Sites for ultrasound scanning

Organ	Position of animal	Area to clip	Applications
Liver and gall bladder	Dorsal or lateral recumbency or standing (may need to reposition to relocate bowel gas if it interferes)	Ventral abdomen from xiphisternum to umbilicus, for several centimetres, to either side of midline	Focal lesions (e.g. tumours) Diffuse lesions (e.g. cirrhosis) Biliary obstruction Portocaval shunts Venous congestion
Liver in deep-chested dogs	Left lateral recumbency	Ventral third of last four ribs on right. Position transducer in intercostal spaces	
Spleen	Dorsal or right lateral recumbency	As for liver but extend further caudally. Locate head of spleen on left then follow body and tail	Focal lesions (e.g. tumours) Diffuse lesions (e.g. venous congestion, tumours)
Kidney	Lateral recumbency with kidney to be examined uppermost (or can use sternal recumbency or standing)	Slightly beneath sublumbar muscles L: behind last rib R: over last two intercostal spaces	Focal lesions (e.g. cysts) Diffuse lesions (e.g. tumours) Hydronephrosis Pyelonephritis Renal calculi
	Dorsal recumbency	Ventral abdomen (but flank approach as above is best)	
Ovary	Lateral recumbency as for kidney	As for kidney. Adrenal located at cranial pole of kidney	Polycystic ovaries Tumours
Adrenal	Lateral recumbency as for kidney	As for kidney. Adrenal located at cranial pole of kidney	Hyperplasia (e.g. Cushing's) Neoplasia
Bladder	Dorsal or lateral recumbency or standing	Ventral midline from umbilicus to pubic brim, or to one side of prepuce in male dogs	Cystic calculi Tumours Cystitis
Prostate	Dorsal or lateral recumbency	To one side of prepuce just in front of pubic brim. Locate bladder then move caudally	Focal lesions (e.g. cysts) Diffuse lesions (e.g. tumours) Paraprostatic cysts
Uterus	Dorsal or lateral recumbency	Ventral midline from umbilicus to pubis	Pregnancy diagnosis Fetal distress/death Pyometra Stump granuloma

Figure 5.33 continues ▶

Organ	Position of animal	Area to clip	Applications
Testicle and scrotum	Dorsal or lateral recumbency	Scrotal testicles rarely require any clipping	Scrotal hernia Tumours Abscesses
Cryptorchid testicle	Dorsal or lateral recumbency	Pubis to umbilicus on appropriate side of midline. Start in front of pubis and work towards bladder and then kidney	Location of intra-abdominal testicle
Pancreas	Dorsal recumbency	Entire ventral abdomen from xiphisternum to umbilicus	Pancreatitis Tumours
Gastrointestinal tract	Dorsal recumbency	Entire ventral abdomen	Bowel wall thickening Intussusception Intestinal tumours
Abdomen	Dorsal recumbency	Entire ventral abdomen	Free fluid Unidentified masses (e.g. mesenteric tumours)
Heart	Left and right lateral recumbency (best to use a table with a hole cut so can scan from beneath; this keeps heart close to chest wall and keeps lung out of the way)	Ventral third of ribs 4 to 6. Transducer placed in intercostal spaces	Pericardial effusion Valvular disease Myocardial disease Congenital defects
Thorax	Left and right lateral recumbency	Over area of interest	Free fluid Masses (e.g. thymic lymphoma, chest wall masses) Diaphragmatic rupture
Eye (most useful if direct visualization obscured)	Use local anaesthetic drops on cornea	Place transducer directly on cornea (can scan through closed eyelids but image not as good)	Retinal detachment Intraocular masses
Orbit	As for the eye	As for the eye	Retrobulbar foreign bodies, abscesses, tumours

particular condition or lesion in the table mean that it will always be detectable using ultrasonography or that the scan will necessarily be able to differentiate it from other lesions that appear similar.

Pregnancy diagnosis

Pregnancy diagnosis is one of the commonest reasons for ultrasonography examination in small animal veterinary practice. Accurate pregnancy diagnosis can be performed from 25 days after the last breeding in the dog, when the gestational sacs will be approximately 1 cm in diameter and heartbeats should be detectable in the embryos. In the cat, accurate pregnancy diagnosis can be performed from 20 days post-breeding onwards. The experienced ultrasonographer can estimate the length of gestation from the size and appearance of the gestational sacs, as well as the number of fetuses, which can be estimated most accurately from day 25 to day 35 of the pregnancy.

Ultrasonography is superior to radiography in this application, avoiding the risk of ionizing radiation to the developing fetuses and allowing much earlier confirmation of a pregnancy. Uterine enlargement becomes visible radiographically at about 35 days but an actual pregnancy cannot be definitely confirmed until skeletal mineralization begins at about 45 days in the dog (a few days earlier in the cat).

Specialized imaging techniques

Fluoroscopy

This technique requires specialist equipment and expertise and its availability is limited mainly to large referral centres with a specialist radiologist. Although new equipment is expensive, second-hand C-arm image intensifiers can sometimes be bought from the National Health Service relatively cheaply. As with all second-hand X-ray sets, the supplier has a responsibility to ensure that the equipment does not emit unnecessary radiation and that it functions properly.

In fluoroscopy, X-rays are used to produce an instantaneous or real-time image over a period of time and so the technique can be used to examine motion. This may be movement of a part of the patient but it may also be used to follow the flow of contrast medium or in some circumstances to aid placement of a needle or catheter in a specific site. The image tones are reversed in fluoroscopy compared with conventional radiography: bone appears black and gas appears white.

Radiation doses are relatively high with this technique compared with conventional radiography and personnel involved with these examinations must be particularly careful to take proper precautions to avoid exposure.

Applications

The clinical indications for fluoroscopy in veterinary work are relatively rare and in some situations the technique can now be replaced by safer techniques such as ultrasonography and endoscopy. Potential uses include:

- Assessment of dysphagia – boluses of food mixed with liquid barium are given to evaluate the process of swallowing
- Assessment of gastric emptying and gastrointestinal motility
- Assessment of animals with suspected portosystemic shunts
- Visualization of removal of oesophageal foreign bodies – endoscopy is preferred by many clinicians
- Monitoring the dilation of strictures (e.g. oesophageal strictures, balloon valvuloplasty in pulmonic stenosis)
- Myelography – to assist in needle placement for lumbar puncture and to check the extent of cranial flow of contrast medium
- Following the passage of contrast medium through various parts of the urinary tract (in incontinence investigations)
- Dynamic evaluation of tracheal collapse (largely superseded by endoscopy, although this requires general anaesthesia)
- Aiding the placement of vascular and cardiac catheters (the need for this has been much reduced by the replacement of angiocardiography with ultrasonography in the majority of cases).

Basic principles

X-rays, produced by an X-ray tube as in conventional radiography and incident on the patient, are transmitted to varying degrees by different parts of the patient according to differences in tissue thickness and composition. The function of an X-ray tube used for fluoroscopy is modified, to allow constant X-ray output for up to several minutes if required, by using very small tube currents and low exposures.

As with conventional radiography, the X-ray photons transmitted through the patient go on to interact with a phosphor screen but in the case of fluoroscopy this is coated on the inside of an evacuated glass envelope, forming part of the image intensifier (Figure 5.34). The absorbed X-ray energy is converted into a pattern of light, proportional in intensity to the pattern of X-ray energies, and this is subsequently converted into a pattern of electrons by a photoelectric screen coated over the phosphor screen. A potential difference (25–35 kV) between the negative input screen of the image intensifier and a positive output screen accelerates these electrons towards the output screen. On their path through the intensifier, they are focused by a series of cylindrical electrodes at intermediate potential. The electrons impinge on the smaller output screen, which also incorporates a phosphor layer to convert the pattern of electrons back into one of light.

The image from the intensifier is intensified, reduced in size and inverted. The intensification and reduction lead to an overall brightness gain in the image, typically of the order of 5000 to 10,000. This is necessary because, due to the low tube current employed, the radiation dose is so small that the image would not be visible without intensification. Contrast in the image is an exact representation of the differential attenuation in different parts of the patient and will be less than in conventional radiography, where the final image contrast also depends on the characteristics of the X-ray film.

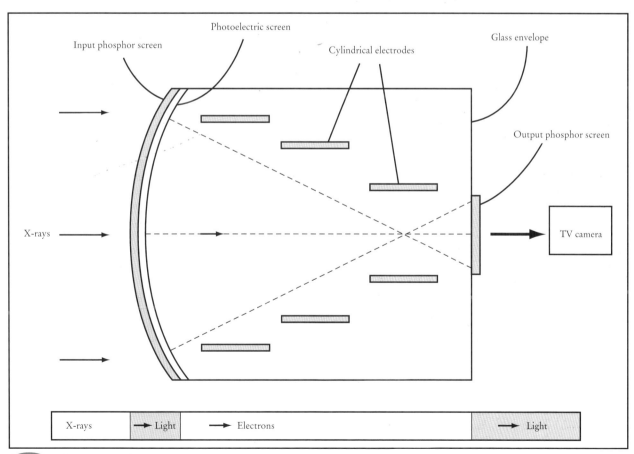

5.34 *The image intensifier.*

Viewing the image

The light emitted from the output screen can be focused on to the input screen of a television camera or transmitted by a fibre-optic cable to the camera. From the TV camera the image is transmitted to a monitor, which is viewed by the radiologist. This output can also be recorded using a video recorder if a permanent record is required.

Alternatively, if a beam splitter is used, 90% of the light from the output screen can be reflected by a partial mirror on to the lens of a 'spot film' camera, which produces a series of rapidly exposed X-ray films, or to a cine-camera. The remaining 10% of the light from the output screen is focused on to the television camera lens so that the image can be monitored at the same time.

Nuclear medicine (gamma scintigraphy)

This method of imaging involves the use of radioactive isotopes (radionuclides) of certain elements. The radioactive decay of these isotopes within the body forms the basis of nuclear medicine.

Like radiography, this technique poses a radiation hazard and special safety precautions are necessary:

- The premises must be registered for the holding and use of radioactive material. Records of the supply, stocks, usage and disposal of radioactive material must be kept for inspection
- Separate areas are required for the preparation and storage of radioactive materials as well as for holding patients after administration of radioactive substances, for imaging and for temporary storage of radioactive waste. Regular monitoring of such areas for contamination needs to be performed
- Personnel should only enter areas where there is radioactivity when it is absolutely necessary. Radionuclides need to be held in shielded containers and drawn up behind a lead barrier, which protects the operator's body and face, into syringes protected by heavy metal or lead glass sleeves. Waterproof gloves are always worn, to avoid any accidental ingestion of radioactive material
- Disposal of containers, syringes, bedding materials and waste material excreted by the patient (this includes respiratory gases, urine, faeces and vomit) must be considered. Solid waste is put into marked bags for incineration; liquid waste must be well diluted with water; bedding can be stored in a protected area until radioactive material has decayed sufficiently for safe release; and gaseous waste can be vented to the atmosphere outside the building.

Applications

Nuclear medicine mainly assesses the physiological function or activity of a particular organ system. It does provide limited information about anatomy and morphology but is much less specific and detailed than other imaging modalities in this respect. However, it is able to demonstrate some lesions much earlier than radiography can, and may detect others that are simply not visible radiographically. It is therefore less specific but more sensitive than radiography. For example, scintigraphy may detect areas of abnormal bone cell activity (such as those caused by metastases to bone from a distant primary tumour or metastases to soft tissues from a primary bone tumour) long before they are otherwise apparent.

A few examples of use of the technique in small animal veterinary practice are as follows:

- Detection of oesophageal and gastrointestinal ulceration and sites of intestinal haemorrhage
- Assessment of oesophageal and gastric motility disorders, including gastric emptying
- Detection and assessment of portosystemic shunts
- Detection of pulmonary embolism
- Detection of active bone tissue (e.g. in tumours, osteomyelitis, fractures) ('bone scan')
- Evaluation of thyroid function (e.g. hyperthyroidism in cats; also used for therapy)
- Evaluation of tissue perfusion of distal extremities (e.g. in traumatized limbs or in cats with embolization secondary to cardiomyopathy).

Basic principles

The atoms of chemical elements have a nucleus made up of protons and neutrons. A nuclide is a specific combination of protons and neutrons. The number of protons is always the same for a particular element and determines its chemical properties, but the number of neutrons is variable. Isotopes of an element have the same number of protons but different numbers of neutrons. Some isotopes are unstable and are known as radionuclides. Unstable nuclei undergo radioactive decay to achieve stability, accompanied by the emission of radioactive particles and radiations.

For imaging purposes, the radionuclide forms part of a compound (the radiopharmaceutical, Figure 5.35), which possesses metabolic properties ensuring that it becomes concentrated in the appropriate part of the body. The radiopharmaceutical is usually administered by intravenous injection and it then concentrates in the organ or tissues under investigation. The decay of radionuclides used in nuclear medicine involves the release of excess energy in the form of gamma rays. Gamma rays are part of the electromagnetic spectrum and have identical properties to X-rays, differing from them only in the way in which they are produced. The emission of gamma rays within the patient signals the location of the radiopharmaceutical within the body.

The gamma rays are detected and the amount of radioactivity from different locations is measured. This can be done in its simplest form using a Geiger counter, which is relatively cheap but provides limited information. The alternative is to use a gamma camera, which can provide much more detailed information. Availability of gamma cameras is limited to just a few of the specialist centres.

The gamma camera has a collimator – a large lead disc drilled with thousands of small holes – which is positioned close to the patient. Each of these holes only accepts gamma rays emitted by the patient along a narrow channel, thus serving to locate the position of any radioactive source within the patient. Behind the collimator is a large phosphor crystal, which absorbs the gamma photons and converts them into flashes of light. The light from the crystal is transferred to an array of photomultiplier tubes that convert the light energy into electrical energy and amplify it at the same time, to produce a voltage large enough to be measured electronically. This information is then processed and stored by a computer and can be displayed on a monitor screen or transferred to a multiformat camera. The brightness of each pixel on the screen corresponds to the number of gamma rays that have been emitted from the corresponding area of the patient. Acquiring a series of separate images in rapid succession performs dynamic imaging that can be used to study the function of, for example, the kidneys, lungs or heart.

Examples of radionuclides and their uses

Body system	Radionuclide	Lesions
Skeleton	99m-Technetium methylene diphosphonate (^{99m}Tc MDP)	Detects increased metabolism (e.g. in bone tumours, infection)
Lung	^{99m}Tc-macroaggregated albumin perfusion studies	Pulmonary embolism Ventilation–perfusion comparison
	^{99m}Tc diethylene triamine pentacetic acid (DTPA) aerosol	Ventilation studies
	^{133}Xenon	Ventilation studies
	^{81m}Krypton	Ventilation studies
Heart	^{99m}Tc erythrocytes labelled in vivo	In humans, assessment of coronary arteries
Brain	^{99m}Tc pertechnetate or glucoheptonate	Tumours, abscesses, vascular disease
Thyroid	^{99m}Tc pertechnetate	Hyperthyroidism
	^{123}Iodine	
Kidney	^{99m}Tc DTPA	Renal function Tumours
Stomach	^{99m}Tc-labelled solids	Gastric emptying
Intestinal tract	^{99m}Tc albumin colloid	Intestinal haemorrhage

Computed tomography (CT)

CT scanning uses X-rays to produce an image of a slice of the patient, usually in the transverse plane (Figure 5.36). This allows a particular structure or area to be imaged without the superimposition of adjacent structures that occurs in conventional radiography. As with conventional radiography, differential tissue attenuation in the patient results in areas in the image that differ in brightness or density. However, smaller differences in contrast that are not apparent with conventional radiographs can be displayed in CT, allowing soft tissues to be differentiated from each other and from fluids (Figure 5.37). Spatial resolution (detail in the image) is not as good in CT, especially when good contrast resolution is required. As in conventional radiography, contrast media can be administered to enhance contrast if required.

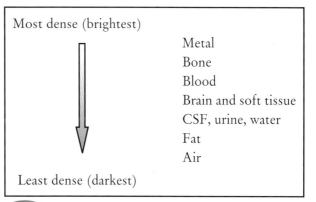

Most dense (brightest)

Metal
Bone
Blood
Brain and soft tissue
CSF, urine, water
Fat
Air

Least dense (darkest)

5.37 *Densities in CT.*

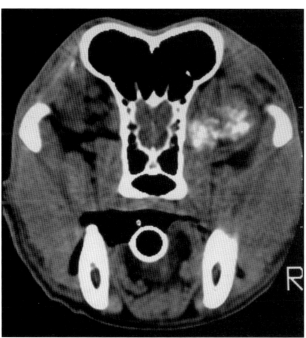

5.36 *CT scan (transverse section) of dog's head showing mineralized tumour affecting the right orbit. Courtesy of D. Habin.*

The radiation dose to the patient is higher in CT scanning than in conventional radiography (it is comparable to that which may be received during fluoroscopy) and it is important that the potential benefits to the patient outweigh the potential risks. General anaesthesia is required, as image acquisition takes quite a long time.

Although second-hand CT scanners are often readily available relatively cheaply from human hospitals updating their equipment, the maintenance and running costs are high. An experienced radiographer is required to perform examinations and these can be quite time consuming. For these reasons, the technique is only available at a few specialist veterinary centres. However, many human hospitals will perform scans on animals during stand-down time by special arrangement. The cost of an individual scan is high.

Applications

The area in which CT scanning has probably been most widely used in the veterinary field is in the detection and evaluation of intracranial lesions. Standard radiographs are usually of no value because of superimposition of the bony structures and lack of contrast between soft tissues. Ultrasonography is similarly unhelpful as there is no suitable acoustic window through which to image (apart from in young animals with an open fontanelle).

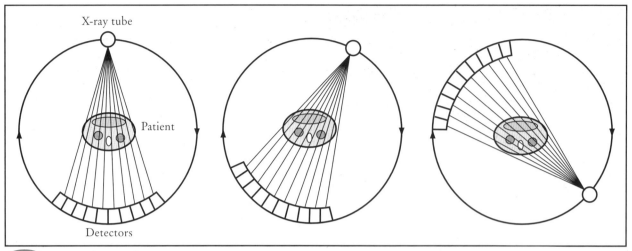

5.38 *Computed tomography scanning.*

There are numerous other potential applications for the technique, including examinations of the spine, thorax and abdomen. A few examples of the use of CT scans in the veterinary field are:

- Detection of brain tumours
- Evaluation of lesions affecting the nasal cavity, sinuses, orbit (see Figure 5.36) and middle ear
- Detection of renal lesions such as cysts and tumours (CT allows earlier detection of such lesions than is possible with conventional radiography)
- Detection of metastatic lesions within parenchymatous organs (e.g. liver).

Basic principles

The position of the transverse sections to be made is chosen from an initial survey scan (usually a sagittal section). The thickness of each slice will normally be about 10 mm but can be altered.

The scanner has an X-ray tube, which needs to have a high heat capacity, as an examination can take up to several seconds. As they leave the tube, the X-rays are collimated into a thin beam, in a fan shape just wide enough to cover the area of the body under examination. The X-rays emerging from the patient fall on an array of several hundred detectors and these convert the photon energy into electrical energy, the size of the current being proportional to the transmitted beam intensity. The tube and detectors are mounted on opposite sides of a ring that rotates 360° around the patient (Figures 5.38 and 5.39). During each complete rotation the X-ray tube produces about 300 pulses of X-rays.

Each time the tube is pulsed, each detector measures the intensity of the radiation that falls on it and the information is stored in the computer. As the tube rotates around the patient, intensity values are stored for each detector at each different position, the values varying according to the tissues through which each X-ray photon has passed.

The computer divides the tissue slice up into a number of squares, known as voxels, which correspond to pixels in the final image, and uses the data acquired to calculate the CT number (a measure of attenuation) for each of these. The computer makes an image from each rotation of the tube and detectors. After a single rotation, the table and patient are moved a specified distance relative to the X-ray tube and detectors to acquire the data for the next image slice.

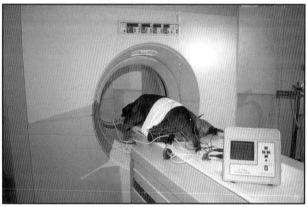

5.39 *Computed tomography scanning: the patient's head is placed within the rotating ring of X-ray tube and detectors for a brain scan.*
Courtesy of J. Mould.

The computer can manipulate the data before they are displayed, to allow production of the best possible image of the tissues of interest. This is done by selecting what is known as a window, which includes all the tissues of interest; for example, it may be chosen to look at bone, soft tissues, lungs or blood. Those structures in the slice that have a CT number that falls outside the selected window appear totally black or white, whereas the tissues of interest are displayed as various shades of grey. The wider the window chosen, the greater is the number of tissue types that will be included in the grey scale but the less specific is the information that will be gained about any particular tissue. By choosing a narrow window, small changes in contrast will be seen more easily.

The window settings only affect the displayed image: the data is retained in the computer and can be manipulated after the scan is completed. This means that the same tissue slice can be examined with different windows if required, without further exposure of the patient. For example, a head scan might be examined with bone, brain or blood windows, depending on the type of lesion present, whereas abdominal scans use mainly soft tissue windows.

Magnetic resonance imaging (MRI)

Like CT, MRI produces images of slices through the patient and therefore has the same advantage of lack of superimposition of adjacent structures (Figure 5.40). As with CT, a computer is used to calculate differences between

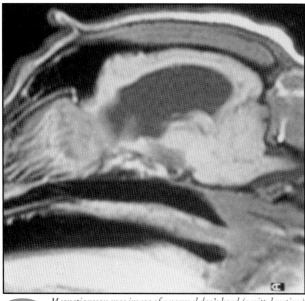

5.40 *Magnetic resonance image of a normal dog's head (sagittal section) demonstrates excellent contrast between soft tissue structures. Courtesy of A. Hotston Moore.*

individual voxels in a slice of the patient and represent these differences as different shades of grey in the pixels on the display screen. In CT the differences are in X-ray attenuation between voxels, whereas in MRI it is the hydrogen content of the tissues that is measured.

MRI compared with CT

- Spatial resolution and soft tissue contrast are superior with MRI
- MRI does not use ionizing radiation and is probably safer than CT
- MRI uses multiplanar reconstruction: images can be viewed in any plane
- MRI is more sensitive to small concentrations of contrast media (though they are rarely required in MRI)
- CT is better for evaluating bone and calcium
- CT is less sensitive to motion artefact caused by patient movement (data acquisition takes a long time in MRI and blurring of images can therefore be a problem; for this reason, the technique is rarely used for thoracic or gastrointestinal imaging because of involuntary movements associated with respiration and peristalsis).

The MRI scanner is a very expensive piece of equipment and installation and running costs are also high. Individual scans are consequently very expensive and availability is even less than for CT scanning. The use of a strong magnetic field in MRI necessitates a special building sited away from structures that may themselves become magnetized (e.g. steel girders), or structures that may distort the magnetic field or cause radiofrequency interference (e.g. power cables). All equipment within the building must be made of non-magnetic materials, as any metal objects will become extremely hazardous projectiles if placed near the magnet. General anaesthesia is required and particular attention has to be paid to the provision of anaesthetic equipment. Obviously, equipment such as anaesthetic trolleys, vaporizers and endotracheal tube connectors cannot be made of metal and all metallic objects (e.g. needles, collars) must be removed from the animal before it is placed inside the magnet.

Applications

To date, MRI has been used predominantly to examine the head and spine in small animal veterinary practice. It is extremely useful in the detection of mass lesions within the brain, and the location and appearance of brain tumours on MRI scans often allow differentiation of tumour type. Its use in examination of the eye and orbit is also described.

In humans, MRI is the technique of choice for most musculoskeletal and articular problems. The excellent soft tissue contrast allows direct depiction of bone marrow, ligaments, tendons and cartilage. There is nothing to prevent it being an equally useful technique in this field in small animals, apart from its cost.

Basic principles

The physics involved in the working of the MRI scanner is complicated and the description offered here is in the most simplistic terms. The patient is placed in a magnet; a radiowave is sent into the patient as a short radiofrequency pulse and is then turned off. The patient's tissues re-emit the radiowaves, which are received by the scanner and used to construct the image. The radiofrequency energy is absorbed and emitted by the nuclei of hydrogen atoms (which consist of single protons) in water and fat in the body. Different tissues contain different amounts of water and therefore display different properties in a magnetic field. Only hydrogen nuclei that are mobile give signals; those that are effectively immobilized (e.g. in bone and calculi) do not. Air contains no hydrogen and therefore produces no signal, always appearing black in images.

Other techniques

None of the following techniques is routinely used in veterinary medicine, although their use is occasionally described in the literature. They are techniques that have emerged only relatively recently in the human field and so are unlikely to be widely used for animal imaging for a considerable time.

Digital radiography

This uses conventional X-rays but data are stored digitally in a computer rather than on X-ray film. This allows windowing of the image to look for specific structures (in a similar way to windowing in CT) and other post-processing of the image.

Digital subtraction angiography

This is used to produce images of blood vessels, filled with contrast medium, in isolation from other tissues. Images of the same region are taken before and after injection of contrast medium, while avoiding any patient movement between images, and the images are stored in the computer memory. The image taken before contrast injection shows normal anatomy and is subtracted pixel by pixel from the contrast image, showing filled vessels superimposed on the normal anatomy. The resulting image shows only the filled vessels.

Single photon emission computed tomography

SPECT is the nuclear medicine equivalent of CT imaging in radiography. A gamma camera rotates slowly around the patient, acquiring a view every 6° of rotation. A computer then uses the data to produce an image of a transverse slice through the patient.

Positron emission tomography

PET is similar to SPECT but, instead of gamma rays, the isotopes used emit positrons (which are like electrons but with a positive rather than negative charge). A positron camera consists of a ring of detectors that surround the patient. It is used for regional blood flow imaging.

Spiral (helical) CT

A conventional CT scanner produces images of slices through the patient with no overlap, by moving in a circle around the patient at each location. A helical CT scanner moves the patient constantly through the tube ring and detectors while the beam spins around the patient at the same time. This produces a spiral of two-dimensional data that can then be manipulated to produce slices in any plane (multiplanar reconstruction, as in MRI) or even three-dimensional images.

Further reading

Barr FJ (1990) *Diagnostic Ultrasound in the Dog and Cat.* Blackwell Scientific, Oxford

Douglas SW, Herrtage ME and Williamson HD (1987) *Principles of Veterinary Radiography*, 4th edn. Baillière Tindall, London

Farr RF and Allisy-Roberts PJ (1997) *Physics for Medical Imaging*. WB Saunders, Philadelphia

Morgan JP (ed.) (1993) *Techniques of Veterinary Radiography*, 5th edn. Iowa State University Press, Ames

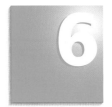

6 Clinical pathology in practice

*Clare M. Knottenbelt
and Kostas Papasouliotis*

This chapter is designed to give information on:

- Setting up the practice laboratory, maintenance and quality control
- Use of automated haematology and biochemistry analysers
- Interpretation of haematology, biochemistry and urinalysis results
- Performance of more advanced haematology techniques such as reticulocyte and platelet counts
- In-house FeLV and FIV tests
- Clotting function tests and tests for immune-mediated diseases
- Basic transfusion medicine
- Collection and interpretation of cytology samples
- Bone marrow aspirates and biopsies
- Biopsy techniques

Introduction

During recent years, the number of in-house laboratories has dramatically increased. Four main reasons account for this phenomenon:

- Desire for faster and more accurate results
- Increase in the number of clinical cases where laboratory data are considered essential
- Increased availability of a wide range of equipment and tests for in-house use
- Veterinary nurses who have the ability and technical skills to perform laboratory procedures.

Setting up the in-practice laboratory

- Designate space
- Designate nurse in charge
- Health and Safety rules – accident book
- Laboratory manual
  - Operating procedures for each instrument
  - Methodology of each analytical procedure
  - Address of companies providing chemicals, reagents, standards, controls

  - Instructions for use of Quality Control Samples (including reconstitution techniques)
  - Acceptable limits for each lot of control solution
- Record results obtained and samples submitted to external laboratories
- Refrigerator and freezer
- Microhaematocrit high-speed centrifuge
- Good quality microscope / glass slides
- Stains: rapid cytology stain (e.g. Diff-Quik™), Leishman's, Gram, new methylene blue
- Good quality centrifuge, automatic pipettes, Pasteur pipettes
- Refractometer with a scale for both urine specific gravity and protein levels (usually g/dl)
- Urine strips, pH paper
- Bins, sharps bins for disposable items.

Test selection
The techniques performed in an in-house laboratory should meet the following criteria:

- Be simple to perform
- Provide rapid and accurate results (in order to be of real benefit to the patient)
- Be cost-effective (both to the client and to the practice).

The following tests can be performed in-house and meet these criteria:

- Blood smears (see Chapter 5 of *BSAVA Manual of Veterinary Nursing*)
- Haematology (automated analyser)
- Biochemistry (automated analyser)
- Serum electrolytes (automated analyser)
- Parvovirus faecal antigen test
- Urinalysis (see Chapter 5 of *BSAVA Manual of Veterinary Nursing*)
- FeLV and FIV (in-house test kits)
- Cytology.

Quality control

To ensure that results obtained from the practice laboratory are accurate it is vital that regular quality control checks are undertaken. All instrumentation (including, for example, the refractometer, microhaematocrit centrifuge and automated analysers) should be subject to quality control. Records of routine quality control checks and instrument servicing should be documented, so that they are performed at the correct time intervals. The simplest method of quality control is to compare results obtained in the practice laboratory with those from an external laboratory.

Haematology

A simple but well designed practice laboratory can provide rapid and accurate haematology results. Considerable information can be obtained with basic equipment such as a microscope and microcentrifuge (see Chapter 5 of *BSAVA Manual of Veterinary Nursing*).

Interpretation of blood smears requires knowledge of normal cell morphology. This can be acquired through practical experience and continuous training.

The availability of relatively inexpensive haematology analysers for the practice laboratory has increased potential for haematological assessment. Although some of the analysers provide quantitative differential white blood cell (WBC) counts, cell types are sometimes grouped together and these should *not* be used in lieu of microscopic evaluation of a properly stained blood smear, because of potential inaccuracies.

Sample collection

This is described in Chapter 5 of *BSAVA Manual of Veterinary Nursing*.

- Blood for haematology should be collected into tubes containing ethylene diamine tetra-acetic acid (EDTA), which prevents coagulation by complexing calcium
- Blood collected into tubes containing heparin must be analysed immediately, because heparin results in poor cell staining
- If blood is not analysed within 3 h, it should be refrigerated at 4°C to minimize haemolysis and degenerative cell changes
  - Red cell parameters remain unchanged if the blood is refrigerated for up to 24 h
  - In contrast, 6–24 h of storage at room temperature (i.e. postage samples) results in red cell swelling, which can increase packed cell volume (PCV), haematocrit (Hct) and mean corpuscular volume (MCV) and decrease mean corpuscular haemoglobin concentration (MCHC)

- The nuclear and cytoplasmic characteristics of white blood cells in EDTA (especially canine neutrophils) can change dramatically within a short time of collection
- At least two blood smears should always be prepared as soon as blood is collected.

Basic in-house haematology

Measurement of packed cell volume (PCV)

Technique
The technique for measurement of PCV is described in Chapter 5 of *BSAVA Manual of Veterinary Nursing*.

This is a reliable test for the evaluation of anaemia (decreased PCV) and/or polycythaemia (increased PCV). It is simple, inexpensive to perform and accurate, provided the sample is collected and handled correctly. Visual examination of plasma in the capillary tube can reveal haemolysis (red), lipaemia (milky) or icterus (yellow). The plasma can subsequently be used for determination of the total protein concentration.

Malfunction of the microhaematocrit centrifuge is uncommon but can result in artificially increased PCVs due to insufficient red blood cell (RBC) packing. The following quality control tests can be performed periodically:

- Measure the PCV of a commercial standard blood sample
- Check the packing time of a sample
- Compare results with those obtained by a diagnostic laboratory.

Interpretation of results
Figure 6.1 gives a guide to normal values for haematological parameters. Figure 6.2 describes the interpretation of abnormal parameters.

6.1 Normal values[a] for haematological parameters

Parameter	Units	Normal range	
		Dogs	Cats
RBC	(x 10^{12}/l)	5.5–8.5	5.5–10
Packed cell volume	(%)	39–55	24–45
Haemoglobin	(g/dl)	12–18	8–14
MCV	(fl)	60–77	39–55
MCHC	(%)	32–36	30–36
WBC count	(x 10^9/l)	6–15	7–20
Neutrophils	(x 10^9/l)	3.6–12.0	2.5–12.8
Immature (band) neutrophils	(x 10^9/l)	0	0
Lymphocytes	(x 10^9/l)	0.7–4.8	1.5–7.0
Monocytes	(x 10^9/l)	0.0–1.5	0.07–0.85
Eosinophils	(x 10^9/l)	0–1	0–1
Basophils	(x 10^9/l)	0.0–0.2	0.0–0.2
Platelets	(x 10^9/l)	200–500	300–600

a *The normal values given in this table should only be used as a guide. Whenever possible use the normal ranges provided by the laboratory or equipment used to perform the test.*

Parameter	High levels	Low levels
RBC and PCV	Erythrocytosis • Dehydration • Polycythaemia	Anaemia
WBC count	Leucocytosis • Inflammation • Infection • Neoplasia • Leukaemia	Leucopenia • Sepsis • Salmonellosis • Bone marrow disease • Chemotherapy
Neutrophils	Neutrophilia • Inflammation • Infection • Neoplasia • Granulocytic leukaemia	Neutropenia • Overwhelming sepsis • Endotoxaemia • Salmonellosis • Parvovirus • FeLV/FIV • Bone marrow disease • Chemotherapy • Immune destruction
Immature (band) neutrophils	Left shift • Inflammation • Infection	Normal (Unless infection or inflammation present)
Lymphocytes	Lymphocytosis • Viral or chronic infections • Stress-associated (cats) • Leukaemia	Lymphopenia • Chronic disease • Steroid administration • Viral infections • FeLV • Hyperadrenocorticism
Monocytes	Monocytosis • Stress (dogs) • Steroid administration • Chronic inflammation • Neoplasia • Necrotic or suppurative diseases • Immune-mediated disease	Monocytopenia • Not significant
Eosinophils	Eosinophilia • Parasitic disease (e.g. fleas, worms) • Allergic disease (e.g. asthma, atopy) • Mast cell disease • Leukaemia	Eosinopenia (may be normal) • Chronic disease or stress • Steroid administration • Hyperadrenocorticism
Basophils	Basophilia As for eosinophils	Basopenia • Not significant
Platelets	Thrombocytosis • Leukaemia • Chronic inflammation	Thrombocytopenia • Platelet clumping (especially if traumatic blood sampling or EDTA used) • Immune destruction • Bone marrow disease • Excessive consumption • Normal in Cavalier King Charles Spaniels

Chronic disease or stress, treatment with corticosteroids and hyperdrenocorticism can all result in a typical white blood cell picture known as a **stress leucogram**. *This comprises:*
  • *Leucocytosis*
  • *Mature neutrophilia*
  • *Lymphopenia*
  • *Monocytosis*
  • *Eosinopenia.*
Recent treatment with corticosteroids can therefore make interpretation of white blood cell levels very difficult. The absence of a stress leucogram in an animal with a chronic illness raises the suspicion of hypoadrenocorticism (a disease that can cause vague clinical signs).

Blood smears

Technique
The technique is described in Chapter 5 of *BSAVA Manual of Veterinary Nursing*. As a matter of routine, at least two smears should be prepared from a fresh blood sample, because anticoagulant will affect blood cell morphology.

Staining
The use of appropriate stains will maximize the benefit obtained from examination of a blood smear:

- Leishman's for routine haematology (see Chapter 5 of *BSAVA Manual of Veterinary Nursing*)
- New methylene blue for reticulocyte counts (see below).

Examination
The finished blood smear has three major areas:

- Start of the smear, which is thick and contains overlapping RBCs, WBCs and platelets
- Monolayer (thinner middle area of major examination) containing RBCs, WBCs and platelets that are well spread and retain their shape
- End of the smear, which contains sparse RBCs that are flattened and distorted, ending in the tail (feathered edge). The tail contains numerous WBCs and clumped platelets, if present. It is not a useful area for examining the morphology of RBCs but can be important for detecting large abnormal cells.

6.3 Assessment of platelet numbers from a blood smear

Average platelet number over ten fields		Equivalent total platelet count
Dog	Cat	(x 10⁹/l)
4	3	100
8	6	200
12	9	300
16	12	400
20	15	500
24	18	600

6.4 New methylene blue stain for reticulocytes

1. Place two drops of whole blood in EDTA in a small tube containing new methylene blue (Merret tube).
2. Gently tap the tube for 10 seconds to mix the blood and stain.
3. Leave tube at room temperature for 15 minutes.
4. Prepare air-dried smears (see *BSAVA Manual of Veterinary Nursing*).
5. Examine monolayer area of the smear under oil immersion (x 100) (see *BSAVA Manual of Veterinary Nursing*)
6. Count the number of reticulocytes present in 1000 RBCs and calculate the percentage of the RBCs that are reticulocytes.

Note: Cat reticulocytes have a prolonged maturation time. Aggregate reticulocytes (Figure 6.6) are released from the bone marrow and mature into punctate reticulocytes after 1 week. Punctate reticulocytes remain in high numbers for up to 4 weeks after regeneration of the bone marrow and therefore should not be included in the reticulocyte count.

Systematic microscopic examination is extremely important (see Chapter 5 of *BSAVA Manual of Veterinary Nursing*). A platelet count is performed by counting the number of platelets in 10 high-power (oil immersion) microscopic fields (Figure 6.3). Absolute numbers for each of the white cell types can be calculated by performing a differential white cell count.

Reticulocyte counts

Technique
New methylene blue stain (Figure 6.4) is routinely used for the identification of reticulocytes. It causes precipitation of intracellular ribosomal RNA into a dense dark blue aggregate (reticulin) (Figures 6.5 and 6.6); mature RBCs appear yellowish or light green. The number of reticulocytes appearing per 1000 red cells is divided by 10 and expressed as a percentage.

Interpretation
A reticulocyte count quantifies the number of immature RBCs present in the blood and therefore helps to determine whether a regenerative response is occurring in an anaemic animal. Normal dogs and cats will have small numbers of reticulocytes in their peripheral blood. The increase in the circulating reticulocytes does not become evident until 2–3 days after the onset of the anaemia.

In anaemic animals the reticulocyte count (%) can be misleading. The low total RBC count results in an artificially increased percentage value. As the anaemia gets more severe, more immature reticulocytes are released from the bone marrow. These immature cells take longer to mature and therefore reticulocytes accumulate in the peripheral blood.

Equations have been developed to improve the accuracy of using reticulocyte counts to determine bone marrow regeneration (Figure 6.7).

6.5 Identification of reticulocytes in the dog and cat

Reticulocyte type	Appearance after staining
Dog reticulocytes and cat aggregate reticulocytes	RBCs containing clusters or chains of granules
Cat punctate reticulocytes	RBCs containing a few (2–10) dark blue granules

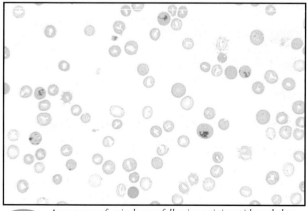

6.6 *Appearance of reticulocytes following staining with methylene blue.*

Parameter	Method	Mild regeneration	Marked regeneration
Reticulocyte percentage (%)	Visual count (see Figure 6.5)	Dogs: >1% Cats: >0.5%	Dogs: >20% Cats: >5%
Corrected reticulocyte percentage	CRP = reticulocyte (%) x (patient's PCV ÷ normal PCV)	Dogs: >1% Cats: >1%	Dogs: >5%
Reticulocyte production index (dogs)	RI = CRP / life span of reticulocytes[a]	Dogs: >1	Dogs: ≥ 3
Absolute reticulocyte count	Reticulocyte (%) x RBC count	Dogs: >150 x 10^9/l Cats: >50 x 10^9/l	Dogs: >500 x 10^9/l Cats: >200 x 10^9/l

a Reticulocyte life span in dogs:

PCV (%)	Reticulocyte life span (days)
45	1
35	1.5
25	2
15	2.5

Automated haematology analysers

A wide variety of haematology analysers are available for the in-house laboratory, although many are specifically designed for the analysis of human samples. The simplest models provide RBC, WBC and platelet counts, and measure the red blood cell mean corpuscular volume (MCV) and haemoglobin (Hb) concentration of the sample. From these values the instrument can calculate:

- Haematocrit (Hct) = RBC x MCV
- Mean corpuscular haemoglobin (MCH) = Hb/RBC x 10
- Mean corpuscular haemoglobin concentration (MCHC) = Hb/Hct x 100.

See Chapter 5 of *BSAVA Manual of Veterinary Nursing* for definitions of MCV, MCH and MCHC.

It should be noted that the terms PCV and haematocrit cannot be used interchangeably:

- PCV reflects the red cell volume following packing
- Haematocrit is the total red cell volume calculated from the number of red cells per litre and the average volume of each red cell (MCV).

Packed cell volumes can be affected by varying centrifuge speed and duration, or by the presence of red cell agglutination.

Instruments utilizing newer technologies can also provide information on the different types of white blood cells and morphological features of RBCs (i.e. nucleated red blood cells). These fully automated analysers are capable of diluting the sample, adding solutions that lyse cells and printing the results.

Coulter counters (electronic resistance analysers)

This technology is based on the principle that cells are poor electrical conductors.

- Blood is mixed with a diluent that conducts electricity and the mixture is passed through an opening in an electrode
- As the cell passes through the opening, the resistance to electrical flow increases

- The machine counts the number of times resistance increases in a given volume of blood, and therefore calculates the number of cells present in that volume
- By measuring the magnitude of the change in resistance, the machine can calculate the size of each cell it has counted
- RBCs and platelets are differentiated by their differing size, while WBC counts are performed after the RBCs have been lysed. Occasionally WBCs may be included in the RBC count, but this problem is usually insignificant unless the high white cell count is extremely elevated (e.g. patients with leukaemia).

Quantitative buffy coat analysis

Quantitative buffy coat (QBC) analysis is based on the principle that various blood cells have different densities, so that when blood is spun in a microhaematocrit tube, cell types are sorted into separate layers.

- Whole blood in EDTA is placed in an oversized haematocrit-type tube and a cylindrical float is used to expand the buffy coat layer (containing the white blood cell and platelet layers), which lies between the red cell layer and the plasma
- The tube is coated with a fluorescent dye (acridine orange) which stains nucleoproteins, lipoproteins, glycosamines and other cellular substances
- The stain causes cellular components to fluoresce in blue–violet light
- The machine distinguishes cell types by detecting differences in the intensity of fluorescence
- This information is processed into a buffy coat profile graph (drawn at the top of a QBC printout).

Interpretation

Interpretation of abnormal parameters is outlined in Figure 6.2. The following points should be borne in mind:

- The normal range given by the machine should always be used, as normal ranges can vary with the technique used
- Microscopic examination of blood smears remains an essential quality control check for WBC counts, platelet counts and WBC differential counts and should always be performed

- The available in-house systems cannot detect the presence of the following, which can only be identified by examination of a blood smear:

  - Immature (band) neutrophils (left shift) (Figure 6.8)
  - Toxic neutrophils (basophilic, granular, vacuolated cytoplasm) (Figure 6.9)
  - Nucleated red blood cells
  - Atypical cells, such as blasts or mast cells
  - Abnormal RBCs, such as spherocytes (small round dense RBCs without central pallor) (Figure 6.10)
  - Heinz bodies (denatured haemoglobin within the RBCs)
  - Blood parasites.

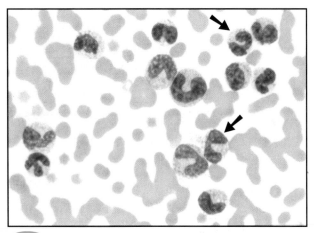

6.8   *Immature (band) neutrophils (arrows).*

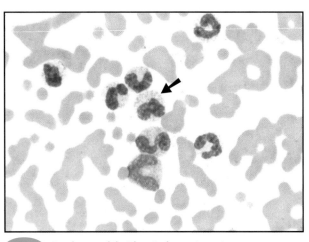

6.9   *Band neutrophil with toxic changes (arrow).*

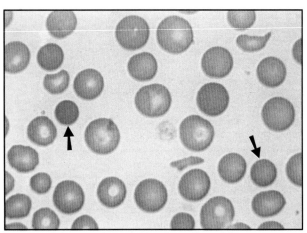

6.10   *Spherocytes (arrows). Note the small round dense appearance of the RBCs. There is no evidence of central pallor.*

Biochemistry

Sample collection

This technique is described in Chapter 5 of *BSAVA Manual of Veterinary Nursing*. Most biochemical tests can generally be performed on either plasma or serum.

- The anticoagulant fluoride oxalate is used to inhibit the glycolytic enzymes in the RBCs. These enzymes are normally responsible for depleting glucose levels in blood samples within hours of collection
- In cases where dry reagent strips are used for glucose measurement, samples containing fluoride must not be used because this enzyme inhibitor will also inhibit the enzymes used in the reagent strips. To avoid this, fresh whole blood or fresh heparinized samples should be used
- Calcium levels should not be estimated on samples collected into EDTA, fluoride or oxalate, because these anticoagulants bind calcium – resulting in falsely low values.

Sample preparation

Plasma is widely preferred to serum, because there is no delay in separation and a greater volume of sample material can be obtained. If samples cannot be tested immediately, serum or plasma should be refrigerated (or frozen if considerable delay is expected). All samples must be allowed to return to room temperature before testing. Preparation of serum and plasma samples is described in Chapter 5 of *BSAVA Manual of Veterinary Nursing*.

Basic in-house biochemistry

Interpretation

Normal values and interpretation of biochemical abnormalities are given in Figures 6.11 and 6.12. Plasma protein levels should be interpreted in conjunction with PCV when assessing anaemia and dehydration. For example: dehydration can mask anaemia by resulting in a normal PCV (due to loss of intravascular fluid). The concurrent elevation in total plasma, however, will identify the presence of dehydration and suggest that, once dehydration has been corrected, anaemia may be significant. Specific profiles are used to detect disease in a particular organ (Figure 6.13) or as a screening test prior to anaesthesia (Figure 6.14).

6.11   Normal values for biochemical parameters in blood

Parameter	Dog	Cat
Total protein (g/l)	58–73	69–79
Albumin (g/l)	26–35	28–35
Globulin (g/l)	18–37	23–50
Alkaline phosphatase (IU/l)	20–60	20–100
Alanine aminotransferase (IU/l)	15–60	15–60
Creatinine (umol/l)	30–90	26–118
Urea (mmol/l)	1.7–7.4	2.8–9.8
Glucose (mmol/l)	3–5	3.3–5.0
Calcium (mmol/l)	2.3–3.0	2.1–2.9
Sodium (mmol/l)	139–154	145–156
Potassium (mmol/l)	3.6–5.6	4–5
Inorganic phosphate (mmol/l)	0.9-1.2	1.4–2.5
Total thyroxine T4 (nmol/l)	15–48	13–48

The normal values given in this table should only be used as a guide. Whenever possible use the normal ranges provided by the laboratory or equipment used to perform the test.

Interpretation of biochemical abnormalities

Parameter	High levels	Low levels
Total protein	Dehydration Infection/inflammation Feline infectious peritonitis (FIP) Some types of neoplasia	Protein loss (kidney, intestines, skin loss) Liver failure Infectious exudate (e.g. pyometra, peritonitis)
Albumin	Dehydration	Protein loss (kidney, intestines, skin loss) Liver failure Infectious exudate (e.g. pyometra, peritonitis)
Globulin	Dehydration Infection/inflammation Feline infectious peritonitis (FIP) Liver inflammation Some types of neoplasia	Overwhelming infection
Alkaline phosphatase[a]	Young growing animal Steroid administration (dogs) Hyperadrenocorticism Liver disease Bone tumours	Not significant
Alanine aminotransferase	Liver disease	Not significant
Bilirubin	Haemolytic anaemia Liver disease Bile duct obstruction	Not significant
Creatinine	Kidney disease Dehydration	Muscle wasting
Urea	Kidney disease Dehydration	Low protein diet Liver failure
Glucose[b]	Diabetes mellitus Stress (cats)	Insulin overdose Insulinoma Liver tumour/failure Sample storage
Calcium	Lymphosarcoma Hypoadrenocorticism Kidney failure Hyperparathyroidism Some tumours	Eclampsia Hypoparathyroidism
Inorganic phosphate	Kidney failure Hypoparathyroidism	Hyperparathyroidism
Potassium	Acute renal failure Urethral obstruction Hypoadrenocorticism	Chronic anorexia Kidney disease
Total thyroxine	Hyperthyroidism	Hypothyroidism Any chronic disease

[a] Treatment with corticosteroids can result in elevations of alkaline phosphatase in the dog. This phenomenon is not seen in the cat.
[b] The stress associated with blood sampling can result in an increase in blood glucose levels in the cat.

6.13 Interpretation of common laboratory profiles

Profile	Conditions highlighted	Interpretation
Kidney Urea Creatinine	Pre-renal (dehydration, shock, hypovolaemia) Renal (chronic or acute renal failure) Post-renal (urinary tract obstruction)	Calculate how significant the increase is in terms of the normal range (e.g. 2 x normal range) Compare the increase seen in urea and creatinine in these terms If urea is proportionally more elevated than creatinine, pre-renal problems are most likely Renal and post-renal problems cannot be accurately differentiated, although in post-renal problems creatinine may be proportionally more elevated than urea
Liver Alkaline phosphatase Alanine aminotransferase Albumin	Liver disease Bile duct obstruction	Alkaline phosphatase is not specific for liver disease. It is elevated by recent treatment with corticosteroids, liver disease and biliary obstruction. Injured liver cells produce this enzyme Alanine aminotransferase is liver-specific. Liver cells that are severely injured or destroyed produce this enzyme The liver produces albumin. Levels fall when liver failure is present

Selection of tests for a preanaesthetic profile

Test	Conditions	Approach to abnormalities
PCV	Dehydration Anaemia	Dehydration should be corrected prior to anaesthesia Anaemia may be exacerbated by surgical procedures. Blood transfusion may be required prior to anaesthesia if anaemia is severe
Total protein and albumin	Dehydration Low protein	Dehydration should be corrected prior to anaesthesia Many anaesthetic agents are bound to protein in the blood stream. Low protein levels can result in more sudden and profound anaesthesia, unless dose rates are reduced
Urea and creatinine	Dehydration Renal disease	Dehydration should be corrected prior to anaesthesia Renal disease may limit the excretion of some anaesthetics. The reduced blood pressures associated with anaesthesia may reduce renal perfusion and exacerbate renal disease unless intravenous fluids are administered
Liver enzymes	Liver disease	The liver is responsible for the metabolism of some anaesthetic agents. Reduced dose rates may therefore be required when liver disease is present
Platelets	Low platelet count	Platelets are vital for normal clot formation. Low platelet counts will predispose the patient to bleeding during surgical or biopsy procedures. Transfusion of platelet-rich plasma or fresh whole blood may be required during surgery
Electrolytes	Secondary electrolyte disturbances	Electrolyte abnormalities can increase risk of cardiac arrhythmia during anaesthesia. Electrolyte abnormalities should be corrected prior to anaesthesia whenever possible

Refractometer

Technique
Although primarily used for urine, the refractometer can also estimate protein concentrations in serum, plasma and pleural or abdominal fluids (Figure 6.15). Cerebrospinal fluid has a very low protein content, which cannot be detected by the refractometer.

Dry reagent strips

Technique
The blood sample is applied to the reagent pad for a short period of time. The pad is either rinsed with water or dried (depending on the type of strip). The colour of the pad is compared to a colour chart. The dry reagent strip for measuring blood urea nitrogen (BUN) has been widely used in veterinary practices; however, it may underestimate blood urea. Blood glucose strips are reliable and can be read in a handheld reflectance meter for increased accuracy and precision (Figure 6.16).

6.15 **Estimation of total plasma protein using a refractometer**

1. Calibrate the refractometer:
   - Place water beneath plastic cover of refractometer
   - Adjust until SG = 1.000
   - Dry refractometer
2. Centrifuge a capillary tube of whole blood in EDTA as described for measurement of PCV (see *BSAVA Manual of Veterinary Nursing*)
3. Break the capillary tube above the buffy coat layer
4. Place a few drops of plasma on the glass plate of the refractometer and firmly close lid
5. View through the lens at the other end and read value from the scale (g/dl)
6. Multiply figure by 10 to get value in g/l.

Note: Lipaemic (turbid, milky) and haemolysed (red) plasma samples can result in erroneously elevated protein concentrations by this method. The refractometer is also inaccurate when total plasma protein levels are markedly reduced (< 35 g/l) (hypoproteinaemia).

6.16 **Using a glucometer to measure blood glucose**

Equipment required: drop of fresh blood, glucose strips, glucometer, swab

1. Check that the glucometer programme number matches the number on the side of the glucose strip container
2. Lay the glucose strip on the swab with pad facing up
3. Open the side of the glucometer (where the stick will be placed) and press the glucometer start button
4. The glucometer will 'beep' when the blood should be applied to the pad – ensure that the whole pad is covered with blood
5. When the glucometer counter starts to 'bleep' again, use the swab to blot the pad dry on the third 'bleep'
6. Place the glucose strip into the port of the glucometer, ensuring that the pad is facing towards the main part of the machine. Close the port before the glucometer countdown has reached zero
7. The result should be given within a matter of seconds of the countdown reaching zero.

Quality control: Normal control fluid can be measured and may be particularly useful when glucose strips are close to their expiry date.

Automated 'dry' chemistry analysers

Analyser type

Individual test analysers
Instruments designed primarily to run individual tests tend to have the largest test menu and greater flexibility, but often carry a higher cost per test. These instruments are best used in cases where single tests or small sets of tests are required. They are unsuitable for practices that perform large numbers of comprehensive health screens.

Profile analysers
The use of predetermined profiles is cheaper and requires minimum technical expertise. They are most suitable for practices with a moderate to high caseload that are primarily performing health profiles for diagnostic or screening purposes. Predetermined profiles reduce flexibility and are costly when only a specific individual test is required.

Individual test and profile analysers
Analysers that allow selection of individual tests or a panel of tests are more flexible than profile instruments. Each individual test costs the same as those performed on an individual test analyser. They are unsuitable for practices that perform large numbers of comprehensive health screens. Combination instruments may require more technical input and can be more expensive to purchase.

Analyser maintenance
Used consumables and discarded blood samples should be disposed of daily. Appropriate cleaning procedures should be performed routinely. The analyser should be calibrated and cleaned on a regular basis according to the manufacturer's instructions. Failure to perform routine cleaning and calibration can result in system failure or inaccurate results. Software upgrades are commonly provided free of charge and the company should therefore be advised of any errors or problems being experienced. Consumables should be stored appropriately and routinely checked to ensure that they have not exceeded their expiry date. Although some analysers will record the results from recent samples, it is advisable to make a permanent record of all results obtained. This record will enable determination of whether the analyser has developed an error in the measurement of any given parameter.

In-house 'wet' chemistry analysers
These systems operate on the same principles as the dry chemistry analysers but use tubes containing liquid reagents. Some wet chemistry analysers are available for in-house use. They are more expensive and more technically demanding than the available dry chemistry analysers but may be cheaper for individual tests.

Quality control
Quality controls are the procedures developed to identify and reduce errors in analysis. Errors can occur in instruments, reagents or operator techniques. The general principle of quality control is to compare the results obtained by in-house testing with those obtained by an external (and presumably more accurate) test centre. This can be achieved in two ways:

- By dividing a fresh sample and testing one half in-house and the other half at an external laboratory. Unfortunately it can be difficult to compare results from in-house and external laboratories as normal ranges may vary significantly. It may also be impractical and costly to perform quality controls on all parameters measured in-house. This method should be considered a good system for assessing the accuracy of the in-house system as a whole and therefore should be used on an intermittent basis as part of the quality control checks
- By assaying a sample of known concentration (usually provided by the manufacturers). This method is cheap and reliable and should form the basis of regular quality control checks. By using the same sample for repeated measurements it is possible to determine both the accuracy and the precision (i.e. the repeatability) of the testing procedure.

In commercial laboratories, control sera of different concentrations (one with values within the normal range) are used routinely with each batch of samples. This is impractical for the in-house laboratory and therefore their quality control programmes are restricted to only one control for each biochemical parameter.

It is important to note that an analyser that appears to be accurate when analysing normal samples may be very inaccurate when samples contain abnormal levels of a particular parameter. Ideally the controls used should comprise a solution with normal parameters and one with abnormal parameters. This should assure reliability of results outside the reference range.

Control solutions must be prepared and stored correctly in order to provide accurate quality control information.

Urinalysis

In-house urinalysis can be performed using a refractometer, urine dipsticks and examination of urine sediment (see Chapter 5 of *BSAVA Manual of Veterinary Nursing*). Although the refractometer is an accurate way of assessing urine specific gravity (SG), it should always be calibrated before use by obtaining a reading for distilled water (SG = 1.000).

Urine dipsticks have been developed for humans and so results in a veterinary context can be inaccurate. The use of dipsticks should therefore be limited to obtaining a rapid result before performing further tests on the same sample, or to minimizing the cost of monitoring a patient (e.g. during the control of diabetes mellitus).

Interpretation of results
When using urine dipsticks it is essential that they are dry and within their use-by date. Care should be taken to ensure that they are read at the correct time and all results (positive or negative) should be recorded. Figure 6.17 describes the interpretation of the results of dipstick urinalysis.

Dipstick parameter	Normal	Abnormality	Causes
Specific gravity (SG)[a]	Dogs: 1.015–1.040 Cats: 1.015–1.050	Hyposthenuria (< 1.010)	Diabetes insipidus Hyperadrenocorticism Hypercalcaemia Hypokalaemia Pyelonephritis Drug therapy Intravenous fluids
		Isosthenuria (1.011–1.018)	Kidney failure
		Hyperosthenuria (> 1.040)	Normal or dehydration
pH[b]	5.5–7.0	Increased pH (urine too alkaline)	Delay in analysis Delay in reading dipstick Recent eating Urinary tract infection Drug administration
		Decreased pH (urine too acidic)	Metabolic alkalosis (due to severe vomiting)
Protein[c]	Negative, or trace if urine very concentrated	Proteinuria (increased protein)	Delay in reading dipstick Urinary tract infection Haematuria Kidney disease Pyometra or vaginitis Prostatic disease Myeloma Lymphosarcoma Nephrotoxic drugs
Glucose	Negative	Glucosuria	Diabetes mellitus Stressed cats Severe bladder haemorrhage Primary renal glucosuria (rare) Fanconi syndrome (rare)
Ketones[d]	Negative	Ketonuria	Diabetic ketoacidosis Prolonged anorexia
Bilirubin	Cats: negative Dogs: trace	Bilirubinuria	Haemolytic anaemia Liver disease causing jaundice Bile duct obstruction
Blood[e]	Negative	Haematuria (RBCs)	Urinary tract infection Prostatic disease Trauma Urinary calculi Neoplasia Vaginitis Renal haemorrhage
		Haemoglobinuria	Haemolytic anaemia Haematuria
		Myoglobinuria	Acute muscle trauma Myositis Hyperthermia

a   Must be interpreted alongside plasma urea/creatinine. Dipstick measurements of SG are unreliable.

b   Changes in urine pH can predispose the patient to crystalluria.

c   Small amounts of protein may be significant if the urine is very dilute. The protein:creatinine ratio is used to determine the significance of proteinuria by taking into account urine concentration. The ratio cannot be used if there is evidence of lower urinary tract inflammation on examination of the sediment (See BSAVA Manual of Veterinary Nursing, Chapter 5).

d   Dipsticks do not detect one of the ketones (β-hydroxybutyrate) and therefore may underestimate the amount of ketones present in the urine of a patient with diabetic ketoacidosis.

e   Dipsticks cannot differentiate between the presence of red blood cells, haemoglobin and myoglobin. Examination of the sediment will determine the presence of red blood cells (See BSAVA Manual of Veterinary Nursing, Chapter 5).

Virology

In recent years, recognition of the clinical importance of feline leukaemia virus (FeLV) and feline immunodeficiency virus (FIV) has led to the development of various test kits for rapid and accurate in-house diagnosis. FeLV and/or FIV testing is performed for cats showing clinical signs suggestive of infection, cats that have been in contact with an infected animal and prior to breeding or FeLV vaccination.

FeLV

Samples required

- Plasma or serum from non-haemolysed blood gives the most reliable results
- Anticoagulated whole blood (not centrifuged) may be used
- The use of whole blood without anticoagulant can cause false positive results
- Saliva tests are associated with a large number of false positive results and each positive result should therefore be confirmed by testing a blood sample.

Tests

The FeLV tests detect virus antigen – specifically a protein called p27, which is identical in all known FeLV strains. Since the FeLV tests detect antigen, they are not affected by the presence of antibodies or by previous vaccination.

There are two types of in-house tests available:

- Enzyme-linked immunosorbent assay (ELISA)
- Rapid immunomigration (RIM)/immunochromatography.

Principle of the ELISA (Figure 6.18)

- Antibodies against the p27 protein are bound to a membrane or well
- Blood is added to the well and any p27 antigen present will attach to the antibodies in the well
- The blood is washed away, but the antigen attached to the antibody remains
- A conjugate (antibody against p27 bound to an enzyme) is then added, which binds to the p27 antigen stuck in the well
- After washing a second time, the conjugate remains fixed to the p27 antigen in the well
- Finally a substrate is added that changes colour when it comes into contact with the enzyme (Figure 6.19).

Principle of the RIM/immunochromatographic tests

This kit comprises a membrane containing antibodies against p27, which are attached to gold or latex particles.

- The blood sample is applied to the membrane, which acts as a filter
- Viral antigen p27 attaches to the labelled antibodies in the membrane
- The diluent is then added, which allows the gold or latex particles to migrate across the membrane to the reaction zone
- The reaction zone is a band of more anti-p27 antibody. This band captures the migrating p27 antibody–antigen complexes, forming an antibody–antigen–antibody sandwich covered in gold or latex particles
- The accumulation of these particles forms a visible band
- Any unbound particles migrate further and form a visible band at the validation zone (Figure 6.20).

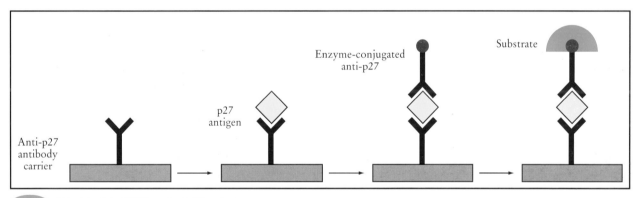

6.18 *Principle of the ELISA test for FeLV antigen.*

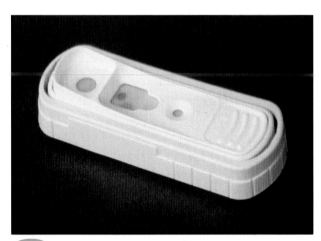

6.19 *A positive ELISA test for FeLV.*

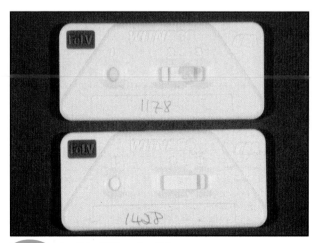

6.20 *A positive RIM test (top kit).*

FIV

Samples required
Plasma or serum from non-haemolysed blood gives the most reliable results.

Test
The FIV tests detect *antibodies* to the virus, as virus particles (antigens) are only present at very low levels in the blood. Detection of antibodies to FIV indicates lifelong infection with FIV.

Principle of the ELISA tests
This is very similar to the FeLV ELISA (Figure 6.18) except that a viral protein (antigen) is bound to the membrane of the well. The viral protein can be a synthetic protein replica or part of a real FIV particle. The antigen–antibody complex that forms when antibodies in blood are added to the well are detected by adding a conjugate comprising the same viral protein bound to an enzyme.

Principle of the RIM/immunochromatographic tests
This is very similar to that described above for FeLV with the difference that the test detects antibodies rather than antigen. The RIM kits currently available detect antibodies to a synthetic protein.

Assessment of clotting function

There are a number of tests available to assess clotting function (Figure 6.21). These tests are usually performed in patients with bleeding disorders or that are to undergo procedures that may result in significant bleeding, such as liver biopsy, nasal biopsy or surgical procedures. Each test assesses a different aspect of the process of clot formation.

The clotting cascade is traditionally divided into three pathways:

- Intrinsic pathway
- Extrinsic pathway
- Common pathway.

Each pathway contains specific clotting factors. By using multiple tests of clotting function it is sometimes possible to identify which pathway and therefore which clotting factors are affected (Figure 6.21). Unfortunately many bleeding disorders eventually cause abnormalities in more than one pathway as other clotting factors are depleted.

6.21 Assessment of clotting function

Test	Principle	Method
Activated clotting time (ACT)	Tests intrinsic and common pathways and platelet number and function.	1. Place 2 ml fresh blood in ACT tube 2. Keep tube at body temperature 3. After 60 seconds, check for clot formation every 10 seconds 4. Clot should form within 90 seconds
Activated partial thromboplastin time (APTT)	Tests intrinsic and common pathways	1. Collect 2 ml of whole blood in potassium citrate anticoagulant 2. Submit to external laboratory 3. Laboratory may require a sample from an age-matched normal for comparison
Prothrombin time (PT)	Tests extrinsic and common pathways	1. Submit whole blood in potassium citrate anticoagulant to an external laboratory
Buccal mucosal bleeding time (BMBT)	Tests platelet and blood vessel function	1. Place patient in lateral recumbency 2. Tie top lip with a gauze bandage to expose mucosal surface 3. Using a Simplet or scalpel blade, make stab incision in mucosa 4. Record time until bleeding stops 5. Collect blood with filter paper, avoiding touching the incision 6. Normal is less than 2.5 min 7. If bleeding for more than 5 min apply pressure to incision This test should not be performed if platelet numbers are significantly reduced.
Platelet count	Tests platelet numbers	1. Make a fresh blood smear and stain with Diff-Quik or Leishman's 2. Count number of platelets in ten high power (oil immersion) microscopic fields 3. See Figure 6.3 **OR** 1. Submit whole blood in potassium citrate anticoagulant to an external laboratory EDTA tends to cause platelet clumping within hours of collection

Tests for immune-mediated diseases

External laboratories usually perform the available tests for immune-mediated disease. The samples required for each test are listed in Figure 6.22, but the type of sample required should always be confirmed with the laboratory performing the test. Figure 6.23 illustrates the principle of the Coombs' test.

Blood transfusions

Blood transfusions are being performed with increasing frequency in veterinary practice. In order to avoid the risk of a transfusion reaction (which can be fatal in some cases) it is necessary to ensure that the donor and recipient have compatible blood groups. This can be achieved by performing a cross-match or by blood typing both donor and recipient. Figure 6.24 identifies the circumstances in which cross-matching and blood typing should be performed.

Cross-matching

Cross-matching assesses the effect that recipient serum antibodies will have on the donor cells (*major cross-match*) and the effect that donor serum will have on recipient cells (*minor cross-match*). Since the main aim of the transfusion is to provide the recipient with red blood cells, it is most important that the recipient's serum antibodies do not destroy donated cells and in so doing evoke a transfusion reaction. Cross-matching will only predict the likelihood of an immediate reaction occurring – it cannot predict whether antibodies could develop in the future. Figure 6.25 describes the procedure for cross-matching.

6.22 Tests for immune-mediated diseases

Test	Detects	Disease	Sample required
Antinuclear antibody (ANA)	Antibodies against the nuclear material of various cell types (joints, skin, etc.)	Many autoimmune disorders	Serum
Rheumatoid factor (RF)	Antibodies against other antibodies	Rheumatoid arthritis	Serum
Coombs' test (Figure 6.23)	Antibodies against RBCs	Immune-mediated haemolytic anaemia	Whole blood in EDTA

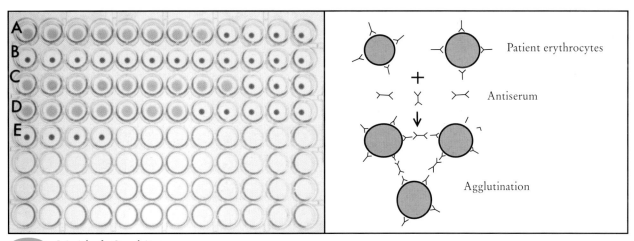

6.23 *Principle of a Coombs' test.*

6.24 Tests to determine donor and recipient compatibility

Species	Recipient status	Minimum tests	Tests required to ensure matching
Dogs	First transfusion	None	Check donor is negative for DEA 1.1 and 1.2
	Subsequent transfusions	Cross-match	Check donor is negative for DEA 1.1 and 1.2 and cross-match
Cats	First transfusion	Blood type	Blood type and cross-match
	Subsequent transfusions	Blood type and cross-match	Blood type and cross-match

Performing a cross-match

Equipment required: heparinized plasma and whole blood in EDTA from the donor and the recipient, test tubes, well plate or slides, saline, automatic pipettes

Technique:

1. Centrifuge both EDTA samples at 3000 rpm for 10 min.
2. Remove the supernatant (plasma and buffy coat layer).
3. Resuspend the erythrocytes in saline.
4. Wash the red cells by recentrifuging the samples at 3000 rpm for 10 min.
5. Remove the supernatant (saline).
6. Resuspend the erythrocytes in saline to make a 3–5% solution.

To perform major cross-match:

7. Mix two drops of donor red cell suspension with one or two drops of recipient plasma, either on a slide or, preferably, in test tubes or well plates.

To perform minor cross-match:

8. Mix two drops of recipient red cell suspension with one or two drops of donor plasma, either on a slide or, preferably, in test tubes or well plates.
9. Ideally tubes should be incubated at 37°C for 60 min.
10. A positive result is recorded if haemolysis (diffuse reddening of solution) or agglutination (granular appearance) is seen.

> The use of slides is less reliable since only serum with high levels of antibody directed against red blood cells will show agglutination. Mixing whole blood from recipient and donor gives a crude indication of compatibility but is unreliable and is not recommended.

Blood typing

Blood typing involves looking for particular antigens on the surface of the red blood cells. It is more accurate than cross-matching as it will predict the likelihood of an immediate or a delayed reaction due to future antibody development. Desktop kits are now available for blood typing cats and for identifying canine donors that possess the antigen most likely to cause a reaction (DEA 1.1).

Cytological samples

Fine needle aspiration

Fine needle aspirates (FNAs) are a rapid and simple method of determining the cytological characteristics of an abnormal mass or organ. A needle is used to detach cells from the organ or mass. A syringe attached to the needle can be used to create suction, which increases the harvest of cells. Suction is particularly useful when aspirating masses that do not exfoliate cells well. The equipment required for this procedure is listed in Figure 6.26. Figure 6.27 describes the two techniques available for collection of FNAs; Figure 6.28 describes making a squash preparation.

Body fluids

Sample collection and preparation

Sample collection is described in Chapter 5 of *BSAVA Manual of Veterinary Nursing* and Chapter 4 of this volume. Body

Sample sites and equipment required for fine needle aspiration

Procedure	Sample site	Equipment required
Needle-only technique	Superficial lymph nodes Superficial masses Palpable internal masses Abdominal organs (liver, spleen, kidney, intestines) Consolidated lung	Clippers and spirit 23 gauge 1¼ inch needle Clean slides (degrease with alcohol)
Needle with suction	Superficial lymph nodes Superficial masses Palpable internal masses	Clippers and spirit 23 gauge 1¼ inch needle 10 ml syringe Clean slides (degrease with alcohol)

Obtaining a fine needle aspirate

1. Lay out at least five slides on a clean surface and draw back an empty 10 ml syringe.
2. Clip the area to be aspirated and clean with spirit.
3. Immobilize the mass if possible (aspirates of body organs should be performed with ultrasound guidance).

Needle-only technique:

1. Insert the needle into the mass and move it rapidly in and out (to ensure cells are broken away from the tissue).
2. Remove the needle and attach to a syringe containing 10 ml of air.

Fine needle aspirate with suction:

1. With the needle attached to the syringe, insert the needle into the mass.
2. Draw back on the syringe to the 5ml mark (this should be quite difficult because of the negative pressure created).
3. Whilst maintaining suction, move the needle around within the mass.
4. Release suction before removing the needle from the mass.
5. Remove needle from end of syringe, draw 10 ml air into the syringe and reattach to the needle.

Making the smear:

1. With the bevel of the needle facing down squirt out the contents of the needle on to one end of a clean slide.
2. Make a smear (*BSAVA Manual of Veterinary Nursing*, Chapter 5) or a squash preparation (Figure 6.28).

Making a squash preparation

1. Place material on a clean slide.
2. Place a second slide over the top of the sample at right angles to the first.
3. Allow material to spread out under the effect of gravity.
4. Rapidly draw second slide along the first.
5. Both slides can be rapidly air-dried and stained.

> It is usually the second slide that provides the best material for examination as the smear tends to be less thick and air-dries more rapidly.

6.29 Interpretation of abdominal and thoracic fluid tests

Fluid type	Appearance	Protein levels	Cell counts (x 10⁹/l)	Predominant cell types
Normal	Clear, straw-coloured	Low (<25 g/l)	Low (<3.0)	Mesothelial cells Macrophages
Transudate	Clear, straw-coloured	Low (<25 g/l)	Low (<0.5–1.0)	Mesothelial cells Macrophages
Modified transudate	Yellow or pink-red turbid fluid	Low (usually <25 g/l)	Medium (1.0–7.0)	Mesothelial cells Macrophages, RBCs Neutrophils
Exudate	Turbid	High (usually >35 g/l)	High (>7.0)	Neutrophils Macrophages Neoplastic cells
Chylous or pseudochylous	Milky fluid	High	High	Lymphocytes Neutrophils

fluids are usually collected to determine the amount of protein and the type and number of cells present. The amount of fluid collected will vary according to the site:

- Cerebrospinal fluid tap and arthrocentesis commonly produce small volumes of fluid
- Abdominal or thoracic paracentesis commonly produces larger fluid volumes.

Direct smear
This technique allows rapid assessment of cell type and a crude assessment of cell numbers and can be performed in-house. It is therefore useful for very small fluid volumes, which would be lost if placed in a container. Unfortunately direct smears often have a low cellularity and multiple smears are required to perform WBC differential counts and to search for neoplastic cells.

Cell counts
Cell counts are usually performed using a Coulter counter (see above). Cell integrity needs to be preserved and samples are commonly placed in anticoagulant (usually EDTA). The addition of anticoagulants and other preservatives may alter cell morphology and make cell differentiation more difficult. Since different preservatives are preferred for different samples, it is always advisable to contact the laboratory before sample collection so that the appropriate samples are submitted.

Cytospin preparations
Cytospin preparations concentrate the cell content of a body fluid without disrupting the cell morphology or integrity. This allows a larger number of cells to be examined on any given smear and therefore makes WBC differential counts and the search for neoplastic cells easier to perform. External laboratories have specialist equipment which centrifuges the sample and drops the cell pellet on to a slide for smearing. A similar effect can be achieved by making a sediment smear in-house (see Chapter 5 of *BSAVA Manual of Veterinary Nursing*).

Cytospin preparations are useful for most body fluids and are mandatory for cerebrospinal fluid, which typically has a low cell count.

Fluid analysis
Analysing the biochemical components of a body fluid is useful for determining the type of disease process present.

Protein levels are particularly important for determining the characteristics of abdominal and thoracic effusions and the presence of inflammation within the CSF.

- Samples that are submitted to an external laboratory for analysis should be placed in a plain tube
- Since myelography is contraindicated in cases with elevated CSF protein levels, measurement of protein levels should be performed, before injection of contrast, using the Protein Square of a urine dipstick
- The protein content of larger fluid volumes can be estimated by placing a few drops of the supernatant into a refractometer (Figure 6.15)
- The measurement of urea and creatinine in abdominal fluid is used to diagnose rupture of the urinary tract.

Interpretation of fluid analysis
The characteristics of the different types of fluid are described in Figure 6.29. The type of fluid present in a body cavity often helps to determine the cause of fluid accumulation (Figure 6.30).

6.30 Causes of abdominal and thoracic fluid

Fluid type	Causes
Transudate	Low blood protein
Modified transudate	Cardiac disease Liver disease Neoplasia Chronic transudate
Exudate	Infection (e.g. peritonitis, pleurisy) Neoplasia
Chylous or Pseudochylous	Cardiac disease (thoracic only) Lymphatic (especially thoracic duct) rupture

Staining cytology samples
Cytology samples can be stained with rapid cytology stain for assessment in-house. If samples are to be submitted to an external laboratory they should be air-dried and despatched unstained.

Interpretation of cytology samples

Cytology samples can be difficult to interpret. Normal cells can have some of the characteristics normally attributed to malignant cells when undergoing multiplication or present in an abnormal location (Figure 6.31).

6.31 Characteristics of malignancy

- Specimen is highly cellular
- Multiple nuclei within each cell
- Multiple nucleoli within each nuclei
- Evidence of dividing cells (mitosis)
- Abnormal nuclear to cytoplasmic ratio
- Large poorly differentiated cells
- Variation in cell characteristics
- Single population of grossly abnormal cells.

Bone marrow sampling

Bone marrow samples are collected to determine the presence of bone marrow disease in cases of abnormal blood cell counts, leukaemia and anaemia. Bone marrow aspiration involves the collection of bone marrow granules containing cells, which are then made into smears (Figure 6.32). Bone marrow biopsy involves the collection of a core of bone marrow tissue for histopathological examination, which is placed in formalin. Figure 6.33 lists the advantages and disadvantages of the two techniques. Figures 6.34 and 6.35 show the equipment required.

Sites of collection

Bone marrow samples are usually collected from the iliac crest. In cats and small dogs, the proximal humerus or proximal femur may be preferable.

6.32 Making a bone marrow aspirate smear

1. Place three slides on a small pile of gauze swabs.
2. Following collection of an aspirate in EDTA in a 10 ml syringe, cover two or three slides with the contents of the syringe.
3. Leave for approximately 1 min to allow the bone marrow granules to settle.
4. Tip each slide slightly to pour off the liquid on to the swabs below.

> Avoid tipping the slides too far as this may result in the granules being removed from the slide.

5. Check for the presence of bone marrow granules (yellow-white firm granules).
6. Draw a clean slide back through the granules at an angle of 45 degrees, collecting some of the granules on the edge of the clean slide.
7. Slide the edge along a clean slide to make a smear.
8. Repeat steps 6 and 7 until a number of bone marrow smears have been produced.

NOTE: Making a bone marrow smear uses the same technique as making a blood smear (see BSAVA Manual of Veterinary Nursing) except that when making a bone marrow smear the drawing back and pushing away are performed on separate slides.

6.33 Bone marrow aspiration and biopsy: advantages and disadvantages

Technique	Advantages	Disadvantages
Bone marrow aspirate	Rapid results	Low cellularity may be due to poor technique or bone marrow disease
Bone marrow biopsy	Preserves architecture of the bone marrow	Sample requires decalcification; therefore results may be delayed

6.34 Equipment required for bone marrow sampling

Technique	Equipment required
Bone marrow aspiration	General anaesthesia or sedation and local anaesthetic Clippers Surgical scrub and spirit Scalpel blade 10 ml syringe containing 2 ml of 3% EDTA solution 15–20 clean glass slides Klima biopsy needle 14–18 gauge (Check that stylet and cap fit if using resterilized needle) Note: EDTA solution is inactivated by daylight and therefore should regularly be made up fresh or stored in a dark cupboard
Bone marrow biopsy	General anaesthesia or sedation and local anaesthetic Clippers Surgical scrub and spirit Scalpel blade Jamshidi biopsy needle (check stylet and cap fit if using resterilized needle) 10% formalin in a container

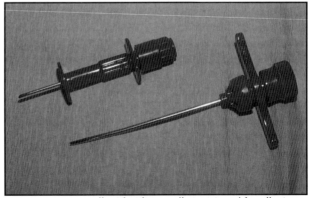

6.35 *Biopsy needles. The Klima needle (top) is used for collecting a bone marrow aspirate. The Jamshidi needle (bottom) is used for bone marrow biopsy.*

Biopsy techniques

Fine needle aspiration

- FNAs (see Figures 6.26 and 6.27) provide a rapid assessment of cell type, but provide no information regarding tissue architecture or local infiltration
- Tissue architecture and infiltration help to determine the tissue or cell of origin and the degree of malignancy.

Trucut biopsy

- A Trucut or similar needle removes a core of tissue from the centre of a mass or organ
- The samples collected are large enough to provide information about tissue architecture, but small enough to minimize bleeding
- This biopsy technique is often used when surgical procedures or general anaesthesia are contraindicated
- It must be noted that patients with clotting abnormalities may bleed significantly after this procedure
- Spring-loaded biopsy guns are available that fire the needle into the tissue to be sampled
- This technique is commonly used for the percutaneous collection of liver biopsies.

Excisional biopsy

- In excisional biopsies, a mass or organ is removed completely
- Excisional biopsies provide information about tissue architecture and have the advantage that the diseased tissue or organ is removed in its entirety
- This type of biopsy is commonly performed on superficial lymph nodes and the spleen
- Inadequate tissue margins may require repeat surgery if the disease process has been identified as malignant.

Incisional biopsy

- In incisional biopsies, only a small part of the mass or organ is removed
- Like Trucut biopsies, they provide information about tissue architecture
- If a malignant disease process is identified, a second surgical procedure will be required to remove the diseased tissue, or the organ is removed in its entirety
- The technique allows collection of both abnormal and apparently normal tissue close to the edge of the mass
- Incisional biopsies are commonly performed on large skin tumours
- Examination of the margin of the mass allows assessment of tumour infiltration
- This method ensures that adequate tissue margins are removed along with the mass or organ when definitive surgery is carried out.

Further reading

Bush BM (1975) *Veterinary Laboratory Manual*. William Heinemann Medical Books, London

Bush BM (1991) *Interpretation of Laboratory Results for Small Animal Clinicians*. Blackwell Science, Oxford

Davidson MG, Else RW and Lumsden JH (1998) *BSAVA Manual of Clinical Pathology*. BSAVA, Cheltenham

Meyer D and Harvey J (1998) *Veterinary Laboratory Medicine. Interpretation and Diagnosis*, 2nd edn. WB Saunders, Philadelphia

Pratt PW (1996) *Laboratory Procedures for Veterinary Technicians*, 3rd edn. Mosby Year Book, St Louis

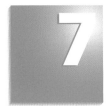

7 General practice management

Carole J Clarke

This chapter is designed to give information on:

- Records the practice must keep
- Staffing and personnel issues
- Managing practice stock
- The practice's responsibility for health and safety
- Improving practice presentation

Introduction

This chapter covers the main management areas in which a veterinary nurse may be involved from day to day. Each section will introduce the topics, give enough detail to understand the issues and prompt further reading. Legal and statutory requirements will be outlined, but the relevant detail should be obtained from the statutory authorities. Titles for further reading in these and other management areas are given at the end of the chapter.

The veterinary practice as a business

The primary concern of veterinary nurses is with animals in their care. To give patients the best treatment, staff need both skills and resources (equipment, drugs, etc.) and practices must supply these by offering adequate facilities and training.

A veterinary practice is a business, offering services and products to the public or to other businesses (e.g. veterinarians or farmers) in return for payment. It must attract and keep clients in order to survive. The money earned by the business is used to pay the costs of running the business and providing the service (overheads and establishment costs), and to pay interest on financial loans taken out to establish and improve the business. Any money left after settling all these costs is the profit, and producing sufficient profit is all important if the business is to prosper. A proportion of the profit should be reinvested regularly to upgrade facilities and purchase new equipment. Loans are also paid off out of profit.

It follows that for a veterinary practice to be successful it must be managed effectively by someone with knowledge of the business aspects of practice. Veterinary surgeons and veterinary nurses frequently find themselves taking on more

7.1 Areas of responsibility in practice management

Marketing the practice	Market research Customer service Advertising Special projects, newsletters, brochures, etc.
Human resources	Planning staff requirements Recruiting staff Duty rotas Performance appraisal Planning and implementing training Payroll
Buildings and equipment	Purchasing/leasing Maintenance Servicing
Overhead costs	Controlling and budgeting costs (e.g. heat, light, cleaning, stationery, bad debts)
Direct costs	Stock control and organization Negotiating with suppliers
Current legislation	Ensuring practice complies with: – Health and Safety and COSHH (Control of Substances Hazardous to Health) regulations – Employment legislation – Medicines legislation – Data Protection Act – Ethical standards
Finance	Negotiate loans, bank and other finance charges

management work, often alongside their clinical responsibilities. Many practices now employ a practice manager or administrator who may have a clinical, financial or business background in another industry or service sector.

In all cases, it is helpful to consider the responsibilities of a manager in the areas shown in Figure 7.1.

One person may take overall responsibility for all areas, or several members of staff (partners, nurses, administrative staff) may share different areas.

Record keeping

Veterinary practices are required to generate and keep many different types of record in the course of their work:

- Client or customer records
- Medical records
- Personnel records
- Financial records
- Health and Safety files.

The principles of record keeping are shown in Figures 7.2 and 7.3. Records may be kept in paper files or on computer and usually a combination of both is used. The important requirements of any filing system are that it should be simple to understand, easy to use and safe. Authorized personnel should be able to access and use the information easily, but confidentiality must be maintained and access denied to any person not entitled to see the files. Other considerations are legal requirements to keep documents for a certain length of time and the Data Protection Act 1984 (see Figure 7.4).

7.2 Principles of good record keeping

To make records easy to use, they should be:

- Conveniently located (e.g. at point of use)
- In a logical order (e.g. numerical, alphabetical or colour-coded
- Clearly labelled
- Returned to file regularly if removed
- Purged regularly (remove old or unused records to keep files a manageable size).

To keep records safe, they should be:

- Protected from day-to-day physical damage (e.g. spilt coffee, dust and dirt)
- Protected from fire and flood damage if possible (e.g. by using a fireproof safe for computer disks)
- Copied if important (e.g. by backing up computer data – Figure 7.3)
- Regularly checked or validated
- Archived when necessary in a logical manner.

To keep records secure from unauthorized access, they should be:

- Locked in filing cabinets or in a safe
- Password-protected on a computer
- Destroyed when no longer needed (e.g. by shredding or burning)
- Only accessed when absolutely necessary.

7.3 Backing up computer files

- Computer file back-up is essential for retaining information in the event of a fire, theft or computer breakdown
- Files can be backed up to a remote server, floppy disk or zip disk, or data or other tape
  - The choice of system is determined by the amount of data backed up, speed of back-up and cost
  - Always purchase the best available back-up option when installing new equipment
- Back-up tapes or disks should be stored in a secure fireproof area, or off the premises
- The back-up routine should be simple, preferably automatic, and checked regularly
- Backed-up data should be verified, ideally at each back-up
- Back-up tapes or disks should be clearly labelled; several should be used in rotation
- Programs and operating systems can be backed up separately from data files, ensuring that the most recent version of software is backed up. Monthly back-up or retention of original disks may suffice
- Data files (medical records, client data, financial and PAYE records) should be backed up more regularly, or every time they are updated
  - In general, PAYE records can be backed up weekly or monthly at every pay day
  - All other records should be backed up daily or twice daily.

Client records
Essential information for contacting clients during and following treatment and for sending accounts includes:

- Correctly spelt name
- Address and telephone numbers (daytime and evening).

Additional notes might include:

- Directions to client's premises or farm
- Any special discount or surcharge rate
- Payment arrangements
- Client preferences.

The client database is also used for proactive marketing, such as mailing booster vaccination reminders and sending newsletters or information about new treatments and products.

Because the database is often used for mailings, taking the trouble to check spelling and address formats is important for maintaining a professional image. Client information is confidential and must never be disclosed to a third party without permission. Comments not intended for clients to see should be avoided, particularly as clients are entitled to see all information held about them on computer under the Data Protection Act 1984 (Figure 7.4). Used computer printouts containing client information should be destroyed, preferably by shredding.

Medical records
Information to be recorded includes:

- Clinical findings
- Diagnoses
- Treatments
- Laboratory results and results of investigations
- Referral letters
- Telephone contacts.

7.4 Data Protection Act 1984

Any veterinary surgeon or partnership holding or controlling personal data (on employees or clients) on computer is required to register with the Data Protection Registrar (Wycliffe House, Water Lane, Wilmslow, Cheshire SK9 5AF). Registration lasts for 3 years.

Failure to register in respect of information that is subject to the Act is a criminal offence, punishable by a maximum fine of £5000 in the Magistrates' Court or an unlimited fine in the Crown Court.

The data protection principles are set out in a code of good information handling practice. Personal data must be:

- Obtained and processed fairly and lawfully
- Held only for the purposes specified
- Used or disclosed only in accordance with these purposes
- Adequate, relevant and not excessive for those purposes
- Accurate and, where necessary, kept up to date
- Kept no longer than is necessary for those purposes
- Accessible to the individual (e.g. owner or client) who has the right to have the information corrected or erased
- Surrounded by proper security.

Accurate and complete records should be kept at the time, and are invaluable when different staff are dealing with a case, or if a client questions treatment or arbitration is necessary. Abbreviations should be standard and agreed, and a list of commonly used ones is useful for new members of staff.

Practices that keep most data on computer often still generate paper records, such as farm visit notes, hospitalization notes, consent forms and anaesthetic records. Legibility is essential if misunderstandings are to be avoided. These notes are still part of the medical record and should be filed in a logical and accessible way.

Within the medical record, it is useful and good practice to record briefly all telephone contacts or significant discussions with owners. This may help if there is any future disagreement over treatment or payment, and lets other practice members know what has been discussed if they take over the case. The Royal College of Veterinary Surgeons recommends that medical records should be kept for a minimum of 7 years.

A bound Controlled Drug Register (available from the Royal Pharmaceutical Society of Great Britain) must be completed and kept for all controlled drugs used.

Personnel records

The following should be kept filed for each employee:

- Contracts or statements of terms and conditions of employment
- Pertinent correspondence
- References
- Tax Office and Benefits Agency papers
- Pay As You Earn (PAYE) records
- Details of Statutory Sick Pay (SSP) and Statutory Maternity Pay (SMP)
- Records of extra payments, such as bonuses and mileage allowances
- Records of other benefits – for example, the provision of a practice car or petrol for private use, which in most cases must be notified to the tax office
- Records of assessments and action related to veterinary nursing training as required by the RCVS (see RCVS Training Centre Handbook).

A personal development file for each employee is a good idea. This should contain staff appraisal notes, continuing professional development (CPD) plans, a record of CPD (RCVS or Veterinary Practice Management Association record card) and college or training reports.

Financial records

There are four main types of financial record:

- PAYE records (see Personnel records above)
- Sales records
- Business accounts
- Purchase invoices and receipts.

7.5 Storage times for financial records

DSS records	3 years after end of tax year
Inland Revenue records	6 years after end of tax year
VAT records	6 years

Sales records
The financial details of every client transaction should be recorded so that cash takings can be reconciled and accounts sent to non-payers. These records can be used to monitor credit control and improve payment rates where this is a problem. Records may be kept in a day book, or as separate paper invoices, or on a till or computer.

Business accounts
Financial accounts are usually prepared annually by an accountant. The ready availability of computer programs for the preparation of accounts means that more and more practices are preparing accounts in-house.

Regular monthly management accounts allow practice owners and managers to monitor performance and respond to changes in income and expenditure, as well as predict the effect of planned changes.

Accounts include:

- Profit and loss account (a record of income and expenditure under various headings)
- Balance sheet (a summary of the practice's financial position) listing:
  - Assets (property and equipment, and money owed to the practice)
  - Liabilities (money owed by the practice).

Purchase invoices and receipts
These documents, together with bank statements, cheque book stubs and similar records, must be kept for 6 years after the end of the tax year to support the accounts in case of inspection or a tax investigation. They should be filed in either date or number order for easy retrieval.

Most practices will be registered for Value Added Tax (VAT) and must complete a regular VAT return for HM Customs and Excise, giving totals of income (outputs) and expenditure (inputs). A VAT inspector may wish to inspect these financial records at any time.

Health and safety records

- *Risk assessments* should be filed for all practice activities and for the standard operating procedures used

- A written *health and safety policy* is a requirement for practices employing five or more people, and is strongly recommended for all practices
- *Equipment maintenance and testing records* are required in some cases – for example, autoclaves, X-ray machines and portable electrical equipment
- A *COSHH* (Control of Substances Hazardous to Health) assessment must be carried out and recorded, and COSHH data sheets filed for each substance used by the practice
- The practice must keep an *Accident Book* and a record of first aid treatments given, and must comply with RIDDOR 1995 (Reporting of Injuries, Deaths and Dangerous Occurrences Regulations).

General information

As well as the categories of records listed above, it is helpful in a busy practice to organize some general information files. These can be looked up readily as the need arises, and might include the following.

Information for clients

To improve customer service and save time in reception, keep information for clients to hand:

- Practice policies on routine health care (e.g. vaccination, worming, neutering)
- Lists of kennels and catteries in the area
- Dog-training classes and groomers
- Details of lost and found pets.

Information for staff

To improve efficiency and safety and to minimize error, keep notes of:

- Useful names, addresses and telephone numbers
  - Practice suppliers
  - Referral centres and practices
  - External laboratories
  - Local police
  - Local doctor and hospital emergency department
- Instructions for practice equipment
- Details of maintenance agreements and repairers for practice equipment
- Service records for practice equipment
- Training checklists to monitor the progress of new staff members and ensure that they have received adequate training
- Memos and notes regarding practice policies and protocols
- Emergency procedures.

This information may be usefully organized into Area Information Manuals (see Figure 7.11) and a Practice Manual (see Figure 7.10).

The pharmacy and stock control

All veterinary practices handle stock. For most, drugs and items for resale are an important source of income and the value of stock on the shelf can be substantial. Other stock requiring control includes stationery, promotional literature and consumables such as cleaning materials.

Organization of the pharmacy

- Medicines should be stored according to the manufacturer's recommendations and should be secure from the public
- All medicines in a veterinary practice should be stored in a pharmacy area where they are safe from physical damage and vermin and arranged logically (e.g. in alphabetical order)
- Stock should be rotated properly, using oldest stock first
- Duplication of similar items should be avoided, to minimize stock levels
- Shelving should be well designed to maximize visibility and minimize damage to stock
- Where a single location is impossible, a system of standard stock levels for each location can help proper stock control, and is useful for maintaining stocks in cars and vans
- Consulting room stock should be kept as low as possible, and public access prevented
- Any storage area should be at the correct temperature; maximum and minimum thermometers are essential for monitoring rooms and refrigerators
- Drugs requiring refrigeration (e.g. vaccines) should never be left out of the refrigerator for prolonged periods. Minimal working stocks should be kept in cars, particularly when the weather is very hot or cold. Portable refrigerated coolboxes may be required
- Pharmacy areas should have impervious working surfaces, a minimum level of equipment for dispensing, and proper handwashing and drying facilities
- Under the Misuse of Drugs Act 1971, Schedule 2 Controlled Drugs must be stored in a locked receptacle (a car is not adequate) that can only be opened by a veterinary surgeon or a person authorized by them to do so. In practice, there should be only one key per veterinary surgeon and this should be kept on the person at all times. A bound Controlled Drugs Register should be used to record all purchases and administrations of these drugs. More detail will be found in the books for further reading at the end of this section and in Chapter 2 of the *BSAVA Manual of Veterinary Nursing*.

It is advisable for a specific veterinary surgeon to be responsible for the overall control of the pharmacy area and stock organization. Working with a senior nurse or other trained staff member with specific responsibilities in this area, this veterinary surgeon can monitor adherence to practice policy and ensure that medicines are stored and used correctly (Figure 7.6).

Stock control

The aim of stock control is to keep adequate stock levels for the day-to-day and emergency needs of the practice without tying up excessive resources. Properly rotated stock is working for the practice and generating income in the form of sales.

- If stock levels are too low, the practice will run out of items. This may be just inconvenient, or it may jeopardize customer service and future sales, or compromise an animal's treatment
- If stock levels are too high, stock may become damaged or go out of date and have to be discarded. Stock on the shelf is tying up money that could be used elsewhere, and so represents a cost to the practice.

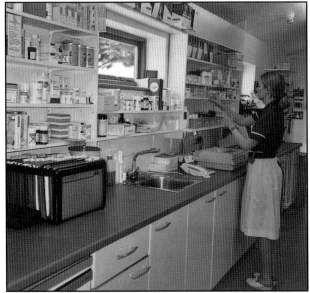

7.6 *A well organized dispensary makes stock control easier and reduces stock wastage.*

All incoming stock should be checked for damage and expiry date and matched to the invoice or delivery note. Price changes should be acted upon either on delivery or on receipt of price updates from the manufacturer or wholesaler. New stock should be placed behind or under existing stock to ensure that older stock is used first.

There are several well established systems of stock control in use in practices, as follows.

Manual reorder
Staff order stock when they feel it is required. This system can be effective in small practices with tight visual control, but frequently leads to overstocking or out-of-stock situations.

Manual stock records
Stock is ordered to a predetermined level, or when a set minimum is reached. Manual systems can be excellent, particularly if a running calculation is used to alter stock levels according to usage (stock control books to do this are available), but they can also be very time consuming.

Computerized stock control

Using a handheld computer
This system can be programmed to allow the user to scan shelves as they are arranged in the practice. From an input of current stock level, an order is generated that can maintain a stock appropriate to level of usage. The system is simple but requires manual input of stock quantity regularly, and may not handle part quantities. If stock is stolen, this may be difficult to pick up.

Using the medical records computer
As items are used or sold and charged for, they are 'destocked' and reordered automatically. Minimum quantities are usually set manually, but more sophisticated programs allow for adjustment of stock and ordering levels according to level of usage. Part quantities may be handled, and the system can be completely automatic, particularly if stock is ordered and added via a modem link to a wholesaler. Controls need to be tight, however, to minimize errors. Fully computerized stock control will highlight problems with undercharging (e.g. by not destocking) or stealing from the pharmacy.

Stock organization
However good an ordering system is, poor stock organization and handling and human error will limit its effectiveness. It is good practice to involve the clinical staff regularly in deciding on stocked lines and adjusting stock to changing or seasonal patterns of use. Good practice discipline is essential and involving staff in setting up standard procedures will help to ensure their support.

If automatic stock control methods are used, these should not be overridden manually or the system will lose its effectiveness. In particular:

- Increasing the frequency of ordering and delivery can help to keep stock levels down (important if space is limited), but will be more time consuming than handling a larger order less frequently
- Minimizing the number of suppliers used will increase efficiency and possibly reduce costs, because discounts are given for large accounts
- An expensive item may be worth keeping at a low level, particularly if it is not likely to be needed in an emergency but can be ordered in when required
- Cheaper items or emergency drugs can be kept at a higher level so that they are less likely to become out of stock
- The minimum stock level of some drugs will be set by the expected dose rate for emergency use, which may be higher than the average rate of use per month
- If the practice sells life-stage diets, a little overstocking may be necessary to cope with extra sales at weekends and to avoid running out of stock and losing repeat custom to a competitor.

Reducing costs
Special offers and large-order discounts can save the practice money, but as a general rule no more than 2–3 months' stock should be ordered at one time. Free gifts and incentives for orders, particularly if new or infrequently used items have to be purchased, should be looked at sceptically. It may be cheaper just to buy the gift instead.

Much more effective in the long term is to negotiate increased discounts or lower prices for normal orders. Wholesalers offer discounts for prompt payment; they often offer other services and help with stock management too. Individual suppliers will often negotiate discounts and special deals, usually through their representatives. All discounts and arrangements should be reviewed regularly and checked to make sure they are being received as expected.

Personnel management

Veterinary practice is a service industry, relying heavily on its people for success. This is also true in referral centres and in academic institutions. In any department, enough staff must be available to provide the services required, but as staff costs are usually one of the highest expenditures of the business, overstaffing can be disastrous and result in lower profits.

A business must gain all it can from wise use of its staff and must continually develop them in line with the aims of the business so that they remain motivated and able to deliver the best possible service to the business and its clients.

Job descriptions
A vital tool to ensure that employees are working within the expectations of the employer and themselves is the job

description (Figure 7.7). Job descriptions are helpful baselines for performance evaluation or appraisal and for planning training. They are also invaluable when recruiting staff (see below).

Job descriptions must be agreed between employer and employee and should contain the following:

- The job title
- The overall aims of the practice or organization
- A brief description of areas or tasks that are the responsibility of the employee
- Details of any supervisory role over other staff
- An indication of expected standards (e.g. by referring to the practice manual)
- To whom the employee reports (their line manager)
- A date for review (usually at least annually).

7.7 Example of a job description

JOB DESCRIPTION
OFFICE MANAGER

It is the aim of the practice to provide a comprehensive and caring service for all our clients and their pets, paying attention to and respecting their needs, and always offering support and understanding as well as technical expertise.

All members of the practice are required to participate regularly in continuing education and keep abreast of modern knowledge and techniques.

The Office Manager assists the Practice Administrator and Partners with administrative and secretarial tasks in the practice. Confidentiality and accuracy are paramount, and all work should be carried out according to the guidelines, rules and protocols contained in the practice manual.

In particular, the Office Manager has responsibility for:

- Credit control (monthly invoicing, handling of accounts)
- Processing insurance claims
- Banking of takings
- Word processing, recording minutes of practice meetings
- Relief reception work when required
- Stationery stock control and ordering
- Filing and archiving
- Photocopying, assistance with preparation of in-house publicity and educational material
- Dealing with incoming and outgoing mail
- Assistance to the Practice Administrator as required
- Cash reconciliation
- Assistance with training of staff in the use and maintenance of the computer systems, other office equipment and credit control
- Coordinating and collating survey results.

The Office Manager reports to the Practice Administrator, although on a day-to-day basis a team approach to problems is encouraged.

The management team currently consists of both Partners, the Administrator, Senior Receptionist and Senior Nurse.

Review date: ....

Signatures: (Employer) ....
(Employee) ....

To write job descriptions for the first time, it is most helpful if the employer and employee each sets out a task list. They can then compare notes and the job description is written by combining the two lists. This exercise can be extremely useful for aligning expectations.

Rotas

Veterinary surgeons, nurses and support staff will often have to work unsocial hours and be available for emergency call. A good rota system enables the practice to have sufficient staff available for the work to be done at all times, whilst still allowing staff adequate time off in a fair manner. Provision must be made for holiday periods and leave due to sickness, and the rota should be flexible enough to accommodate necessary changes caused by out-of-work commitments. To assess staffing needs, it may be helpful to note down all the tasks to be done each day, marking those that have to be done at a certain time and dividing the day into sections. By working out how many staff members are needed to cover the workload in each section, and devising a plan for absence cover, guidelines for staffing needs at each time of the day can be formulated. Very often, once the staffing guidelines have been set, it may be most effective for work groups to set their own rotas, as they are likely to be more committed to making them work.

Staff appraisal

Staff appraisal need not be an onerous paper exercise. Employees need to know how well they are doing, and employers need to know they are gaining the best value from their staff. With proper advance preparation, an agenda-based interview (Figure 7.8) can be invaluable in maintaining motivation, developing and encouraging employees, and ensuring that everyone is working towards the same overall aim.

It is essential that staff appraisal is a two-way process, with plenty of opportunity for discussion on both sides. The experience should be a positive one for both employee and manager (Figure 7.9).

Staff should be appraised at least annually and their job description reviewed as part of the process. Short mini-appraisals with smaller goals may be helpful for new or junior staff, particularly those in formal training (e.g. student veterinary nurses).

Staff should be encouraged to prepare for appraisal by making notes first, and gathering evidence of good work and achievements. The appraisal itself is a private interview, held preferably on site but on neutral ground (i.e. not the line manager's office). Interruptions are forbidden and the employee should be encouraged to do most of the talking. The whole process should ensure that the expectations of both parties are clear and in line, and should set out an agreed action plan for the coming period.

7.8 Suggested agenda for staff appraisal

- Review job description
- Achievements over the period
- Training and CPD completed, and how this has benefited the employee and employer
- Any problems or difficulties encountered
- Action plan – aims and targets for the next period
- Training to be concentrated on in the next period (usually tied to aims).

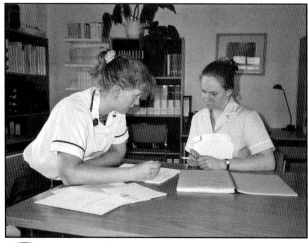

7.9 *Staff appraisal should be a positive experience.*

Appraisal is usually performed by the immediate line manager of the employee concerned (e.g. senior nurse, in the case of a student nurse) but the employer may wish to be involved too and this can be helpful. Appraisal is a skilled task and should not be attempted without specific practical training.

Training and continuing professional development (CPD)

Planning training

Training should continue throughout the working life of an individual, but the format and amount will vary at different times. Training should be regarded by the practice as an investment, not a cost, as staff development is essential to the growth and success of the practice.

Training must be focused and relevant to the aims of the practice, as well as tailored to the individual. Important considerations are:

- Need – what training is needed, and is it going to benefit the individual and the practice?
- Objectives – what is to be achieved by the training, and does this tie in with the individual's development plan and practice objectives?
- What specific problems will the training solve? For example: is there a high level of client complaints; or are nurses having difficulty operating specific equipment?
- Style – what is the individual's specific learning style, and what are we trying to achieve? Would a lecture course or one-to-one training be more appropriate?
- Source – is expertise available to train within the practice or is external training necessary?
- Cost effectiveness – is the training value for money, and are the returns immediate or longer term?

These questions can be used to compile an analysis of training needs across the practice, which is invaluable for planning training.

Evaluation

After the training, evaluation should take place to see whether the training was relevant and effective. An action plan may be drawn up to follow up on the training and ensure that new skills are put into practice. Training should be evaluated not only at the time but also at the end of each programme, again after 2–3 months, and finally after about a year (often at annual appraisal). Useful questions to ask are:

- What new skills have been gained?
- What can the employee do now, that they were not doing before?
- How will this benefit the practice?
- Can this benefit be measured?
- Is the training suitable for other staff?

The benefits of training and development include better motivated and more focused staff, with increased self-esteem. This means:

- More efficient use of resources; increased productivity
- Improved quality standards and greater proficiency; better customer service
- Better use of equipment and instrumentation
- Better time management
- Reduced accidents, absenteeism and lateness
- Reduced staff turnover.

All of these can be measured to assess results.

External versus internal training

Internal training is often the best option, as it can be more tailored to the needs of the practice and the individual, can be team-building, and increases the self-esteem of the trainer. Most practices have huge untapped sources of expertise within the staff, and there are now a number of courses available to give staff the skills they need to be trainers. In-house training can be more cost-effective, particularly if a number of staff are being trained, but devoting adequate time to sessions is a problem for most practices. Another useful source for training in-house is visiting representatives from pharmaceutical or pet food manufacturers.

External training gives access to expertise not available in the practice and has the important benefit of social interaction with colleagues from other practices and the exchange of ideas which may follow. Cost can be a limiting factor for some. Maximum benefit can be gained from external training if individuals report from their courses to the rest of the team, and share notes and new skills in-house.

Induction training

Settling in new staff quickly and familiarizing them with their job and the practice policies and protocols is vital to long-term success for the new employee. A new staff member must be made to feel welcome (a welcome card is a nice touch), with uniforms, name badge, locker key and other personal work items all ready when they arrive on the first day. All staff members should be aware of the appointment, and appointing a mentor to help through the first weeks or months is a good idea.

On the first day, new recruits should be introduced to all the staff, shown round the premises and introduced to the aims and philosophy of the practice. They should be shown where to find information, and who to approach with different types of query. Sessions with their supervisor should cover health and safety issues, fire rules, and employment rules and procedures (for example, how to apply for leave of absence or notify sickness). These issues should ideally be contained in a practice manual (Figure 7.10), which is issued to the employee but also explained face to face.

To avoid information overload, a planned induction programme is essential, with regular reviews to check progress. A system of checklists, particularly for reception training, is helpful, and readily available area information manuals will aid training (Figure 7.11).

7.10 Suggested contents for a practice manual

- Practice mission statement or aims (see Figure 7.7)
- List of personnel and their job titles and responsibilities
- Overtime and absence policies
- Disciplinary and grievance procedures
- Equal opportunities policy
- Sexual harassment policy
- Training and development policy
- Dress and behavioural code
- Health and safety written statement
- COSHH assessments
- Practice rules and guidelines for working, including security policy
- Practice clinical policies and protocols, e.g. worming and neutering policies
- Confidentiality and ethical guidelines
- Information (important telephone numbers, practice handouts and literature).

7.11 Area information manuals

Area information manuals might contain:

- Name of person responsible for the area
- Health and safety risk assessments
- COSHH risk assessments
- Health and safety rules and standard operating procedures
- Fire rules
- Detailed instructions for procedures carried out in the area
- Reference information
- Equipment instruction booklets
- Guarantees and maintenance contracts, instructions for repair of equipment
- Equipment service records.

Recruitment

An effective recruitment programme is vital if a practice is to maintain high quality and motivated staff. Stages in the process are:

- Attract a large number of suitable applicants, by advertising
- Select a shortlist of applicants who fit the selection criteria
- From the shortlist, select the ideal candidate for the position, usually after interview
- Successfully integrate the new recruit into the culture and environment of the practice.

Advertising

Although an overwhelming response to an advertisement can be off-putting, it is far better than too small a pool of candidates.

- Before placing the advertisement, compile a list of essential and desirable attributes of the ideal candidate. These are the selection criteria (Figure 7.12). Use work colleagues and the job description to help. Essential selection criteria must be measurable
- Advertise vacancies as widely as possible, and look in unusual places. (Good student nurses have not necessarily always wanted to nurse – they may not be in your files already)
- Do not skimp on advertising – a good new recruit may be with you a long time, and may bring the practice a healthy level of profit

7.12 Some selection criteria for recruiting a qualified veterinary nurse

Essential:

- VN qualification
- Good health and attendance record
- One year post-qualifying experience
- Competent surgical and medical nursing skills
- Available for duty rota.

Desirable:

- Pet health counselling experience
- City and Guilds Certificate in Small Animal Nutrition
- Three years post-qualifying experience
- Experience of training student nurses
- Experience of Schedule 3 procedures
- Local residence
- Ability to work in a team
- Enthusiasm and self-motivation
- Professional appearance
- Access to own transport
- Organized approach
- Good customer service skills
- Experience with horses.

- Make sure the right people will be attracted by the advertisement by considering carefully its style and where it is to be placed. Radio advertising can be useful to reach those workers not actively looking for a job in 'situations vacant' columns
- Try to include the main selection criteria (e.g. minimum age, academic qualifications) within the advertisement to discourage unsuitable applications, and remember to avoid discrimination on the grounds of sex, race or ethnic origin
- The advertisement must be legal, decent, honest and truthful
- Always acknowledge every applicant, particularly if there will be some delay between application and interview, and thank them for their interest in the position. This is an opportunity for good practice presentation.

Shortlisting

Shortlisting must be fair and efficient, particularly if effective advertising has attracted a good field of applicants.

- Interview as many promising candidates as possible but, to avoid confusion, do not interview too many on one day
- Use standard application forms and request a supporting handwritten letter, to assist the process of sorting first from second choice candidates (using the list of essential and desirable requirements mentioned above)
- If necessary, using the list of essential and desirable characteristics, score each applicant to maintain objectivity, then place them in order
- Write or telephone shortlisted applicants with an interview time, and be prepared to be flexible – the best candidates may be working elsewhere and may be reluctant to take time off
- Confirm the arrangements and let the candidate know how long the process is expected to take.

Interviewing

Interviewing candidates is a skilled task and even the most experienced recruiters make mistakes. The selection criteria should always be kept in mind, together with the attributes the new recruit will need to fit into the team. Ways to avoid common pitfalls are:

- Use aptitude tests to check cognitive and written skills (a number are available commercially). This is particularly useful to assess mathematical ability and concentration
- Use as many staff as possible within the interviewing process. They can show the candidate around or take part in the formal interview
- Follow the same format for each interview
- Try to avoid interviewing across a desk – maintain a relaxed atmosphere
- Always use open questions (those that do not attract a 'yes' or 'no' answer). If you find this difficult, start questions with the words 'Tell me about…'
- Do not ask personal questions that could be construed as sexual discrimination (e.g. regarding plans to have a family or arrangements for childcare)
- Follow up inconsistencies, gaps or ambiguities on the application form
- Avoid common interview questions, which professional interviewees answer very well; instead, ask questions they are not expecting. Good examples are:
  - 'Situational' questions, using scenarios from practical experience. These are the 'What would you do to sort this out?' questions
  - 'Experience' questions, asking candidates how they actually dealt with a situation. These are the 'Tell me how you dealt with the last…' questions
- If possible, a day or two's work trial can be helpful, but is not always practical
- Make all the working conditions clear to the interviewee and do not oversell the job – this will only lead to disappointment later
- Give the interviewee plenty of opportunity to ask questions.

Using these techniques, the best candidate is selected by concentrating on attitude and enthusiasm rather than experience alone. Staff can be trained in technical skills, but attitude and enthusiasm cannot be trained into an unsuitable employee.

Obtaining references is an essential part of the process of selection.

- Poor or ambiguous references should not be ignored. Telephoning or writing for clarification may be advisable
- Written references can be obtained from previous employers and school or college tutors before the interview, or can be followed up later
- Frequently, a telephone call to a referee will tell you more than a written reference. Ask specific questions, and check that the applicant's description of their experience matches the referee's
- Always ask why an applicant is leaving their current job and confirm this if possible. Remember that a good reference may be given to enable a poor employee to be moved from a dissatisfied employer.

Once the decision is made, the candidate should be offered the position and given the opportunity to ask further questions. Written confirmation should follow, and the unsuccessful candidates should be informed as soon as possible.

The position may be offered for a trial period first, with progress reviewed at the end of this period. It is important that, if a mistake has been made and the new employee is not suitable for the job, this issue is addressed early on. As long as dismissal cannot be seen to be unfair or discriminatory, a clean break at this stage is better than an unhappy employer and employee several months or years later.

Statutory obligations of employers

A number of legal requirements apply to employers, including veterinary surgeons in practice. Those discussed here fall into two main areas: employment legislation; and health and safety issues. Some requirements vary with the numbers of staff (including partners and principals) employed. A comprehensive account of legislation relating to employment and to health and safety is beyond the scope of this chapter, but some of the main provisions are outlined here.

Employment legislation
All employers must:

- Register with the Inland Revenue and the Department of Social Security (DSS)
- Take out employer's liability insurance cover and display the current certificate in the workplace
- Under the Employment Rights Act 1996, give all employees a written statement of terms and conditions – irrespective of the number of hours they work – within 2 months of employment commencing (Figure 7.13)
- Issue itemized pay statements
- Inform employees individually and in writing within one month of any change to contract conditions taking effect
- Make documents referred to in the terms and conditions of employment readily accessible to employees
- Not discriminate on the grounds of sex or race. This has a particular implication for part-time workers (the majority are women) who, if discriminated against, could argue that they are suffering discrimination on the grounds of their gender.

Disciplinary and grievance procedures
All employers should have a grievance procedure. Practices with more than 20 employees must have their disciplinary procedures included in contracts of employment. In all cases, the procedures should be clear and easy to understand and include procedures for appeal. These procedures may be essential to prevent claims for constructive or unfair dismissal, and good notes must be kept of all actions taken.

Maternity rights

- Expectant mothers are entitled to paid time off for antenatal appointments
- A minimum period of maternity leave of 14 weeks is provided for, during which all terms and conditions other than remuneration must be preserved. No qualifying period of service or number of hours per week are required
- For those with two years' qualifying service at the 12th week before the baby is due, an additional 29 weeks of leave as above are allowed, providing for up to 40 weeks absence

The Employment Rights Act defines the following points, which must be included in every written statement of terms and conditions. The written statement is not in itself a contract, but it is evidence of the contract of employment.

1. The full names of employer and employee

2. The date of commencement of employment and whether this is part of a continuous period of employment

3. The job title and job description (can be brief)

4. The job location

5. Pay, including details of:
   – Bonus schemes
   – Overtime rates and when they apply
   – Other benefits
   – Deductions from pay
   – Methods of payment
   – Standby arrangements and payments

6. Hours of work, including flexible or shift-working arrangements

7. Holidays, including public holidays and holiday pay, and how holiday is accrued. Sufficient detail should be given to enable calculation of ongoing holiday entitlement and entitlement accruing on termination

8. Sickness absence (entitlement to sick pay, statutory sick pay, waiting days)

9. Pension scheme. If there is no scheme, this should be stated. It should also be clear whether or not a contracting-out certificate for National Insurance Contributions is in force (e.g. if the practice pension scheme is contracted out of the State Earnings Related Pension Scheme – SERPS)

10. Ending the employment. There should be provision for reasonable notice on either side to terminate the contract:
    – In the case of temporary employment, the expected period for which the employment is to continue
    – For a fixed-term contract, the date of expiry of the fixed term

11. Disciplinary rules. This section must include the name or description of the person to whom the employee can appeal against disciplinary action or decisions, and details of how such an appeal should be made

12. Name or description of the person to whom the employee can apply if they have a grievance.

Items 1–7 must be included in a single document, the 'principal statement'. If there is no provision for any of these items, this should be made clear.

Items 8–12 can be contained in other documents issued with the principal statement or issued in instalments within 2 months of the date of starting work.

The written statement may also contain non-compulsory clauses. For example:

• Restrictive covenants – to stop ex-employees working for competitors or within a geographical distance of their old workplace. These must be reasonable
• Requirements for confidentiality
• Relocation terms
• Frequency of salary reviews.

• Part-time workers have the same rights under the Employment Protection (Part-time Employees) Regulations 1995
• Dismissal for reasons connected with pregnancy is automatically unfair, and no qualifying period is required
• Employees taking 14 weeks' maternity leave are entitled to continue their existing terms and conditions at the end of the period
• Employees returning from extended maternity leave have the right to return to a job with terms and conditions 'not less favourable' than those that would have applied had they not been absent
• Full-time workers do not have a right to return to work part-time after maternity leave
• The right to return to work is more restricted for small employers with fewer than five employees.

Women have a right to paid suspension from work on maternity grounds because of health and safety reasons. Examples include exposing their unborn child to increased risks of infection from zoonoses, work involving heavy lifting, or contact with substances known to present a risk to pregnancy. However, the employer may offer reasonable alternative duties instead of paid suspension and, in practice, most veterinary practices manage to find work for pregnant employees in non-risk areas of the practice for the duration of their pregnancy.

Health and safety regulations prevent women from returning to work within 2 weeks of childbirth.

Current regulations and information booklets should be consulted for more details of notice periods and of the certificates and statements that must be prepared.

Disability Discrimination Act 1995

This wide-ranging Act defines disability and makes it unlawful for an employer to discriminate against a disabled person (for example, by refusing to offer or deliberately not offering employment, or offering less favourable terms of employment), as long as the person can do the job. The Act also includes a duty on the employer to make reasonable adjustments to prevent a disabled person being put at a disadvantage, and makes discriminatory advertisements unlawful. Employers with fewer than 20 employees are exempt from the provisions of the Act, but this may be reviewed.

Sexual harassment

This is defined as unwanted conduct of a sexual nature or other conduct based on sex affecting the dignity of men and women at work. Developing a policy to prevent sexual harassment and deal with it if it arises is recommended, to prevent accusations under the Sex Discrimination Act 1975.

Health and Safety at Work (HSW) etc., Act 1974

Every year, about 500 people are killed at work and several hundred thousand more are injured or suffer ill health. The Health and Safety at Work (HSW) etc. Act 1974 covers anyone who is at work in any situation or location (except domestic servants), and it puts a duty on every employer and employee to fulfil every aspect of the law as far as is reasonably practicable. It is all embracing and provides for regulations to be made under the Act. Some of these regulations are listed in Figure 7.14 and all are available in detail from the Health and Safety Executive (HSE). The HSE also publishes Approved Codes of Practice, which can be useful resources when formulating a policy.

Under the HSW Act, employers must ensure the health and safety of themselves and others who may be affected by what they do or fail to do. This includes workers, subcontractors, visitors, clients and trainees, and also people who use the employer's equipment, any products made or supplied and services. The self-employed and employees also have responsibilities under the Act. Employees have a duty under the Act to take reasonable care for their own health and safety and that of others who may be affected by their acts or omissions at work.

7.14 Health and safety legislation

The regulations under the Health and Safety at Work (HSW) etc., Act 1974 deal with specific areas of health and safety. The following regulations are of relevance.

- *Management of Health and Safety at Work Regulations 1992*
  - Risk assessment
  - Health and safety arrangements and procedures
  - Health surveillance
  - Informing and cooperating with employees
  - Training
  - Duties of employees

- *Health and Safety (Young Persons) Regulations 1997*
  - Ensuring that risk assessments are made for risks to those under 18 years old before they start work
  - Taking account of inexperience and immaturity
  - Taking account of lack of awareness of existing or potential risks
  - Information must be provided to parents of school-age children (e.g. children on work experience)

- *Workplace (Health and Safety and Welfare) Regulations 1992*
  - Condition and design of buildings, lighting, workstations, facilities and cleanliness
  - Prevention of slips and trips (e.g. on wet floors)

- *Health and Safety (Display Screen Equipment) Regulations 1992*
  - Definition of users (usually only administrative staff or some receptionists in practice) who must have well designed work areas with suitable lighting and adjustable seating

Employers must:

- Have a written up-to-date health and safety policy if they employ five or more people
- Carry out a risk assessment
- Record the main findings of the risk assessment and the main arrangements for health and safety if five or more people are employed
- Notify occupation of premises to the local health and safety inspector
- Display a current certificate as required by the Employers' Liability (Compulsory Insurance) Act 1969 if anyone is employed
- Display the 'Health and Safety Law' poster for employees, or issue the leaflet
- Notify certain types of injuries, occupational diseases and events (RIDDOR 1995)
- Consult union safety representatives (if applicable) on issues such as changes affecting health and safety and provision of information and training
- Take account of the special needs of workers who are new or expectant mothers.

Help with writing a health and safety policy statement is available from consultants and from publications issued by the HSE and the Stationery Office (HMSO). The risk assessment (Figure 7.15) is fundamental to health and safety management, and must be carried out by a competent person. Involving employees in risk assessment can be very effective, and increases awareness of safety issues. Training in risk assessment is often available at local colleges.

  - Breaks or changes of activity to be planned
  - Users' entitlement to eye tests and spectacles, if required, for VDU work only, at employer's expense

- *Electricity at Work Regulations 1989*
  - Suitability of plugs, sockets and fittings for the working environment
  - Maintenance in good repair, and regular inspection of, electrical connections and portable equipment

- *Provision and Use of Work Equipment Regulations 1992*
  - Safety issues related to equipment in use

- *Manual Handling Regulations 1992*
  - Lifting and carrying loads
  - Training of staff to use proper lifting techniques and to use equipment (e.g. stretchers and trolleys) to help with lifting

- *Construction (Design and Management) Regulations 1994*
  - Duties of principal contractors, clients, designers and planning supervisors (important if extensions or alterations to premises are planned)

- *Noise at Work Regulations 1989*
  - Action required if noise reaches 85 dB(A)

- *Ionizing Radiations Regulations 1985[a]*
  - Appointment of a Radiation Protection Advisor
  - Use of standard schemes of work and exposure charts
  - Involvement of only designated persons

Figure 7.14 continues ▶

- Appointment of a Radiation Protection Supervisor within the practice
- Use of radiation dosimetry in most practices
- Keeping of records of exposure
- Copy of 'The Guidance Notes for the Protection of Persons Against Ionizing Radiations arising from Veterinary Use (1988)', published by the National Radiological Protection Board, to be available in the practice

a – Regulations and new Guidance Notes are expected during 1999

- *Pressure Systems and Transportable Gas Containers Regulations 1989*
  - Requirement for a Written Scheme of Examination for all autoclaves and compressors in the practice

- *Control of Substances Hazardous to Health Regulations 1994 (COSHH)*
  - Assessment to be made for all substances used in the workplace
  - Holding of data sheets for hazardous substances
  - Standard operating procedures to mimimize risk in use and in case of spillage
  - Replacement of hazardous substances by less hazardous alternatives wherever possible (if this is impossible, specific precautions to be taken)
  - Approved occupational exposure standards for substances such as halothane and isoflurane (Booklet EH40, 'Occupational Exposure Limits')
  - Regular monitoring of staff exposure levels (expressed as Time Weighted Average figures) in some instances
  - Good hygiene precautions concerning bacteria and viruses (of particular importance as zoonoses in veterinary practice)
  - Requirements for clear and standard labelling of different classes of hazardous substances

- *Environmental Protection Act 1990 (Duty of Care); Controlled Waste Regulations 1992; Collection and Disposal of Waste Regulations 1988; Control of Pollution (Special Waste) regulations 1980*
  - Procedures to be adopted by the practice for handling, storing and disposing of clinical and special waste
  - Clinical waste is defined as:
    * Any waste which consists wholly or partly of human or animal tissue, blood or other body fluids, excretions, drugs or other pharmaceutical products, swabs or dressings, or syringes, needles, or other sharp instruments, being waste which unless rendered safe may prove hazardous to any person coming into contact with it
    * Any other waste material arising from medical, nursing, dental, veterinary, pharmaceutical or similar practice, investigation, treatment, care, teaching or research, or the collection of blood for transfusion, being waste which may cause infection to any person coming into contact with it.
  - Such waste includes animal carcasses and must be placed in appropriately marked polythene bags (sharps into approved sharps containers at point of use) and disposed of by incineration in an approved manner

- The duty of care for correct disposal of clinical and special waste rests with the producer of the waste

- *Health and Safety (First Aid) Regulations 1981*
  - Arrangements for first aid in the workplace, requiring an appointed person available whenever people are at work
  - First aid box(es) and notices indicating the name of the appointed person and the location of the first aid box
  - Determination (at risk assessment) of the number of first-aiders and the training they require, according to the type of work being carried out
  - Requirement for first aid arrangements for lone workers and self-employed people working alone

- *Reporting of Injuries, Diseases and Dangerous Occurrences Regulations 1995 (RIDDOR)*
  - Reporting of work-related accidents, diseases and dangerous occurrences (even when no injury occurred)
  - Application to all work activities, but not all incidents
  - Requirement for a copy of the guidance notes and report forms to be kept in the clinic
  - Immediate reporting of certain injuries (e.g. death, loss of limb) to the enforcing authority (generally, the area office of the Health and Safety Executive). In other cases (e.g. injury resulting in an employee being admitted to hospital for more than 24 hours, or being unable to do their normal job for more than 3 days), a report to be sent within 7 days

- *Personal Protective Equipment at Work Regulations 1992*
  - Use of personal protective equipment (PPE) only as a last resort (where possible, controls and safe systems of work should be used instead)
  - PPE, if needed, to be provided free by the employer, of good quality, suitable for the wearer, properly maintained and used by trained personnel (examples of PPE used in veterinary practice are face masks and safety spectacles during ultrasonic dental scaling, and gloves to protect hands when dealing with infected material).

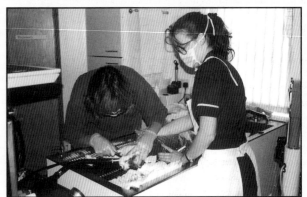

Personal protective equipment, such as the gloves, face masks and spectacles worn here for dentistry, must be readily available, suitable for the task and kept in good condition.

Performing a risk assessment

A *hazard* is something with the potential to cause harm (can include substances, machines, infectious organisms, or methods of work and other aspects of work organization).

Risk expresses the likelihood that the harm from a particular hazard is realized. The extent of the risk covers the number of people who might be exposed and consequences for them. Risk therefore reflects both the likelihood that harm will occur and its severity.

To perform a risk assessment:

1. Look for hazards – walk around, talk to staff, look at accident reports
2. Decide who might be harmed and how – not just staff but also consider visitors and clients
3. Evaluate the risks arising from the hazards and decide whether current precautions are adequate or whether more should be done
4. Record your findings, particularly if five or more staff are employed
5. Review your assessment regularly and revise it if necessary.

Practice presentation

The way a practice presents itself to its clients is of paramount importance. Clients must be made to feel welcome and want to return in future. The clinical abilities of the team and the medical and surgical facilities must be marketed to prospective and existing clients for the practice to be a successful business and maintain sufficient client support and profitability to reinvest on an ongoing basis. Marketing is a huge subject, and further reading is recommended, but here are a few areas to consider.

Matching presentation to practice aims

The practice must attract the types of clients it is aiming to serve. This means matching presentation and marketing activities to the aims of the practice, its current facilities and staff, and the client base in the locality. Trying to market a high-cost clinic in a low-income area will be less successful than in an area where there is a high proportion of higher income households. The specific needs of the client base must be considered. For example, commuters may need availability of late-night or weekend appointments, or the option to drop pets off early in the morning. Farm clients may not appreciate carpeted floors, soft lights and music, but may prefer quick service at a reasonable cost and a coffee machine when collecting prescriptions.

There are no fixed guidelines to practice presentation, but by starting with the practice business plan, looking at the demographics of the local area and asking existing clients, a good picture can be built up to help to match what the practice offers with client expectations.

Client surveys are particularly useful and should always include an option for freely given comments so that maximum information can be gained. Encouraging clients to make suggestions and making it easy for them to complain about services is also helpful.

Practice presentation must be consistent, and all parts of the facility and all written material should convey the same impression. Staff must be involved as they are a major part of the overall impression given to the client.

First impressions

Clients' first impressions of a practice will form their picture of the practice as a whole. 'Perception is reality' to a client, and medical and surgical expertise may often be judged on the cleanliness of a pet after the procedure, and the confidence the client has in the veterinary surgeon. Similarly, the most brilliant clinical facilities will not appear to be so good if the reception area is dirty, the telephone is answered badly or the receptionist fails to smile.

External appearance of the practice

The practice building and its surroundings will give the first impression. It should be easy to find, clearly marked with professional signage and kept in good repair.

- Professional name plates should be clean, polished if necessary and up to date
- Regular maintenance and repainting is essential, windows should be kept clean, and graffiti removed
- Grounds should be swept and kept clear of litter and dog faeces (Figure 7.16). Any gardens or planted areas should be weed-free and attractive and parking areas should be clearly marked.
- Adequate lighting is essential after dark and to improve security.

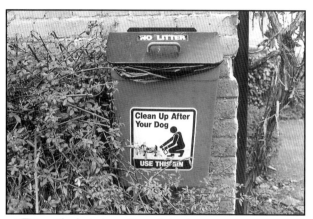

Clearly sited wastebins and shovels encourage owners to remove unsightly deposits of dog faeces in the surgery grounds.

Reception

As a matter of routine, all staff members should make a point of sitting in reception for a few minutes to spot deficiencies in presentation and procedure.

- The reception area should always be clean, tidy and odour free. Because odour is difficult to assess whilst working in an area, encourage staff to come on duty through the day by walking into reception first – they are likely to notice any deficiencies. Commercially available air fresheners and extraction or forced ventilation may be helpful
- Seating should be clean and comfortable
- Displays should be current and interesting (no dog-eared posters)
- Merchandise should be clearly priced
- There should be a supply of relevant and current magazines for waiting clients to read
- A corner for children's toys and books is a great help to young families, which make up a high proportion of clients for small animal practices (Figure 7.17)
- A friendly touch is a photograph board which can include a photo and introduction to each member of staff

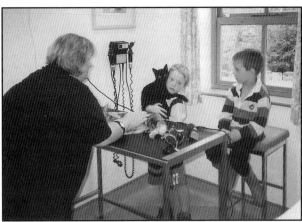

7.17 *Catering for children is important to young families and can make visits to the surgery less stressful*

- The receptionists or nurses should be accessible (not hidden behind an excessively high desk or wall hatch) so that eye contact can be made as soon as a client enters the practice
- The use of too many long instructional notices should be avoided – it is better to include information on fees, payments, procedures for appointments and repeat prescriptions in a practice information sheet that the client can take away
- Clients should be greeted immediately they arrive and made to feel welcome. Good receptionists and nurses will get to know regular clients and recognize them and their pets. Greeting the pet always makes the pet owner feel good, too
- Service in reception should be friendly and efficient, with waiting times kept to a minimum and reasons given for any delay. Keeping a client informed if things are not going according to plan will often defuse a difficult situation.

Staff

Practice staff should be selected for their presentation and customer service skills as well as clinical experience. Standards of dress and behaviour should match the impression the practice is trying to give, and all members of staff must present the same image. Well trained staff with a genuine interest in people will be more motivated and knowledgeable, and will be an asset to the practice.

Telephone skills

The telephone is a powerful marketing tool for the practice. Very often, a client's first contact with the practice is with the person who answers the telephone. This person represents every member of the practice team, and must have good telephone skills.

People calling to enquire about practice services are all potential clients, and these calls must be handled well if they are to result in new business for the practice. It is better to ask a few questions about the pet and explain what is involved in the service requested rather than simply offer prices. Offering to send a practice brochure or other information can be helpful to a new client.

- The telephone must be answered promptly but not immediately, as this can surprise the caller – after two to three rings is ideal
- The initial greeting should be clear, including the name of the veterinary practice and the identity of the staff member if possible

- Enquiries should be dealt with efficiently
- The hold button should be used as infrequently as possible, and never without asking the caller and waiting for a reply
- Where required, clear messages should be taken, ideally using a specific message pad
- If a call back is arranged, give an expected time and follow through to ensure that it happens
- Consider answering calls away from reception if possible, to reduce disruption.

Written material

- All the promotional and educational material used by the practice should be of high quality, current and useful for the clients
- Headed notepaper style should mirror the practice image. A logo or common style can help to project this
- Practice invoices, receipts, consent forms and medical record sheets should also project this image
- Consider the colour and quality of the paper and envelopes used as well as the printed image
- Practice brochures can now be produced in colour relatively cheaply and offer the opportunity to display 'behind the scenes' photographs
- A regular newsletter is of interest to clients. Staff members can be involved in writing articles on veterinary topics and practice news
- Individual information sheets on pet or herd health topics and further information on disease conditions can be very useful. They are now available commercially and through some computer system companies
- When sending correspondence (including booster reminders and recalls for other treatments) the contents should convey the right impression. A large number of leaflets may detract from the main message, and a poorly written or wrongly spelt address, or a label printed badly, will not give a professional look
- Franking machines are available that advertise the practice name or logo. To avoid the impression of mass mailing, individual stamps may be preferred.

Practice activities

There are many other ways in which a practice can promote its services.

- Most powerful is a tour 'behind the scenes', either on an individual basis or as part of an open evening or open day. These are always popular and can be a good team-building exercise for staff and clients
- New puppies and their owners can be invited to a 'puppy playgroup' for early socialization and training. Clients who have attended such a group often return to the practice more frequently for advice and their pets are easier to handle
- Other services, such as weight loss clinics, dental home care consultations and help with prescription diets, can be offered by experienced veterinary nurses
- Involving the practice in the community can be very rewarding. Visits by children's groups and by special interest groups are always popular
- Veterinary surgeons and nurses are often in demand to give talks (for example, to local Women's Institutes and Rotary Clubs) or to participate in charity events. These are ideal opportunities to promote the practice and its staff.

Development of the role of the veterinary nurse within the practice

The opportunities available to veterinary nurses in practice are wide ranging and include clinical and administrative or management responsibilities. The way a particular practice is organized will have a bearing on career direction for the veterinary nurse, but there is plenty of scope for a motivated and skilled individual to develop and progress within any number of areas. Some of these are suggested below.

- In-patient clinical nursing – skilled nurses can do much to drive continuous improvement in nursing care and monitoring of patients. Responsibilities may include:
  - Developing intensive care and nutritional protocols
  - Physiotherapy
  - Developing and maintaining hospitalization records
  - Evaluating treatment plans
  - Ensuring that thorough patient assessment is carried out, communicated and acted upon
- Offering consultations in 'well pet' clinics, advising on health care, weight reduction, dental care, behavioural development and socialization
- Staff development and training of student nurses and support staff. The assessment qualifications D32/33 and D34 are relevant and will become a requirement for the Scottish/National Vocational Qualification (S/NVQ) scheme
- Staff management and motivation
- Marketing and client education
- Practice administration and practice management.

Training is available within the veterinary sphere, particularly to prepare nurses for increased responsibility in clinical areas. Regular reading of journals and books as well as attending meetings and congresses will be invaluable and are an integral part of every nurse's continuing professional development.

Courses are available in training and assessment skills and in marketing and general management; local colleges often run suitable courses, though these may not be veterinary-based. Nurses wishing to pursue a career in practice management will benefit from courses in bookkeeping and accountancy as well as supervisory management studies.

There are a number of S/NVQ qualifications available in business administration, customer service and management studies, and the Veterinary Practice Management Association offers the Certificate in Veterinary Practice Management (CVPM) examination for managers with experience.

Further reading

General practice management

Bower J, Gripper J, Gripper P and Gunn D (1997) *Veterinary Practice Management*. Blackwell Science, Oxford

Jevring C (1996) *Managing a Veterinary Practice*. WB Saunders, London

Sheridan JP and McCafferty OE (1993) *The Business of Veterinary Practice*. Pergamon Press, Oxford

Pharmacy and stock organization

NOAH (1995) *Animal Medicines: A User's Guide*. National Office of Animal Health, Enfield

RCVS (1996) *The Guide to Professional Conduct* (1996) Royal College of Veterinary Surgeons, London

Employment legislation and staff management

ACAS Publications Advisory Handbooks and Booklets are available from:
  ACAS Reader Ltd
  PO Box 16
  Earl Shilton
  Leicester LE9 8ZZ
  (tel. 01455 852225)

Clarke CJ (1997) How to get the most from chat with your boss. *Veterinary Nursing Journal* **12** (5), 162–165

Health and safety and COSHH

Health and Safety Executive publications are available from:
  HSE Books
  PO Box 1999
  Sudbury
  Suffolk CO10 6FS
  (tel. 01787 881165)

Stationery Office publications are available from:
  Publications Centre
  PO Box 276
  London SW8 5DT
  (tel. 0171 873 9090)

8 Small mammal, exotic animal and wildlife nursing

Sharon Redrobe and Anna Meredith

This chapter is designed to give information on:

- The principal aspects of hospitalization of the exotic pet and wildlife patient
- The common diseases of these animals
- The main points of perioperative care of these species
- Zoonoses of these species and how to minimize the risks associated with their handling
- The correct administration of medicines to these species

Introduction

This chapter will deal with the group of small animals commonly presented for veterinary treatment that are 'not cats or dogs'. This includes common pet small mammals, birds and reptiles. The reptile group includes snakes, lizards and chelonians. The term chelonian refers to those reptiles that possess a shell (turtles, terrapins and tortoises). Some native UK wild animals that are brought into the veterinary surgery by the public will also be considered.

All these animals require a different approach to inpatient care from that given to dogs and cats. Correct veterinary nursing forms a vital part of the care of these patients and affects whether treatment is successful or otherwise.

Hospitalization

- Weigh patients daily to evaluate body condition and clinical progress and to ensure accurate treatment dosage
- Handle correctly to minimize stress, trauma and injury to both handler and animal
- Minimize handling to reduce stress (tame social species are an exception)
- Offer correct feed to stimulate the animal to eat and to prevent gastrointestinal upset and dietary deficiencies
- Ensure that each individual animal can be identified from the moment it is admitted to the veterinary surgery. A description of the animal is sufficient in some cases; stickers with names may be affixed to reptile shells; and cages should be clearly labelled. Some species may be microchipped for permanent identification (Figure 8.1).

 8.1 **Suggested sites for identification microchip** (based on guidelines of the British Veterinary Zoological Society)

Animal	Suggested site
Fish	Midline, anterior to dorsal fin
Amphibians	Lymphatic cavity
Reptiles	It is recommended that tissue glue is placed over the needle entry site in all reptiles
Chelonians	Subcutaneously in left hindleg (intramuscularly in thin-skinned species)
	Subcutaneously in the tarsal area in giant species
Crocodilians	Cranial to nuchal cluster
Lizards	Left quadriceps muscle, or subcutaneously in this area (all species)
	In very small species, subcutaneously on the left side of the body
Snakes	Subcutaneously, left nape of neck placed at twice the length of the head from the tip of the nose
Birds	Left pectoral muscle
	Exceptions: ostriches – pipping muscle; penguins – subcutaneously at base of neck
Mammals	Large: left mid neck subcutaneously
	Medium and small: between scapulae

Clinical parameters

It is important to be able to distinguish the normal from the abnormal animal. The level of activity or stress should be taken into account when evaluating whether the rates for vital signs are within the normal range.

It is also important to examine the animal and gain an appreciation of body condition (e.g. obese, very thin) rather than rely on absolute figures for body weight.

Mammals

Examples of the clinical parameters of common mammal species are presented in Figure 8.2.

Birds

Examples of the clinical parameters of common bird species are presented in Figure 8.3. The body condition of a bird may be gauged by feeling for the prominence of the breastbone (keel) and giving a condition score ranging from 0 to 5:

- A very prominent keel with no muscle cover is given a score of 0

- If the keel can only be palpated with pressure, due to prominent muscles and fat, the score is 5
- Most birds in good condition have a score of 3–4 and tend to be leaner if they have free flight.

Reptiles

Examples of the clinical parameters of common reptile species are presented in Figure 8.4.

- The snout–vent length (SVL) is an important measurement in the examination of a reptile. This is the straight distance from the nose to the vent
- Weight will obviously depend upon the size of the animal; for example, a young boa constrictor with an SVL of 10 cm might weigh only 15 g, compared with an older boa with an SVL of 2 m which might weigh 15 kg
- The body length of chelonians is taken as the straight-line distance between the front and back edge of the shell, not including the head or tail.

8.2 Clinical parameters of common mammal species (adults)

Mammal	Weight range (g)	Rectal temperature (°C)	Approximate pulse rate/minute	Approximate respiratory rate/minute
Badger	10000–15000	38–39	50–80	15–45
Chipmunk	100–250	38	200	100
Chinchilla	400–600	35.4–38	100	45–65
Ferret	500–2000	38.8	180–250	30–36
Fox	5000–10000	38	40–80	30
Guinea-pig	500–1100	38	230–380	70–100
Hamster	85–120	37–38	280–500	50–120
Hedgehog	800–1100	35.1	100–250	40–60
Mouse	20–60	37.4	300–700	150–200
Rabbit	1000–5000	38.5–40	130–320	30–60
Gerbil	50–90	39	260–600	70–120
Rat	250–400	38	300–500	80–100

8.3 Clinical parameters of common bird species (adults)

Bird	Approx. weight range (g)	Rectal temperature (°C)	Approximate pulse rate/minute	Approximate respiratory rate/minute
African Grey Parrot	300–400	40–42	100–300	15–45
Blue-fronted Amazon Parrot	300–500	40–42	125–200	15–45
Budgerigar	30–60	40–42	260–400	60–100
Canary/finch	12–30	40–42	300–500	60–100
Chicken	2000–4000	40–42	80–100	20–50
Cockatiel	100–180	40–42	150–350	40–50
Umbrella Cockatoo	450–750	40–42	100–300	15–40
Lesser Sulphur-Crested Cockatoo	250–400	40–42	100–300	15–45
Duck	2000–3000	40–42	100–150	15–30
Kestrel	150–300	40–42	150–350	15–45
Lovebird	50–70	40–42	250–400	60–100
Blue and Gold Macaw	900–1300	40–42	115–250	15–30
Greenwinged Macaw	1000–1500	40–42	100–250	15–30
Pennant's Parakeet	180–200	40–42	150–300	30–60
Peregrine Falcon	550–1500	40–42	100–200	30–60
Pigeon	260–350	40–42	150–300	30–50
Quail	20–40	40–42	300–600	60–100
Sparrowhawk	150–300	40–42	150–350	15–45
Sparrow	25–30	40–42	250–600	100–150
Swan	5000–7000	40–42	60–100	15–30

8.4 Clinical parameters of common reptile species (SVL = snout–vent length of adult)

Common name	Species	Typical SVL (cm)	Weight range (g)	Environmental temperature range (°C)	Approx. pulse rate/minute	Approx. respiratory rate/minute
Boa Constrictor	*Boa constrictor*	200–400	10000–18000	25–30	30–50	6–10
Cornsnake	*Elaphe guttata*	100–180	150–250	25–30	40–50	6–10
Day Gecko	*Phelsuma cepediana*	10–15	15–40	23–30	40–80	6–10
Garter Snake	*Thamnophis* sp.	50–120	50–100	22–26	20–40	6–10
Green Iguana	*Iguana iguana*	100–150	900–1500	26–36	30–60	10–30
Leopard Gecko	*Eublepharus macularius*	10	25–50	23–30	40–80	20–50
Royal Python	*Python regius*	80–150	400–800	25–30	30–50	6–10
Red-eared Terrapin	*Trachemys scripta elegans*	20 (shell length)	800–1200	20–30	40–60	2–10
Mediterranean (spur-thighed) Tortoise	*Testudo graeca*	20–30 (shell length)	1000–2500	20–35	40–60	2–10

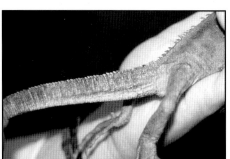

8.5

The tailbones are readily visible in this emaciated Green Iguana.

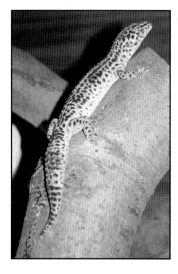

8.6

The tail of this well-fed Leopard Gecko is wider than the pelvis.

When calculating drug dosages, the whole weight of the chelonian is used. A common mistake is to attempt to deduct the weight of the shell. The shell is part of the skeleton – trying to ignore this weight is similar to trying to deduct the weight of a dog's skeleton from its body weight when calculating doses and is clearly not sensible.

Body condition is estimated from the soft tissue (muscle) covering the pelvis and tail bones – these bones should be barely visible. Figure 8.5 illustrates the tail of an emaciated green iguana. Some animals store fat in the tail (e.g. leopard gecko) and so the tail base should be thicker than the pelvis width if the animal has adequate fat storage (Figure 8.6).

Reptiles regulate their internal body temperature by moving between hot and cool areas in their enclosure. The temperatures listed reflect the normal temperature range to which the animals should have access in order to regulate successfully.

Note the high variation in 'normal' rates; for example, these are low when basking but higher when exercising or stressed. The level of activity or stress should be taken into account when evaluating whether the rates are within the normal range.

Amphibians

Amphibians can tolerate a wide range of environmental temperatures but the lower temperatures may be immunosuppressive. Clinical parameters for common pet amphibian species are given in Figure 8.7.

8.7 Clinical parameters of common amphibian species (SVL = snout–vent length of adult)

Common name	Species	Typical SVL (cm)	Weight range (g)	Environmental temperature range (°C)	Approx. pulse rate/minute	Approx. respiratory rate/minute
Crested Newt	*Triturus cristatus*	10	5–15	18–22	40–80	10–40
Tiger Salamander	*Ambyostoma tigrinum*	10	100–150	15–25	40–80	5–40
Leopard Frog	*Rana pipiens*	8	50	15–25	60–80	50–80
Tree Frog	*Hyla arborea*	3	20–50	15–25	60–80	50–80

Fish

Fish should be examined initially in the tank or pond, where their behaviour should be noted. For closer examination, individual fish may then be transferred with some water into a small clear plastic bag.

Checking the water quality is an important part of the investigation of disease in fish. Clinical parameters evaluated in the examination of fish are presented in Figures 8.8 and 8.9 along with the water parameters required to ensure fish health.

8.8 Signs of health in common ornamental fish

- Swimming upright
- Smooth scales
- No evidence of skin lesions
- No rubbing
- No petechiation

8.9 Water quality for common ornamental fish

Group	pH	Temperature (°C)	Ammonia level (mg/l)
Cold water	6.5–8.5	10–25	
Tropical	6.5–8.5	23–26	
Marine	6.5–8.5		< 0.05
Salmonids	6.5–8.5		< 0.002
Non-salmonids	6.5–8.5		< 0.01

Special techniques

Bandaging techniques

Bandages are not required to cover lesions or wounds in all cases. They should be used only after due consideration of the advantages and disadvantages of bandage application in a particular situation.

In some cases the use of dressing or bandages can create a problem: for example, the stress of repeated restraint to perform regular bandage changes can be detrimental to the welfare of a captive wild animal. Some animals will consistently chew a bandage but would not interfere with the underlying lesion if it were left uncovered.

Mammals

Many of the bandaging techniques used for domestic mammals can be applied to exotic mammals. Some individuals will not tolerate bandaging and will self-traumatize in an effort to remove the bandage. Certain rabbits will tolerate an Elizabethan collar, whereas others will not; the use of these appliances should be judged on a case-by-case basis.

Birds

Most birds will not remove subcutaneous sutures and so bandaging may not be necessary. Bandages should be placed so as not to restrict chest movements, or respiration will be compromised. The use of strong adhesive tape on the skin should be avoided as avian skin is easily torn.

Reptiles

Most reptiles tolerate bandages well. Care should be taken to use lightweight materials in animals with poor skeletal density (e.g. cases of metabolic bone disease), since fractures may be caused by the weight of the bandages. Snakes provide a unique challenge to bandaging technique but finger or stockinette bandage materials may be used. Plastic drapes or condoms with the tips cut off make useful occlusive bandages (Figure 8.10). Strong adhesive tape should not be used on the thin-skinned geckos as the skin may easily tear on removal of the bandage.

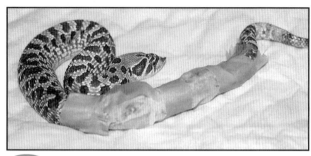

8.10 *An occlusive bandage in a snake.*

Amphibians

Bandaging of amphibians is impractical and adhesive tapes will easily damage the thin skin. The use of human oral ulcer barrier creams on the skin will protect underlying lesions and seal the skin to prevent secondary infection.

Fish

Bandaging of fish is impractical. The use of human oral ulcer barrier creams on the skin will protect the underlying lesions and reduce osmotic stress on the fish.

Assisted feeding and oral therapy

If the animal is bright and alert, warmed oral fluids may be given. Oral rehydration fluids may be given daily equal to 4–10% of body weight initially. Liquidized feed may be used once the animal is rehydrated. The general points concerning assisted feeding of animals are:

- A small amount of the food should also be available to tempt the animal to self-feed
- To prevent digestive disturbances, an appropriate food substance should be used – i.e. vegetable-based diets for herbivores, meat-based diets for carnivores.

Mammals

Most mammals have a strong chewing response and will readily feed from a syringe placed gently into the corner of the mouth. Appropriate food substances should be given; feeding the incorrect diet can lead to digestive disturbances that may severely compromise the health of an already sick animal.

The use of a nasogastric tube for assisted feeding is a useful technique in the supportive care of larger mammals that tolerate an amount of handling (e.g. rabbits, ferrets) (Figure 8.11).

 Rabbits are obligate nose breathers, so avoid placing a nasogastric tube in those animals already showing signs of respiratory distress, or they may be further compromised.

8.11 How to place a nasogastric tube in mammals

1. Sedate the animal or restrain safely
2. Instil topical local anaesthetic drops into the nose and allow to take effect
3. Measure the distance from the nose to the position of the stomach externally and mark the length on the tube
4. Lubricate the tube with lubricant gel
5. Gently introduce the tube into the ventral medial aspect of the nostril and advance it into the nose
6. If resistance is detected: stop, withdraw the tube, relubricate and reposition
7. Gently advance the tube until it is in the stomach as indicated by the mark on the tube
8. Check the tube is in place
9. Glue the tube to the head using a flap of tape and tissue glue
10. Some animals will require a restriction collar to prevent them pulling out the tube.

Never administer fluids into any nasogastric tube without first checking that it is in place. Many sick rabbits will passively inhale the tube. Check that the tube is in the stomach: either use radiography (if a radiopaque feeding tube has been used) or quickly inject 5 ml of air into the tube whilst listening over the stomach area with a stethoscope for a 'pop' noise. Figure 8.12 describes how to use a nasogastric tube safely.

8.12 How to use a nasogastric tube safely

* Carefully calculate the safe volume to instil each time
* If the animal shows signs of discomfort: stop, withdraw some fluid and inform the attending veterinary surgeon
* Many sick rabbits develop ileus (gastrointestinal stasis), thus decreasing stomach emptying time. This will require a reduction in oral fluid volumes and medical therapy to treat the ileus.

 Rabbits are unable to vomit and their stomach is relatively non-distensible. It is possible to rupture the stomach by giving too large a volume of fluid.

Birds
With birds, oral tube feeding is often called crop tubing, as the liquid is instilled into the distal oesophagus or crop, not the equivalent of the stomach. However, not all birds possess a true crop. Those with a well defined crop include parrots, pigeons, and raptors; those with a poorly defined crop include most waterfowl.

* Parrots have strong beaks and large fleshy tongues that can make inserting the gag difficult
* Pigeons have small tongues and the beak can be held open with a finger
* Raptors have small tongues but it is wise to use a gag to keep the beak open
* Do not fight with a struggling patient: many of the birds are very ill and easily stressed. It is possible to injure the choana (the slit on the roof of mouth) or crop if the bird is not restrained properly.

The technique for crop tubing is described in Figure 8.13 and illustrated in Figure 8.14. The approximate volumes and frequency of crop tubing will vary with the size of bird; guidelines are given in Figure 8.15.

8.13 How to crop tube a bird

1. Warm fluids to 38–40°C
2. Restrain bird upright
3. Extend neck
4. Insert gag if using plastic crop tube, or use metal crop tube
5. Insert crop tube into mouth at left oral commissure and angle into right side of neck
6. Palpate placement in crop
7. Infuse fluid slowly
8. Check during infusion for regurgitation, if seen release bird immediately and allow bird to swallow

8.14 Crop tubing a parrot

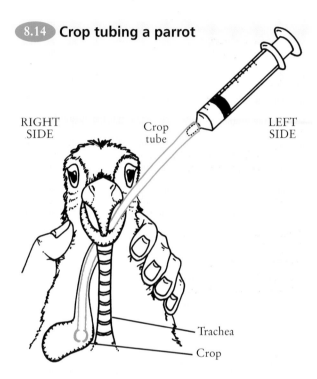

RIGHT SIDE   Crop tube   LEFT SIDE

Trachea

Crop

8.15 Suggested volumes and frequency of crop tubing of selected species

Bird species	Volume (ml)	Frequency (times per day)
Finch	0.1–0.5	6
Budgerigar	0.5–3	4
Lovebird	1–3	4
Cockatiel	1–8	4
Small conure	3–12	4
Large conure	7–24	3–4
Amazon parrot	5–35	3
African grey parrot	5–35	3
Cockatoo	10–40	2–3
Macaw	20–60	2–3

Reptiles
Liquids may be instilled directly into the reptile stomach. Figure 8.16 gives the method for stomach tubing, Figure 8.17 suggests appropriate tube sizes and Figure 8.18 describes the position of the stomach in reptiles.

When the head of a tortoise is retracted, the oesophagus has an S-bend. Thus the neck of a tortoise must be fully extended before a tube is introduced (Figure 8.19) or the tube may be accidentally pushed through the wall of the oesophagus.

8.16 How to stomach tube a reptile

1. Select flexible feeding tube of appropriate size and length (Figure 8.19)
2. Measure distance to stomach so that appropriate length is inserted, to ensure end of tube is in stomach (Figure 8.18)
3. Lubricate tube well (a small amount of lubricant can also be placed at the back of the mouth)
4. Insert gag gently into mouth (avoid damaging the delicate teeth of snakes and lizards)
5. The reptile glottis and trachea lie rostrally in the floor of the mouth thus the whole of the back of the oral cavity is oesophagus
6. Insert tube to stomach distance – stop if resistance is detected
7. Slowly infuse warmed fluid
8. If fluid is seen coming back into the mouth: stop immediately and note the volume already given (for future reference)
9. Once the animal starts to eat or drink by itself, less will be required by stomach tube
10. The stressed reptile will regurgitate food immediately after instillation. Tube the animal whilst holding it vertically and hold it so for about a minute after tubing to prevent immediate regurgitation
11. Avoid handling the reptile for 24 hours to prevent regurgitation.

8.17 Reptile stomach tube: suggested sizes and volumes

Species	Bodyweight	Size of feeding tube (Fr)	Approx. volumes (ml) twice daily
Mediterranean tortoises	> 1 kg	8	10
Juvenile iguanas	100–400 g	6–8	2–8
Adult cornsnake	200 g	8–10	5–10

8.18 Position of stomach and methods of orally dosing reptiles

Reptile	Stomach position	Method of orally dosing
Lizard	Caudal edge of the ribcage	Some will take fluids straight from the syringe Many will open their mouths defensively if the snout is tapped Gentle traction on the dewlap (if present) may also be used
Chelonian	Middle of the abdominal shield of the plastron (lower shell)	Fully extend the neck To extract the head, push in the rear limbs and tail, placing the fingers around the back of the mandibles, and maintain traction
Snake	At the beginning of the second third of the body length	The snake may disarticulate its jaws if the mouth is prised open; this is a normal response

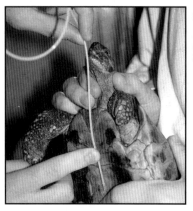

Measuring the mouth-to-stomach distance in a tortoise.

- When orally dosing or force feeding reptiles, the use of sharp objects to push the item into the mouth should be avoided as they may lacerate the oesophagus
- If the operator is scratched by a reptile's teeth, the hands should be thoroughly washed and the incident reported appropriately
- Care should be taken to avoid damaging a reptile's teeth, as this may lead to osteomyelitis of the jaw. If a snake's teeth are damaged, ensure that the animal is checked again 2 weeks and 4 weeks later and that appropriate therapy is initiated

- If tube feeding is required over a long period, consider placing a temporary pharyngostomy tube to prevent oesophageal damage from repeated stomach tube placement
- For most snakes, force feeding means using a whole dead rodent of appropriate size (Figure 8.20)

8.20 How to force feed a snake

1. Choose a food item equivalent to the diameter of the snake
2. Lubricate the food item with a water-based lubricant
3. Hold the snake vertically
4. Gag open the mouth
5. Gently introduce the food item to the back of the mouth
6. 'Milk' the food item to the stomach region (approximately halfway down snake)
7. Retain snake in vertical position for 1 minute
8. Gently return snake to vivarium.

- A general guide to the type of food to be force fed to reptiles is given in Figure 8.21
- The amount and frequency of feeding required in reptiles depends on the age, size and species of the reptile; guidelines are given in Figure 8.22.

Type of food for assisted feeding of reptiles

Species		Products for assisted feeding	
Group	Examples	Diet	Examples
Snakes	Boas, pythons, rat snakes, gopher snakes, bull snakes, vipers, garter snakes, water snakes, racers, vine snakes	Meat-based	Proprietary liquid meat products for dogs or cats
Lizards Herbivores Carnivores	 Green iguanas Monitors, geckos, anoles, skinks, chameleons	 Vegetable-based Meat-based	 Purees, baby food Meat-based products
Chelonians Carnivores Herbivores	 Turtles and terrapins Tortoises	 Meat-based Vegetable-based	 Meat-based products Purees, baby food

8.22 **Guide to feeding frequency for reptiles**

Reptile	Frequency
Small snakes and lizards	Once or twice/week
Young of boas and pythons	Three times/week
Herbivores	Daily
Large snakes	Once/2–4 weeks

Amphibians

Food may be placed directly into the mouth of an amphibian. It will usually be swallowed if it is placed at the back of the mouth. Care must be taken not to damage the delicate skin when attempting to open the mouth to introduce feed.

Administration of medicines

Oral route

The methods described above for assisted feeding are also applicable to individual oral dosing of animals. These are the most accurate methods of oral administration of drugs.

Administering drugs in the drinking water is of limited use. Success of treatment using this method depends upon:

- The amount of water consumed – most psittacines and reptiles drink too little to make this a useful option
- The oral bioavailability of the drug – if the drug is not absorbed from the gastrointestinal tract then it can only be used to treat gut infections using this method.

Birds

Proprietary medicated seed is available to treat birds. It is difficult to assess an accurate dose for the bird as not all the seed offered may be eaten. This method is obviously not suitable for the anorexic or non-seed-eating bird.

Amphibians

Amphibians may be dosed from a syringe placed directly into the mouth.

Fish

Some types of medicated fish feed are commercially available. Homemade medicated feed can be produced by combining fish flakes and the required drug with gelatine. A dose of medicine per fish is calculated and the amount of food the fish will eat is assessed. The concentration of drug to be used in the feed is then calculated. The necessary amount of gelatine is made up with water to which the drug has been added. Fish flakes are then added to the liquid mixture; the mixture is allowed to set and then grated for feeding to the fish at the required dose.

Intravenous route

Figure 8.23 lists accessible intravenous sites. These may be used for the introduction of fluids and drugs or for withdrawing a blood sample.

8.23 **Intravenous injection and blood sampling sites**

Animal	Site(s)
Small mammal	Jugular (ferret, rabbit, chinchilla) Marginal ear vein (rabbit) Cephalic (rabbit, chinchilla, guinea-pig) Lateral tail vein (rodents)
Bird	Jugular, brachial, medial metatarsal
Snakes	Ventral tail vein, jugular vein, cardiac
Lizard	Ventral tail vein, jugular vein
Chelonian	Jugular vein, dorsal tail vein
Amphibian	Central ventral abdominal vein, cardiac
Fish	Caudal vein

Mammals

The use of the intravenous site to deliver fluids or drugs in small mammals is arguably only practical in the rabbit, where access to the marginal ear veins is relatively simple (Figures 8.24 and 8.25). It is useful to apply a local anaesthetic cream to the skin prior to venepuncture to minimize discomfort.

Birds

Three main intravenous sites are used in birds. The brachial vein is readily identified in the medial elbow (Figure 8.26) but is prone to haematoma formation after sampling. The medial metatarsal vein (Figure 8.27) is less fragile and can be used in larger birds. The right jugular vein is larger than the left. Each jugular vein is located in a featherless tract on the neck and so is easily visualized.

8.24 How to place an intravenous catheter in a rabbit

1. Shave the lateral ear over the vein and prepare the site aseptically
2. Apply local anaesthetic cream and leave for appropriate amount of time
3. Insert catheter of suitable size and glue in place, using cyanoacrylate adhesive
4. Flush with heparin saline
5. Pack inside of ear with roll of gauze and tape in place
6. Connect catheter to giving set or mini extension set
7. Apply Elizabethan collar to the rabbit if required.

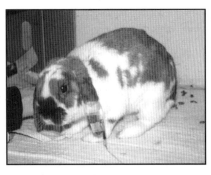

8.25 *Rabbit with an intravenous infusion line in place.*

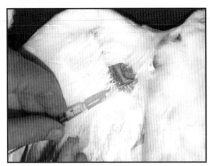

8.26 *Brachial vein of a pigeon.*

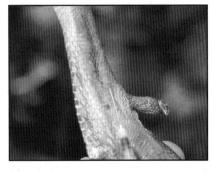

8.27 *Metatarsal vein of a swan.*

Reptiles

The choice of vein used for the intravenous sites depends upon the type of reptile under consideration. The jugular vein is useful in chelonians (Figures 8.28 and 8.29), but access to this vein requires a surgical cut-down in snakes and lizards; the ventral tail vein is useful in snakes and lizards (Figures 8.30, 8.31 and 8.32). Care must be taken if injecting into the dorsal tail vein of a chelonian (Figure 8.33) as the injection may be inadvertently placed in the epidural space and may produce hindlimb paresis or paralysis. Intracardiac catheters may be placed in snakes to access the circulation if the peripheral veins are too small for ready access. Aseptic technique is required when accessing the veins or heart.

8.28 How to access the jugular vein in the chelonian

1. Extend the neck fully by using continuous traction, placing fingers behind head. Sedation may be required for strong patients
2. The vein runs from the tympanic membrane to the base of the neck
3. The vein may be raised by placing a finger at the base of the neck
4. Insert the needle parallel to the neck into the vein
5. After access, apply pressure to the site for a few minutes to limit haematoma formation.

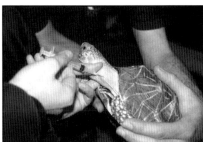

8.29 *Obtaining a jugular blood sample from a tortoise.*

8.30 How to access the ventral tail vein in a lizard or snake

1. Restrain the animal and hold the tail with the ventral aspect facing the operator
2. Insert the needle in the exact midline at a point distal to the vent and hemipenes (if present)
3. Advance to touch ventral aspect of the tail vertebra (at right angles to tail in snake, at 45 degree angle in lizard)
4. Aspirate slowly and withdraw slightly until blood is seen in the hub of the needle.

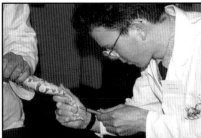

8.31 *Obtaining a ventral tail vein blood sample from a snake.*

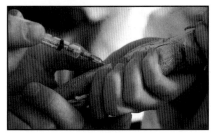

8.32 *Obtaining a ventral tail vein blood sample from an iguana.*

8.33 How to access the dorsal tail vein in a tortoise

1. Fully extend the tail
2. Insert the needle into the exact midline of the dorsal tail close to the shell
3. Advance the needle to touch the vertebrae
4. Aspirate the syringe and withdraw it slightly until blood is seen in the hub of the needle.

Amphibians

The only accessible vein in amphibians is the central ventral abdominal vein. The heart may be accessed for blood sampling in the anaesthetized animal. The lymphatic system is a useful site for injection in amphibians and appears to be effective in delivering parenteral therapy. The site is dorsal, just off the midline of the body.

Fish

The caudal vein in fish is accessed on the ventral aspect on the midline, just cranial to the tail and caudal to the anal fin. The vein lies immediately ventral to the vertebral column. The method is similar to accessing the ventral tail vein of the snake or lizard.

Intramuscular route

Figure 8.34 suggests sites for intramuscular injection.

8.34 Intramuscular injection sites

Animal	Site(s)
Small mammal	Quadriceps (rabbit, ferret) Lumbar (rabbit, ferret)
Bird	Breast (pectoral) muscles
Snake	Intercostal muscles of body in middle third of snake: insert needle just deep enough to cover bevel, shallow angle
Lizard	Triceps (forelimb), quadriceps (hindlimb), tail muscles in some species (not geckos)
Chelonian	As lizard, also pectoral muscle mass at angle of forelimb and neck. A short needle should be used and the head extended to avoid injecting the structures of the neck or penetrating to the lung/heart. The needle should only be inserted to the depth of the bevel
Amphibian	(Fore)limb muscles
Fish	Dorsal lateral musculature

Mammals and birds

A relatively large volume injected into the muscle causes unnecessary pain to small animals. Drug reactions and myositis have been associated with this route in rabbits and rodents. Studies have also shown that the uptake of subcutaneous or intraperitoneal injections in small rodents is as fast as from the intramuscular site.

This is, however, a useful site for dosing birds (Figure 8.35).

8.35 How to give a bird an intramuscular injection

1. Palpate and identify the breast bone (keel) as a ridge running down the centre of the two breast muscles and identify the edge of the sternum
2. Divide the breast muscles into four imaginary parts (top right, top left, bottom right, bottom left)
3. Inject deeply into the muscle in alternate sites
4. After injection, place a finger over the puncture site for a minute to minimize bleeding. Normally, there should be no or very little bleeding.

Reptiles

Reptiles have a renal portal venous circulation. This means that, in theory, blood from the caudal half of the body can flow through the kidneys before returning to the heart. Thus drugs injected into the hindlegs or tail may be lost via the kidneys before being distributed around the body, or may damage the kidneys if the drugs are potentially nephrotoxic. There is still debate as to whether this significantly affects drug distribution. It is generally accepted, however, that injections should be given in the cranial half of the body whenever possible.

Care needs to be taken in giving intramuscular injections to reptiles:

- Some lizards can shed their tails and so the injection of substances into the tail should be avoided
- It is good practice to alternate sides or sites where possible
- Some chameleons may show a temporary or permanent colour change at the injection site.

Amphibians

Amphibians also possess a renal portal system (see considerations for reptiles, above). The front limb muscles may be injected but these are usually small and so large volumes should be avoided.

Fish

Abscess formation and drug leakage out of the needle track is common in fish after intramuscular injection.

Subcutaneous route

The subcutaneous route (Figure 8.36) is an impractical route in chelonians. Larger volumes may be given via the subcutaneous route than intramuscularly in small lizards and snakes.

8.36 Subcutaneous injection sites

Animal	Site(s)
Small mammal	Dorsal body (scruff)
Bird	Dorsal body between wings
Snake	Dorsal lateral third of snake, over ribs
Lizard	In loose lateral skin fold over ribs
Chelonian	Some loose skin on limbs
Amphibian	Dorsal area over shoulders
Fish	Not used

Intraperitoneal/intracoelomic route

This route (Figure 8.37) generally allows for a large volume to be given. The fluids must be warmed to the body temperature appropriate to the species.

Birds

The peritoneal space in birds is merely a potential one and cannot be accessed for injection unless ascites is present. Attempted injection into the abdominal space in birds will usually result in injection into the air sacs, severely compromising respiration, and is often fatal.

Reptiles

Reptiles do not possess a diaphragm and so the injection of large volumes of fluid into the coelom can compromise respiration.

8.37 Intraperitoneal/intracoelomic injection sites

Animal	Site(s)
Small mammal	Off midline, caudal to level of umbilicus
Bird	⚠ Not possible in healthy animal – avoid as attempts may drown animal
Snake	Immediately cranial to vent on lateral body wall
Lizard	Off midline, caudal to ribs, cranial to pelvis
Chelonian	Extend hindlimb, inject cranial to hindlimb in fossa
Amphibian	Ventrolateral quadrant
Fish	Immediately rostral to vent on ventral surface

Intraosseous route

The intraosseous route is a useful one for parenteral therapy, especially in small animals, because:

- Placing an intraosseous catheter or needle into a bone enables fluids to be given into the medullary cavity, where absorption is as rapid as the intravenous route
- Small veins are fragile and easily lacerated by catheters or 'blown' when introducing fluids, whereas an intraosseous catheter is stable in bone
- If the animal displaces or damages the intraosseous catheter, it is unlikely to haemorrhage from this site compared with intravenous catheterization.

Figure 8.38 describes how to place an intraosseous catheter; suggested sites for intraosseous catheters are given in Figure 8.39 and illustrated in Figure 8.40. The management of an intraosseous catheter (Figure 8.41) is similar to the technique used to manage an intravenous catheter.

8.38 How to place an intraosseous catheter

1. Prepare site aseptically
2. Inject local anaesthesia into site (unless animal is under general anaesthesia)
3. Introduce spinal needles or plain needles of appropriate size into the bone (needle size sufficient to enter medullary cavity, based on knowledge or guided by radiographic image of cavity)
4. Flush with heparinized saline to ensure patency
5. Secure in place with surgical cyanoacrylate adhesive or suture
6. Attach short extension tube
7. Bandage area to maintain cleanliness and reduce mobility of limb.

8.39 Suggested sites for intraosseous catheters

Animal	Site
Small mammal	Proximal femur, proximal tibia
Bird	Distal radius, proximal tibiotarsus
Reptile	Proximal or distal femur, proximal tibia; bridge between carapace and plastron in chelonians

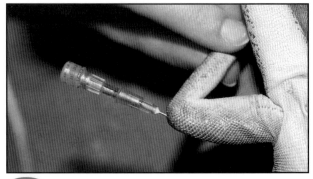

8.40 *Intraosseous catheter in femur of a Green Iguana.*

8.41 How to manage an intraosseous catheter

- Use aseptic technique when giving drugs/fluids
- To prevent clot formation, fill catheter with heparin or heparinized saline between use
- Flush three times daily with heparinized saline if not used for drug or fluid administration.

Nebulization

This is a useful technique for delivering drugs to the respiratory system. Drugs given by nebulization are not systemically absorbed and so potentially nephrotoxic or hepatotoxic drugs may be used relatively safely. This technique is especially useful in the treatment of respiratory tract disease in birds and reptiles, where adequate drug levels may not reach the respiratory tract following oral or parenteral dosing. It also minimizes the stress of handling and potential damage caused by repeated injections. The animal is placed in a chamber and nebulized with the drug for an appropriate length of time (Figure 8.42). The nebulizer must generate particles of less than 3 microns in order to enter the lower respiratory tract of birds.

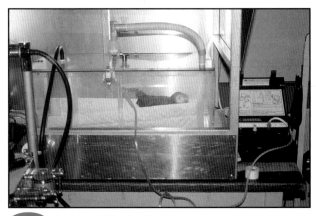

8.42 *Bird in nebulization chamber.*

Via the water environment

This route can be used for fish, amphibians and aquatic invertebrates.

- Antibiotics should not be administered via the water if a biological filtration system is in use
- The calcium present in hard water may chelate some antibiotics and so reduce their availability
- Many of the drugs used are toxic in high doses
- Calculations of water volume and drug required must be made accurately

- If possible, test the solution using a few animals before dosing a large number
- Mix the water thoroughly to ensure that the drug is evenly dispersed
- Starve the animal for 24 hours before treatment.

There are two methods of administering drugs using the water:

- Dipping the animal into a strong solution for a short period (usually administered in a separate 'hospital tank', then the animal is returned to its home environment)
- Bathing the animal in a weaker solution for a longer period. If the animal shows any signs of distress, the treatment should be stopped. This may be performed in the home tank to minimize disturbance, or in a separate 'hospital tank'.

Topical application of medicine

Mammals
Mammals commonly groom off any topical treatment, reducing its effectiveness. Any medication applied to the skin should be non-toxic if ingested. Collars may be used to prevent the animal from removing the topical medication.

Birds
Topical medication should be applied to the skin, not feathers, of a bird. Collars may be tolerated by some animals and can be used to prevent ingestion of the medicine.

Reptiles
Most reptiles will tolerate topical therapy without grooming or licking the medicine. It is useful to bandage the area after application to prevent the animal rubbing the medicine off; this is especially important in snakes.

Amphibians
Most topically applied medications will be systemically absorbed by amphibians and so any wound dressings should be applied with care. This route may therefore be used to administer medicines. The dose should be carefully calculated. Ophthalmic drops are often used for this purpose.

Fluid therapy

- Volumes required are usually 1–2% of bodyweight
- The advantages and disadvantages of subcutaneous, intramuscular and intraperitoneal routes have been described above
- Placement and maintenance of intravenous catheters is as for larger domestic animals (see Figure 8.23 for description of accessible veins)
- Intraosseous catheters are useful to administer fluids to smaller animals or those in which a vein is not readily accessible (see Figure 8.39 for suggested sites and Figure 8.38 for method of placement).

Blood sampling
See Figure 8.23 for blood sampling sites.

- Up to 10% of the blood volume may be safely taken from an animal. This must be carefully calculated using an accurate weight when dealing with small animals (Figure 8.43 gives examples)
- EDTA may lyse some avian and reptile cells
- A fresh blood smear is useful when examining cell morphology and checking for blood parasites
- The laboratory should be contacted for guidance on (minimum) sample volume and tubes required.

Common diseases

Common diseases for various animals, along with their causes and treatment, are described in Figures 8.44–8.50.

8.43 Guide to small animal weights and maximum blood volume that may be taken safely

Weight of animal (g)	Maximum safe volume of blood to take (ml)
500	5
200	2
100	1
50	0.5

8.44 Common conditions of small mammals

Problem	Species	Possible causes	Treatment	Comment
Anorexia	All	Urolithiasis	Surgery when stable	
	All	Renal disease, liver disease	Supportive	Especially older animals
	Guinea-pig, young rabbit, hamster	Change in diet or environment	Reduce stress Probiotics	Very common in new pets
	Guinea-pig, chinchilla, rabbit	Dental disease	Burring/removal of affected teeth	Usually due to lack of dietary fibre or genetic factors
	Guinea-pig, rabbit	Pregnancy toxaemia	Corticosteroids Dextrose Emergency surgery	Especially in obese animals
	Rabbit	Viral haemorrhagic disease	None (fatal) Vaccinate in-contact animals	Routine vaccination recommended

Figure 8.44 continues ▶

Problem	Species	Possible causes	Treatment	Comment
Diarrhoea	All	Dietary change, stress, enteritis (bacterial, fungal, viral)	Increase fibre intake Probiotics Antibiotics Fluid therapy	Address underlying cause
	Rabbit	Lack of fibre, coccidiosis	Increase fibre intake Probiotics Coccidiostats Fluid therapy	Look for and prevent associated myiasis
	Hamster ('wet tail' or proliferative ileitis)	*Campylobacter jejuni* *Escherichia coli* *Chlamydia tracheomatis* *Desulfovibrio* spp.	Oral antibiotics and fluid therapy	Very common Poor prognosis Predisposing factors: stress, dietary change
	Guinea-pig, rabbit, hamster	Inappropriate antibiotics	Increase fibre intake Probiotics Stop antibiotics Fluid therapy	Avoid penicillins, cephalosporins
Respiratory disease	All	Viral, bacterial	Supportive therapy Appropriate antibiotics Mucolytics	'Chronic respiratory disease' in rats may require long-term treatment
Dermatitis	All	Ectoparasites	Ivermectin	Treat underlying cause and in-contact animals Separate animals
		Bacterial	Antibiotics	
		Fungal (e.g. dermatophytosis)	Griseofulvin	
		Viral	None	
		Self or cagemate trauma (barbering)	Separate animals	
	Hamster	Neoplasia (lymphoma; mycosis fungoides)	Euthanasia	
	Guinea-pig	Scurvy	Vitamin C	Always add vitamin C to the diet and/or water
Myiasis (fly strike)	Rabbit	Maggots	Removal of maggots, ivermectin, antibiotics, corticosteroids (shock)	Investigate underlying cause of debilitation (e.g. obesity, arthritis, dental disease)
Haematuria	All	Urolithiasis	Surgery	Investigate individual cause
		Cystitis	Antibiotics	
		Neoplasia, bladder	Surgery/none	
		Neoplasia, uterus	Surgery (spay)	
		Renal infection	Antibiotics	
	Rabbit	Normal red pigments	None required	
Neurological signs	Rabbit	Pasteurellosis (middle ear or brain)	Antibiotics	
	Rabbit, ferret	Parasites in brain (*Encephalitozoon cuniculi*, aberrant migration of nematodes, *Toxoplasma*)	Supportive/none	
	All	Trauma	Supportive/none	
	Rabbit, ferret	Heat stroke	Supportive/cool slowly	
	All	Lead toxicity	Drugs to chelate lead, surgery to remove source if lead ingested	Usually due to ingested lead foreign body (i.e. lead in gut); rarely results from lead shot in muscle tissue
Lameness, weakness	Ferret	Insulinoma	Glucose, surgery	
		Lymphoma	Cancer therapy	

Figure 8.44 continues ▶

Problem	Species	Possible causes	Treatment	Comment
Lameness, weakness *continued*	Ferret *continued*	Anaemia	Specific therapy	Common in entire unmated female ferrets who develop persistent oestrus. May not respond to mating with vasectomized male
		Aleutian disease (viral)	None, supportive	
		Canine distemper	None, supportive	Vaccinate with canine vaccine
	All species, especially rat and rabbit	Pododermatitis ('bumblefoot')	As above, husbandry, bandaging feet	May progress to amyloidosis and renal failure
	All species, especially rat and rabbit	Arthritis (limbs, spine)	Analgesia, anti-inflammatories	
	All	Fractures, intervertebral disc protrusion	Supportive, surgery if fractures, euthanasia if spinal	
Subcutaneous masses	Rabbit, rodents, ferret	Abscess	Lance, drain, antibiotics, treat underlying cause	Facial abscesses in rabbit often related to dental infection or osteomyelitis
	Guinea-pig	Cervical adenitis (*Streptococcus zooepidemicus*)	Surgical removal of infected lymph node(s), antibiotics, euthanasia	
	All	Lipoma, other neoplasia	Surgery	
	Rabbit	Myxomatosis	Supportive, vaccinate other animals in contacts	Usually fatal
	Guinea-pig	Sebaceous adenoma	Surgery	
Corneal ulcer	All	Trauma, entropion	Antibiotics, surgery	
	Rodents	Viral infection of lachrymal glands (SDAV)	None; supportive (eye may perforate)	
	Rodents	Calcification of cornea	None	
	Ferret	Distemper, influenza	Supportive	
Ocular discharge	Rabbit	Dacryocystitis (infection of tear duct)	Flush ducts, antibiotics	Check molar roots not impinging on duct (radiography required to evaluate)
	Chinchilla, rabbit	Overgrown molar teeth roots impinging on duct	Dental treatment	Poor prognosis
Red staining tears	All	Stress, concurrent disease	Treat underlying cause	Known as porphyria/ chromodacryorrhoea

8.45 Common conditions of birds

Problem	Common clinical condition	Treatment
Skin/face		
Periocular swelling	Ocular or sinus disorder	Investigate and treat appropriately
Epiphora, conjunctivitis	Ocular or sinus disorder, partial lid paralysis (cockatiel), psittacosis (cockatiel, duck)	Investigate and treat appropriately
Scabs, scars, pustules	Pox virus	Vaccination of in-contacts
Brown hypertrophy of cere	Endocrinopathy (budgerigars)	None
Hyperkeratosis Crusting of cere	*Cnemidocoptes* spp. (mites)	Ivermectin

Figure 8.45 continues ▷

Small mammal, exotic animal and wildlife nursing   **183**

Problem	Common clinical condition	Treatment
Nares		
Discharge (rhinitis)	Sinusitis, air sacculitis	Based on sensitivity, flush out sinuses, infuse antibiotics
Rhinoliths Enlarged orifice	Hypovitaminosis A Severe rhinitis (bacterial, fungal), atrophic rhinitis(African greys)	Vitamin A therapy Improve diet Rhinoliths: remove with needle point, treat underlying cause
Oral cavity		
Excessive moisture	Inflammation	Investigate and treat appropriately
Blunting choanal papillae	Hypovitaminosis A	Vitamin A therapy Improve diet
White plaques (removable)	Hypovitaminosis A	Vitamin A therapy Improve diet
White/yellow fixed plaques	Pox, bacterial ulceration, *Candida*, *Trichomonas*	Investigate and treat appropriately
Feathers		
Dystrophic	Psittacine beak and feather disease (PBFD) virus, polyoma virus	None
Broken, matted, chewed, plucked, missing	Self-trauma (discomfort, psychological); cage too small, seizures, by cagemate (bullying, mating), endocrinopathy	Investigate and treat appropriately
Beak		
Overgrowth, malocclusion	Cnemidocoptic mange, PBFD, hypovitaminosis A	Investigate and treat appropriately
Crop		
Dilatation	Thyroid hyperplasia (budgerigars); bird 'clicks' and sits forward to breathe	Iodine deficiency if fed cheap loose seed Add iodine to water and give good diet
Thickening	Inflammation – *Candida*, *Trichomonas* spp.	Antifungal therapy
Regurgitation	Behavioural	Bonded to owner or toy/mirror – remove toy
	Proventricular dilation syndrome	Supportive
Abdominal enlargement		
Enlargement	Liver enlargement, egg retention, excess fluid, neoplasia or granuloma of internal organ (gonad, liver, spleen, intestines)	Investigate and treat appropriately
Miscellaneous		
Abnormal position of limbs	Neoplasm, fracture (require radiography to differentiate), trauma	Investigate and treat appropriately
Distortion of limbs	Distortion may be due to incorrect diet, fracture, neoplasia, arthritis, articular gout	Investigate and treat appropriately
External vent – soiled	Gastrointestinal tract disease; differentiate between prolapse, impaction and tumour Papillomatosis, cloacoliths	Investigate and treat appropriately
Increased size of preen gland	Squamous cell carcinoma, adenoma, abscess (note: gland absent in some birds)	Surgery
Nails overgrown, deformed	Hypovitaminosis A, liver disease	Correct diet, investigate cause
Digits – necrosis, abnormal shape	Constriction by wire, etc: frostbite, cnemidocoptic mange, bumblefoot	Amputation, ivermectin, antibiotics, bandaging, surgery as appropriate

Common toxicities of birds

Toxicity	Diagnosis and signs	Treatment	Typical source(s)
Zinc > 2 ppm probable > 10 ppm commonly toxic level	Feather chewing, green diarrhoea	EDTA	New wire, new cages, coins, jewellery
Warfarin	History Bleeding	Vitamin K	Access to rodenticide or poisoned rodents
Vitamin D toxicity	Dietary history Cholecalciferol rodenticide Mineralization of soft tissues	Charcoal, fluid therapy, frusemide, calcitonin, prednisolone, low calcium diet	Access to rodenticide Oversupplementation of diet
PTFE (Teflon®)	Collapse Seizure activity History of cooking in house Often presents as acute death	Oxygen therapy, prednisolone, dexamethasone, fluids, antibiosis	Overheated 'non-stick' pans, oven papers
Lead > 0.2 ppm suggestive > 0.5 ppm very likely	CNS signs, green diarrhoea Radiographic findings	EDTA, surgical removal, D-penicillamine	Ingestion of foreign body, e.g. fishing weight, curtain weight, lead shot/pellets (rarely from shot in muscle tissue)

Common conditions of reptiles

Problem	Clinical signs	Possible causes	Treatment	Comment
Anorexia	Not eating	Most diseases, stress, inappropriate husbandry, seasonal/physiological decrease in appetite	Fluid therapy with glucose, force feeding, treat underlying cause	Requires rapid diagnosis and treatment to avoid hepatic lipidosis Number of feeds missed is more important than total time anorexic with regard to assessing nutrient deficit
Dysecdysis (slough retention)	Dull skin, incomplete shedding (snakes), retained spectacle (snakes), loss of digit (geckos)	Most diseases, stress, inappropriate husbandry (including low humidity), seasonal/physiological decrease in appetite	Soak animal in warm water and rub off loose skin with wet towel. May require several soakings over 4–6 days Treat underlying cause	Take care with retained spectacle to avoid damaging underlying cornea Can lead to loss of digits or tail (dry gangrene of extremities)
Infectious ulcerative stomatitis	Oral petechiation, excess salivation, oral abscessation	*Aeromonas hydrophila* (and other Gram-negative bacteria) May be associated with oral trauma	Early cases: topical povidone–iodine solution Advanced cases: correct antibiotic selection Vitamins A and C for healing	May progress to pneumonia, osteomyelitis
Abscesses	Subcutaneous swelling	Trauma. Check for underlying cause, especially septicaemia	Inspissated pus produced in reptiles requires surgical removal	Commonest cause of swellings in reptiles
Burns	Open wounds, necrotic tissue	Access to unguarded heat source	Clean, debride, suture where necessary Fluid therapy, antibiosis, antifungals, analgesia Plastic adhesive drape useful to keep site clean and avoid excessive water loss	Reptiles will lie on extremely hot surfaces and sustain deep burns (even penetrating coelom). Must be prevented access to heaters

Figure 8.47 continues ▶

Problem	Clinical signs	Possible causes	Treatment	Comment
Nutritional osteodystrophy/ metabolic bone disease	Pathological fractures Lameness, weakness Fibrous osteodystrophy Muscle tremors Seizures Tetany	Calcium deficiency Improper calcium:phosphorous ratio Lack of vitamin D_3 Lack of ultraviolet light Protein deficiency (disease of kidneys, liver, small intestine, thyroid or parathyroid – rare)	Correct diet and husbandry, minimal handling, calcium injections with fluid therapy	Educate owner in proper husbandry of animal
Vitamin A deficiency	Swollen eyes	Deficient diet (meat only)	Vitamin A (correct dose for weight) Correct diet	Common in terrapins Renal damage may be fatal Overdosage results in skin sloughing
Vitamin B_1 deficiency	Neurological signs (fitting, twitching)	Deficient diet (e.g. fed frozen fish without supplementing with B_1)	Thiamine Correct diet	Common in garter snakes Nervous system damage may be fatal Cardiomyopathy may develop
Respiratory disease	Nasal discharge, open-mouth breathing, extended neck/head, cyanosis	Poor husbandry Lack of exercise Poor ventilation Incorrect temperature Bacterial, fungal	Appropriate antimicrobial Nebulization Coupage (hold upside down and tap body to expel debris from lungs) Correct husbandry	Reptiles do not possess diaphragms so cannot cough to expel debris
Dystocia	Straining, lethargy Cloacal discharge	Lack of nesting site Oviduct infection Oversized eggs Debilitation	Stabilize Provision of nest site Calcium Oxytocin if not oversized egg Surgery	Common in captivity (lack of nesting site, poor husbandry)
Pre-ovulatory follicular stasis	Swollen abdomen, constipation, anorexia	(Unknown) Lack of nesting site Poor nutritional status Poor husbandry for nesting	Supportive care in early stages and animal may ovulate, Advanced cases: stabilize and ovariectomize	Common problem in captive iguanas and some other lizards Prophylactic ovariectomy to be recommended for these species
Shell disease	Pitted shell to large shell defects with underlying osteomyelitis	Poor husbandry Trauma Infection (bacterial, fungal)	Debride, appropriate antimicrobial, bandage, fibreglass reconstruction Correct husbandry	Extensive defects must be repaired with acrylic
Cloacal prolapse	Part of distal intestinal tract everted	Calculi Parasitism Polyps Infection Diarrhoea Obstruction of the lower intestinal tract	Treat underlying cause Clean and replace prolapse Amputate necrotic tissue Retaining sutures	
Post-hibernation anorexia	Anorexia on emergence from hibernation	Any concurrent disease Frost damage to retina Aural abscess Rhinitis Pneumonia	Glucose saline i.p., i.v. or i.o. Treat underlying cause	PHA is *not* a diagnosis Requires further investigation to find underlying cause

8.48 Common conditions of amphibians

Problem	Clinical signs	Possible causes	Treatment
Bloat	Swollen body	Gastric fermentation Air swallowing Peritoneal effusions (infection, neoplasia)	If air: remove by aspiration If fluid: treat underlying cause
Cloacal prolapse	Organ protruding from vent	Foreign body, parasites, masses, gastroenteritis	Treat underlying cause Replace prolapse
Diarrhoea	Increased faecal output	Bacterial infection Parasites Toxins (e.g. lead, rancid feed)	Treat underlying cause Supportive care
Masses	Masses in skin or internal organs	Parasites Bacteria *Mycobacterium* Neoplasia	Investigate cause Surgery or medical therapy Spontaneous tumours caused by Lucke tumour herpes virus
Corneal oedema	Cloudy eye(s)	Poor water quality Trauma Ocular infection	Improve husbandry Treat underlying cause
Corneal keratopathy	White patches on cornea	Lipid keratopathy (high fat diet) Trauma Poor water quality	Evaluate diet and husbandry and amend as required
Metabolic bone disease	Curved limb bones Spinal deformities Poor growth Fractures	Poor diet (low calcium, calcium:phosphorus imbalance, vitamin D deficiency) Lack of UV light	Correct diet and husbandry
Poor condition	Weight loss Poor growth	Parasites Bacterial/fungal systemic infection	Treat underlying cause

8.49 Common conditions of fish

Problem	Clinical signs	Possible causes	Treatment
Cataract	Opacity of lens	Nutritional deficiency (e.g. zinc, copper, selenium) Eye fluke	None – treat underlying cause
Corneal opacity	Eye appears cloudy	Trauma Gas bubble trauma Poor water quality Nutritional imbalance Eye fluke	Treat underlying cause
Exophthalmia	Enlarged eye	Spring viraemia of carp (see below) Swim bladder inflammation Systemic infection	None – treat underlying cause
Vertebral deformity	Deviation in spine, fish swimming in circles	Nutritional deficiency (e.g. phosphorus, vitamin C)	None – treat underlying cause
Respiratory distress	Gasping, crowding at inlets	Low dissolved oxygen Gill disease Toxins in the water Anaemia	Treat underlying cause
Skin irritation	Jumping, rubbing	Ectoparasites Toxins in water	Treat underlying cause
White spots or cotton wool patches on skin	As described	*Ichthyophthirius* infection *Saprolegnia* infection *Cytophagia* infection	Treat underlying cause
Skin ulceration	Loss of scales, deep or superficial defect, underlying muscles exposed	Nutritional imbalance Trauma Ectoparasite Bacterial/ fungal infection (*Aeromonas salmonicida*) Systemic infection	Treat underlying cause Surgically debride ulcer, apply barrier cream and administer parenteral antimicrobials as required

Figure 8.49 continues ▶

Problem	Clinical signs	Possible causes	Treatment
'Hole in the head disease'	Large erosions in head	*Hexamita*	Metronidazole
Fin rot	Ragged fins, loss of fins	Trauma *Cytophagia* infection *Saprolegnia* infection *Aeromonas/Pseudomonas* infection Ectoparasite Nutritional imbalance	Treat underlying cause
Spring viraemia of carp	Lethargy, dark skin, respiratory distress, loss of balance, abdominal distension, petechial haemorrhages	Virus (*Rhabdovirus carpio*)	None. Notifiable in UK under the Diseases of Fish Act 1937 (as amended)

8.50 Common conditions of invertebrates

Problem	Clinical signs	Possible causes	Treatment
Trauma	Lost or damaged limbs Damaged body	Mishandling Attacks by others	If losing haemolymph, surgical glue can be used to seal the defect Limbs may regenerate Minor injuries will heal at the next slough
Alopecia	Loss of hairs (especially spiders)	Overhandling Stress Incorrect husbandry	Reduce handling Provide hiding places in enclosure Correct husbandry
Infectious disease	Larvae become wet Adults have diarrhoea, exudates, discharges	Bacteria Fungi Viruses	Isolation of diseased stock Improve husbandry Quarantine new arrivals
Parasites	Weight loss 'Eaten alive' by parasites Death	Parasitic wasps and flies Nematodes Mites	Improve husbandry Use effective barriers Mite treatment licensed for bees
Nutritional	Weight loss Death Poor growth	Incorrect food Too little food Incorrect humidity, temperature	Provide correct feed and conditions
Toxicity	Death	Accidental use of insect sprays or powders near invertebrates	Remove toxin by ventilation, dust off animal, give bathing facilities

Zoonoses

Diseases that can be transmitted from animal to human (zoonoses) are found in common domestic as well as 'exotic' species. It is therefore wise to adopt appropriate precautionary measures with all species. Note that an animal can appear perfectly healthy but be carrying a disease that may affect humans. Figure 8.51 lists some zoonoses and their symptoms in animals and humans.

Steps to decrease the risks of exposure to potential zoonoses include the following.

- Appropriate protective clothing (e.g. hats, masks, gloves) should be worn
- Animals should not be 'petted' unnecessarily
- Hands should be washed after handling an animal or its faeces
- Care should be taken to rinse thoroughly any cuts, scratches or bites incurred and they should be reported appropriately
- It should be ensured that staff tetanus and other appropriate vaccinations are up to date
- The doctor should be made aware of staff contact with animals.

If an animal is suspected of, or confirmed to have, a zoonotic disease:

- Euthanasia of the animal for public health reasons may be considered and submission of its body for post mortem to check for the zoonotic disease under consideration
- The animal may be treated (only after careful consideration of the first point)
- A minimal number of people should have contact with that animal
- Only suitably trained staff should have contact with that animal
- Appropriate precautions should be taken when in contact with that animal
- If a zoonosis in a human is suspected, or staff have been in contact with a zoonosis, the doctor should be informed as soon as possible
- Some diseases must be reported to the appropriate authorities.

Disease	Causative agent	Common animal hosts	Signs in animal	Symptoms in humans	Precautions required
Ringworm	*Microsporum canis* *Trichphyton gypseum*	Hedgehog Hamster (All rodents, rabbits) Ferret	Scaly patches, hair loss	Scaly patch of skin, may be pruritic	Wear gloves, change clothes between animals
Scabies	*Sarcoptes scabiei*	Ferret, fox, rodents	Dermatitis, pruritus	Dermatitis, pruritus	Wear gloves
Cestodiasis/tapeworm	*Hymenolepis* spp.	Mouse, young rat	Weight loss, constipation	Diarrhoea, constipation	Caution when handling animal or its faeces
Salmonellosis	*Salmonella* spp.	Reptiles Fox, badger, ferret Birds Invertebrates	None, diarrhoea	Diarrhoea	Caution when handling animal or its faeces
Cryptosporidiosis	*Cryptosporidium* spp.	Reptiles Ferret	None, diarrhoea Thickening of stomach mucosa causing regurgitation in snakes	Diarrhoea	Caution when handling animal or its faeces (especially if human is immunocompromised)
Giardiasis	*Giardia* spp.	Reptiles Birds Ferret	None, diarrhoea	Diarrhoea, abdominal pain, septicaemia	Caution when handling animal or its faeces
Psittacosis	*Chlamydia psittaci*	Birds	None, respiratory, lethargy	Headache, fever, confusion, myalgia, non-productive cough, lymphadenopathy	Wear mask/respiratory apparatus, gloves, change of clothing Reportable in some areas
Influenza ('flu)	Orthomyxovirus	Ferret	Sneezing, nasal discharge, fever, lethargy	Sneezing, nasal discharge, fever lethargy	Mask More commonly from human to ferret
Leptospirosis	*Leptospira* spp.	Ferret, rodents Amphibians	None	Severe 'flu-like symptoms	Avoid contact with urine Wear mask and gloves
Tuberculosis	*Mycobacterium bovis*, *M. tuberculosis*	Ferret, badger, deer Fish Amphibians	None, wasting, pneumonia	Pneumonia, cough	Wear mask and gloves Notifiable
Lymphocytic choriomeningitis	Arenavirus	Rodents	None, respiratory signs, CNS signs	'Flu-like, choriomeningitis	Very rare Wear mask and gloves
Hantavirus	Hantavirus genus	Small mammals, rodents	None	Fever, vomiting, haemorrhages, renal failure	Very rare Reported in wild rats in UK
Rabies	Rhabdovirus	All mammals	CNS signs None	CNS signs	Not endemic in UK Vaccinate staff if at risk Full barrier protection if suspected Notifiable
Campylobacteriosis	*Campylobacter*	Birds	None, diarrhoea	Diarrhoea	Caution when handling animal or its faeces

Perioperative care

Preoperative care

- Every effort should be made to minimize the anaesthetic time
- Prior to anaesthetizing the animal, all equipment, personnel and drugs should be prepared
- The postoperative recovery area should be set up in advance.

Anaesthesia is required for humane restraint, muscle relaxation and analgesia. There are particular factors to be taken into account when considering anaesthetizing exotic and wild animals. These factors include species, age, weight, percentage of body fat, environmental temperature, and the presence of concurrent cardiovascular or respiratory disease. Any animal that is compromised by dehydration, blood loss, cachexia, anorexia or infection will pose a greater anaesthetic risk than a clinically normal animal. Complete preanaesthetic assessment and stabilization are therefore especially important for wild animals for which no prior history is available.

- A thorough clinical examination is carried out to ensure that the animal is free from clinical disease, especially with regard to respiratory and cardiovascular function
- Food and water intake should be measured preoperatively and used to assess postoperative recovery
- An intravenous or intraosseous catheter may be pre-placed for intraoperative and postoperative care
- The patient should be weighed immediately before surgery to enable the correct dosing of the animal
- The patient should be handled correctly to minimize trauma and stress.

Mammals

- Preanaesthetic fasting is not required in rodents as they do not vomit and there is a risk of hypoglycaemia with prolonged starvation
- Food (not water) may be withheld from rabbits and guinea-pigs for 3–6 hours to reduce the amount of ingesta in the gut
- Fasting may significantly alter the body weight of the animal
- It is beneficial to administer subcutaneous fluids as a routine at a rate of 10 ml/kg Hartmann's fluid before surgery.

Birds

- Assessment of the hydration status, blood glucose level and liver function is particularly important
- Preanaesthetic starvation is restricted to the time required to empty the crop (in those species that have one). This can be easily palpated as full or empty. In emergency cases, the crop can be manually evacuated once general anaesthesia has been induced.

Reptiles

- Premedication is not considered necessary
- Reptiles should be maintained at their correct temperatures prior to anaesthesia and during recovery

- Fluid therapy is essential to maintain hydration, especially if the recovery period is prolonged (e.g. following ketamine anaesthesia)
- Preoperative starvation is generally not considered necessary, provided no food is present in the oesophagus or live insects in the stomach
- Larger chelonians and lizards may be starved for 18 hours, snakes for 72–96 hours, to ensure digestion is completed.

Amphibians and fish

Amphibians and fish should be starved for 24–48 hours prior to anaesthesia.

Anaesthetic agents and methods of administration

Inhalation anaesthesia

Inhalation is a relatively simple method of anaesthetic induction and maintenance of most species. Rapid variations in depth and rapid recoveries are possible. Induction of anaesthesia can be achieved via a face mask or by placing the whole animal in an anaesthetic chamber. Endotracheal intubation should be used whenever possible to allow scavenging of waste gases, to reduce the amount of gas used and to allow positive pressure ventilation if required. In general, isoflurane is the preferred agent, at 4% for induction and 1–2% for maintenance of general anaesthesia. Many reptiles can breath-hold, making induction by mask or chamber impractical.

Mammals

The technique of endotracheal intubation in the larger mammals is essentially similar to that for a similar-sized domestic animal (e.g. badger and dog). Endotracheal intubation, however, is technically difficult in rabbits and small rodents: these animals have a relatively large tongue and big teeth, small oral cavities and a small deep larynx that make visualization of the laryngeal opening difficult.

- Techniques for endotracheal intubation in the rabbit are given in Figures 8.52 (visual technique) and 8.53 (blind technique). Tube sizes and equipment required are given in Figure 8.54
- Unsuccessful intubation attempts can produce laryngospasm in rabbits, which is often fatal. The animal should be sufficiently anaesthetized so that swallowing and coughing reflexes are abolished
- Most rodents can be intubated using the blind technique (Figure 8.53). Endotracheal tubes may be made out of infusion set tubing or plastic intravenous catheters.

Birds

- An uncuffed tube should be used, as birds possess complete tracheal rings that may be ruptured by inflation of a cuff
- Ensure that the bird is anaesthetized by mask inhalation or an injectable regime before attempting intubation
- Use a gag to keep the beak open in those with powerful beaks (e.g. parrots). A finger may be used to keep open the mouth of some birds (e.g. pigeons)
- Visualize the glottis (Figure 8.55). This is easy to see in passerines and raptors but difficult in psittacine species, due to their fleshy tongue – use a tongue depressor to allow visualization of the glottis.

8.52 The visual method of endotracheal tube placement in rabbits

1. Place the animal in sternal recumbency with the head lifted up and extended, or in dorsal recumbency with the neck extended
2. Use a laryngoscope or an otoscope to visualize the larynx
3. Place an introducer (e.g. 4 Fr cat urinary catheter) into the trachea, thread the endotracheal tube over it into the trachea and remove the introducer.

8.53 The 'blind' method of endotracheal tube placement in rabbits

1. Estimate externally the position of the larynx
2. Advance the endotracheal tube until it is at the position of the laryngeal opening
3. Listen for the breath sounds and advance the endotracheal tube into the larynx on inspiration
4. Alternatively, use a transparent endotracheal tube – this will show condensation within the tube when it is near the larynx, when each expiration will fog the tube. Advance the tube on inspiration.

8.54 Endotracheal tube sizes and laryngoscope types required for rabbit intubation

Weight of rabbit (kg)	Size of endotracheal tube (mm O/D)	Type of laryngoscope
1–3	2–3	Wisconsin blade No. 0
3–7	3–6	Wisconsin blade No. 1

> **Tip**
> Endotracheal tubes for birds and reptiles may be made from appropriate gauge intravenous plastic catheters or intravenous drip tubing.

Reptiles

- An uncuffed tube should be used, as reptiles possess complete tracheal rings that may be ruptured by inflation of a cuff
- A gag should be used to keep the mouth open
- The glottis of the snake is easily visualized on the floor of the mouth
- The lizard glottis (Figure 8.56) is positioned at the back of the tongue and is sometimes difficult to visualize in animals with a large fleshy tongue. To aid visualization, pressing beneath the chin externally may raise the glottis
- The chelonian possesses a large fleshy tongue that obscures the view of the glottis. Pressing upwards below the chin raises the glottis; fully extending the head will aid visualization
- Many chelonians have a very short trachea. A long endotracheal tube should not be used, as intubation of one bronchus may occur – resulting in ventilation of only one lung.

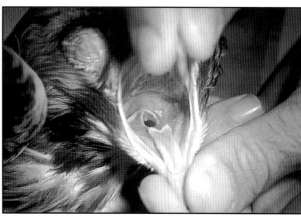

8.55 *The glottis of a raptor. Courtesy of N. Forbes.*

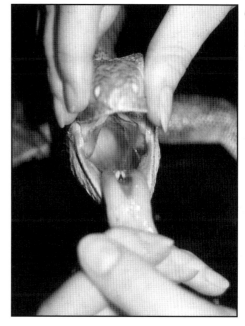

8.56 *Glottis of an iguana.*

Amphibians

Amphibians may be intubated using plastic tubing of an appropriate size.

Injectable agents of anaesthesia

Agents of anaesthesia for the various animals are described in Figures 8.57–8.62. If an injectable agent is used to induce anaesthesia it is always good practice, and in some cases essential, to provide supplementary oxygen via mask or endotracheal tube, with or without the addition of gaseous anaesthesia.

Via the water

This method is used for amphibians, fish and aquatic invertebrates.

- Two containers of water should be available – one to make up the anaesthetic solution and one to recover the animal
- The animal should be anaesthetized and recovered in water taken from its tank or pond, to prevent any stress due to temperature, pH or other differences
- The anaesthetic agent is added to the water at a low dose initially and mixed thoroughly
- The animal is introduced to the anaesthetic mixture
- Once the righting reflex is lost, the animal may be taken out of the anaesthetic solution and placed on a wet towel

8.57 Anaesthetic agents for use in mammals

Drug	Dose per species and route				Duration of anaesthesia (minutes)
	Mouse	Rat	Guinea-pig	Rabbit	
Fentanyl/fluanisone (Hypnorm; Janssen)	0.2–0.5 ml i.m. 0.3–0.6 mg/kg i.p.	As mouse		0.2–0.4 ml	Sedation only 30–45
Fentanyl/fluanisone (Hypnorm; Janssen)/ diazepam	0.4 ml/kg 5 mg/kg	0.3 ml/kg 2.5 mg/kg	1 ml/kg i.m. 2.5 mg/kg	0.3 ml/kg i.m. 2 mg/kg i.p.	45–60
Fentanyl/fluanisone (Hypnorm; Janssen)/ midazolam[a]	10 ml/kg[a]	2.7 ml/kg[a]	8 ml/kg[a]	0.3 ml/kg i.m. 0.5–1 ml/kg i.v.	45–60
Ketamine/medetomidine	200 mg/kg 0.5 mg/kg	90 mg/kg 0.5 mg/kg	40 0.5	35 0.5	20–30
Propofol	26 mg/kg i.v.	10 mg/kg i.v.	–	10 mg/kg i.v.	5
Atipamazole	1 mg/kg i.m., i.p., s.c., i.v., to reverse any combination using medetomidine				

a One part fentanyl/fluanisone (Hypnorm; Janssen), one part midazolam (5 mg/ml), two parts water

8.58 Anaesthetic agents for use in birds

Anaesthetic	Dosage (mg/kg)	Comments
Isoflurane	Induction 4%, maintenance 2%	Swift induction, rapid recovery
Halothane	Induction 1%, increase to 3%, maintain at 1.5–3%	Cardiac failure if too rapid induction, unexpected deaths commonly reported
Ketamine + diazepam or midazolam	25 ketamine; 2.5 diazepam or midazolam i.m.	20–30 min deep sedation
Ketamine/medetomidine	Raptors 3–5 Ket/50–100 Med i.m. Psittacines 3–7 Ket/75–150 Med i.m.	Reversed by atipamazole 250–380 µg/kg i.m.
Propofol	3–5 i.v.	Wears off very quickly Care with transfer to gaseous anaesthetic

8.59 Anaesthetic agents for use in reptiles

Drug	Dosage (mg/kg)	Site
Alphaxalone/alphadolone (Saffan; Coopers Pitman Moore)	6–9 9–15	i.v. i.m.
Ketamine	20–100 (larger dose to smaller animals)	s.c. i.m. i.p.
Propofol	Tortoises 14 Lizards 10 Snakes 10	i.v. (agent of choice for induction)
Halothane	1–4%	Inhalation
Isoflurane	1–6%	Inhalation (agent of choice for maintenance)

8.60 Anaesthetic agents for use in amphibians

Anaesthetic agent	Dosage for amphibians			Comments
	Tadpoles, newts	Frogs, salamanders	Toads	
Methanesulphate (MS222)	200–500 mg/l	500–2000 mg/l	1–3g/l	To effect (begin with low concentration)
Ethyl-4-aminobenzoate (benzocaine)	50 mg/l	200–300 mg/l	200–300 mg/l	Must be dissolved in methanol then added to water, as not very soluble. Stock solution may be kept in dark bottle for up to 3 months
Ketamine	50–150 mg/kg			
Isoflurane, halothane	4–5% bubbled through water			Animals may be intubated using small tubing and placed on moistened towels
Doxapram hydrochloride	Empirical dosage (one drop)			Useful to stimulate breathing

8.61 Anaesthetic agents for use in fish

Anaesthetic agent	Dosage (into water)	Comments
Methanesulphate (MS222)	100 mg/ml	Only licensed product in UK
Ethyl-4-aminobenzoate (benzocaine)	40 g into 1 l methanol; 11 ml of this solution into 9 l water	Must be dissolved in methanol then added to water, as not very soluble Stock solution may be kept in dark bottle for up to 3 months

8.62 Anaesthetic agents for use in invertebrates

Anaesthetic agent	Dosage	Comments
Inhalational anaesthesia in induction chamber or bubbled through water	Halothane (5–10%) Carbon dioxide (10–20%)	Recovery may take hours but is well tolerated
Tricaine Methanesulphate (for aquatic species)	100 mg/l water	Recover in fresh water
Benzocaine (for aquatic species)	Dissolve in acetone, add 100 mg/l water	Recover in fresh water

- Fish and amphibians should be handled with wet gloves at all times
- Anaesthesia may be maintained by syringing the stock anaesthetic solution over the gills in fish or over the skin in amphibians, as required.

To recover, the fish is placed into the clean water and moved in a slow circle until voluntary swimming movements commence. Fish should never be dragged backwards through the water as this will damage the gills.

Amphibians may be recovered in a similar way, or by running the clean water over the animal until it regains voluntary and respiratory movements.

Monitoring anaesthesia

Monitoring anaesthesia in fish and amphibians is limited to observing the heart beat and gill movements. Monitoring in invertebrates is limited to observations of movements.

Temperature

A common reason for perianaesthetic deaths in small animals is hypothermia. A decreased core temperature leads to prolonged recovery times, increases the potency of anaesthetics and may lead to death during anaesthesia or on recovery. The heat sources should be monitored to avoid hyperthermia or burns. All electronic monitoring equipment must be able to measure the heart rate, respiratory rate and volume and core temperature of the particular species being monitored. The standard equipment used for dogs and cats will often not accurately measure these parameters in small mammals (Figure 8.63), birds or reptiles (Figure 8.64).

Methods to minimize heat loss

- Heat loss via respiration and a cold flow of gas should be avoided by using humidifiers and warming the air in the anaesthetic circuit
- Hair/feather removal over surgical area should be minimized
- Excessive wetting of the patient should be avoided
- The use of alcohol-based antiseptics should be avoided, as these will chill the animal
- Anaesthetic time should be minimized by adequate preparation; prolonged surgery should be avoided
- Areas of the body away from the surgical site should be insulated
- A regulated heat source should be provided
- Core temperature should be monitored constantly.

 Avoid excessive feather removal in birds, as many only moult once or twice a year. The extent of feather loss is especially important when assessing whether wild birds are fit for release.

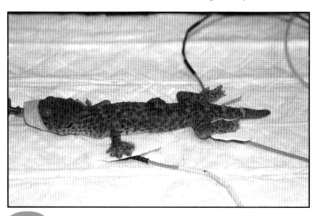

8.63 *Reptile under anaesthesia.*

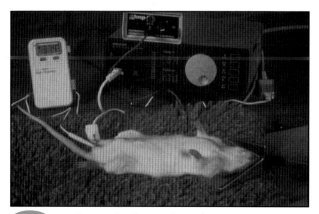

8.64 *Small mammal under general anaesthesia.*

Assessment of anaesthetic depth

Figure 8.65 offers a guide to monitoring the depth of anaesthesia in animals.

Monitoring respiratory and cardiovascular systems

The respiratory rate, depth and pattern may be monitored by direct observation of chest wall, movement of reservoir bag or electronic monitors. The heart rate can be monitored by direct observation of the beating heart or palpation of a pulse (Figure 8.66), using an ECG (Figure 8.67) or indirectly by using a pulse oximeter (Figure 8.68). Capillary refill times, mucous membrane colour and a peripheral pulse may be used to assess cardiac output and tissue perfusion as in larger domestic animals.

General management of animals under general anaesthesia

Mammals

Intraoperative care is as for domestic mammals.

Birds

- Rapid induction/recovery is possible with gaseous anaesthetic agents
- Restriction of ribs/sternal movement by weight on the sternum (e.g. surgeon's hands, instruments, heavy drapes, bandages) can lead to suffocation
- The bird should be positioned in sternal (ideal) or lateral recumbency, as dorsal recumbency compromises respiration by 10–60%
- Force ventilate with 100% oxygen every 5 minutes, as birds easily become hypercapnic (excess carbon dioxide)
- Rapid position changes of the anaesthetized bird should be avoided, as this can lead to a severe drop in blood pressure
- If the bird has ascites, it should be placed in upright or head-elevated position to avoid impairment of respiration and fluid entering the lung during surgery
- Some birds become apnoeic after approximately 30 minutes of anaesthesia and require positive pressure ventilation and careful monitoring during this period.

8.65 Monitoring depth of anaesthesia

Depth	Small mammals	Reptiles and amphibians	Birds	Fish	Invertebrates
Light plane	– Absence of righting reflex – Absence of tail pinch reflex – Intact pedal withdrawal	– Absence of righting reflex – Intact pedal withdrawal – Snakes still respond to stroking of ventral surface	– Absence of righting reflex – Intact corneal palpebral and pedal reflexes	– Erratic swimming – Loss of reactivity	Loss of righting reflex
Surgical plane	Absence of pedal withdrawal	– Absence of tongue withdrawal (snake) – Absence of limb withdrawal – Absence of palpebral reflex	– Eyelids closed – Pupils dilated	– Absence of righting reflex	No response to surgical stimulus
Too deep	Rabbit – palpebral reflex lost	– Fixed dilated pupils – Slow heart rate	– Loss of corneal reflex – Slow shallow respiration – Respiratory arrest	– Very shallow opercular movements – Gasping – Cessation of operculum movements	Difficult to assess

8.66 Sites for manual monitoring of heart rate/pulse

Site	Mammals	Reptiles			Birds	Amphibians	Fish
		Chelonians	Snakes	Lizards			
Carotid artery	✓	✓	✓ (rare)	✓	✓		
Heart beat	✓		✓	✓		✓	✓
Other arteries	Ear (rabbit) Mandibular Tongue Femoral				Medial metatarsal		

8.67 Lead attachment sites for ECG monitor

In general
Red electrode – place on the right foreleg
Yellow electrode – place on the left foreleg
Green electrode – place on the left hindleg
Black electrode – place on the right hindleg.

Special considerations
Large mammals – attach to body wall
Small mammals – attach to feet
Birds – attach pads or clips to wing web and feet
Reptiles – attach to the feet or space out along length of a snake.

> Care must be taken with interpretation: the electrical impulse does not always equate with an adequate cardiac output.

8.68 Pulse oximeter sites and application

- Apply to:
  - Tongue, ears, tail, nail bed and footpads in mammals and reptiles
  - Wing web or tibiotarsal bone in birds
- Not validated for reptiles and so the trend rather than absolute figures should used to monitor the patient
- Allows measurement of the oxygen saturation of the blood and is an indication of respiratory depth, respiratory obstruction or equipment failure
- Displays the pulse rate to give an indication of cardiovascular depression (if low and at a fast rate, may indicate that anaesthetic plane is too light)
- Pulse signal is also evidence that blood is flowing through the tissues

Reptiles

- Many reptiles can maintain apnoea for a prolonged period when conscious; thus induction by inhalation anaesthetic is not recommended
- Many reptiles will require intermittent positive pressure ventilation (IPPV) continuously throughout the operation, as apnoea is common
- The respiratory rate required to maintain gaseous anaesthesia is often greater than the normal respiratory rate of the conscious animal, but should be based on this rate initially and the depth of anaesthesia monitored
- If the reptile had been maintained or induced with a long-acting injectable agent (e.g. ketamine), the animal may take hours to regain consciousness completely
- IPPV with oxygen should not be stopped until the reptile has begun to breathe spontaneously.

> **Tip**
> The careful use of dry heat (e.g. from a hairdryer) on the recovering reptile will speed the time taken to regain spontaneous breathing and voluntary movement. Monitor the heat to avoid overheating the reptile.

Anaesthetic emergencies
Figures 8.69 and 8.70 describe how to recognize and treat respiratory and cardiovascular failure, respectively.

8.69 Respiratory failure

Causes
- Overdose of anaesthetic
- Blocked or displaced endotracheal tube
- Equipment failure
- Lack of oxygen
- Pain
- Laryngeal spasm (rabbits)
- Weight on thorax (e.g. surgeon's hands).

Signs
- Respiratory rate less than 40% of conscious rate
- Cyanosis of mucous membranes (iris in albino animals) (note that oxygen saturation must fall to < 50% before cyanosis is seen in mammals)
- If oxygen saturation falls by:
  - \> 5% = mild hypoxia
  - \> 10% = emergency
  - \> 50% = severe life-threatening hypoxia.

Action
- *If under gaseous anaesthesia*, check oxygen is still supplied, check patency of circuit, check endotracheal tube is not blocked, decrease the plane of anaesthesia
- *If using injectable anaesthesia*, reverse anaesthesia if at convenient stage of procedure, provide oxygen by endotracheal tube (preferable) or face mask
- *In all cases:*
  - Provide oxygen
  - Begin chest compressions to aid ventilation
  - Administer doxapram (respiratory stimulant) every 15 minutes as required
- *Rocking* or gently swinging the small animal is often an effective method of ventilating, especially in small mammals
- *If stable*, continue anaesthesia; if not, continue manual ventilation and recover animal.

8.70 Cardiovascular failure

Causes
- Overdose of anaesthesia
- Hypoxia/hypercapnia
- Blood loss (15–20% = hypovolaemia and shock)
- Hypothermia (body temperature of < 25°C leads to cardiac arrest in mammals).

Signs
- Increased capillary refill time, cyanosis, pallor
- Decreased body temperature (slow change)
- Gradual decrease in blood pressure or pulse rate
- Change in heart rate/rhythm.

Action
- Administer 100% oxygen via endotracheal tube or mask and ventilate
- Administer fluids at a rate of:
  - 10–15 ml/kg per hour for *maintenance*, or
  - 50 ml/kg over 1 hour in emergency due to *hypovolaemia*
- *If cardiac arrest*, start chest compressions at rate appropriate for heart rate of animal
- Reverse anaesthesia.

Postoperative care

- The animal should be monitored until full recovery is noted
- Animals should always be recovered individually in a quiet dimly lit area
- The recovery area should be at the correct temperature for the species
- The animal's core temperature should be monitored until it has recovered fully
- Fluids (including glucose) should be administered if the animal does not begin to eat and drink within a reasonable period for the species

- Analgesia should be administered routinely after a procedure or if assessment on recovery indicates pain (Figure 8.71 describes signs of pain or discomfort in animals)
- The animal should always be given the benefit of the doubt. Analgesics administered appropriately will not harm the animal.

Postoperative analgesia is often overlooked when exotic animal or wildlife surgery is conducted. This is not a humane approach. Animals in pain will reduce their food and water intake and suffer from stress-related disorders. Inadequate analgesia can seriously compromise postoperative recovery. Figure 8.72 suggests analgesic regimes in animals.

8.71 Signs of pain or discomfort

Small mammals	Reptiles	Birds	Amphibians	Fish
Aggression	Immobility	Immobility, collapse	Immobility	Loss of appetite
Overgrooming/lack of grooming	Anorexia	Increased aggression	Anorexia	Hollow sides or underparts
Inactivity	Abnormal locomotion or posture	Abnormal posture or locomotion	Abnormal locomotion or posture	Fins folded
Hiding at back of cage	Increased aggression	Less 'talking' or singing	Increased aggression	Poor skin colour
Hunched posture	Dull colouration	Less response to human if previously tame and interactive	Dull colouration	Sluggish swimming
Increased respiratory rate		Picking or plucking over painful area		Unusual swimming action, e.g. jerkiness, imbalance
Polydipsia				Rubbing on stones or ornaments
Anorexia				
Hyperthermia/ hypothermia				
Tooth grinding				
Self-trauma over painful area				
(*Note:* vocalizing is rare)				

8.72 Analgesia (many of these doses are anecdotal and approximate and may not be licensed for the species)

Drug	Small mammals (e.g. rat)			Larger mammals (e.g. rabbit, badger)		
	Dosage (mg/kg)	Route	Frequency (hours)	Dosage (mg/kg)	Route	Frequency (hours)
Buprenorphine	0.05–0.1	s.c.	6–8	0.01–0.05	s.c.	6–8
Butorphanol	1–5	s.c.	4–6	0.1–0.5	s.c.	4–8
Carprofen	5	s.c.	8–12	1–5	s.c.	8–12
Meloxicam	0.2	s.c.	12–24	0.1–0.2	s.c.	24

Drug	Birds			Reptiles		
	Dosage (mg/kg)	Route	Frequency (hours)	Dosage (mg/kg)	Route	Frequency (hours)
Buprenorphine	0.02	i.m.	2–4	Not established (use mammalian dosage?)		
Butorphanol	3	i.m.	1–4	Not established (use mammalian dosage?)		
Carprofen	5–10	s.c.	4–8	5	s.c.	12–24
Meloxicam	0.2	s.c.	12–24	0.2	s.c.	24

Method of euthanasia	Mammals	Reptiles	Birds	Amphibians	Fish	Invertebrates
Overdose of anaesthetic via:						
Intravenous route (conscious or sedated animal)	✓	✓	✓	✓	✓	–
Intraperitoneal route	✓	✓	–	✓	✓	–
Intrarenal or intrahepatic injection	✓	✓	–	✓	✓	–
Intrahepatic injection *only*	–	–	✓	–	–	–
Intraosseous route	✓	✓	✓	✓	–	–
Cervical dislocation (< 500 g body weight only)	✓	–	–	–	–	–
Overdose of inhalational anaesthetic in chamber	✓ (not diving species)	–	✓ (not diving species)	–	–	✓ (terrestrial species)
Overdose of anaesthetic in water	–	–	–	✓	✓	✓ (aquatic species)
Concussion by striking back of head, followed by destruction of the brain	–	–	–	✓	✓	✓
Overdose of anaesthetic via intracardiac injection after sedation or induction of anaesthesia by other methods	✓	✓	✓	✓	✓	–

Methods of euthanasia

The various methods used to euthanase animals humanely are described in Figure 8.73.

- Do *not* euthanase animals by chilling or freezing. This is not a humane approach: research has shown that animals perceive freezing as painful
- Do *not* use ether to anaesthetize or euthanase animals. It is an irritant substance to the animal and to humans. It is also a fire hazard
- Do *not* attempt to perform an intraperitoneal injection in a bird. The peritoneal cavity is only a potential space in the healthy bird. Injection into the body cavity will result in injection into the air sac and will drown the bird.

Additional considerations for the wildlife patient

Many of the aspects of treating wild animal species can be adapted from the techniques used to treat their domestic counterparts. Poisoning is perhaps seen more often in wildlife but can also occur in captive species (see Figure 8.46). This section will deal with the extra information needed to treat wildlife effectively, safely and legally.

Assessment

On accepting a wildlife patient, an assessment should be made as soon as possible as to whether the animal should be treated or humanely euthanased. This aspect of treating wildlife is perhaps the most difficult, but for the animal's sake this hard decision should be made as soon as possible.

Questions to consider when assessing the wildlife casualty are:

- Will the animal benefit from any form of medical or surgical therapy?
- Will it ever be fit for release?
- Will the prolonged rehabilitation period in itself cause suffering to the animal?

It is important to record, in as much detail as possible, where and when the animal was found. This will aid its release to an appropriate area and will also help to gather information on the prevalence of native wildlife in certain areas.

The animal should be correctly identified as to species and age so that the appropriate husbandry can be provided. Some species are covered by legislation that may require specific action or may affect how or if the animal is to be released.

An assessment should be made of whether the practice facilities and staff are able to deal with the species concerned. It is useful to make contacts with local wildlife centres and discuss which facility would best deal with certain situations.

Nursing

Important points when nursing the wildlife casualty are:

- Accurate daily records should be kept of body weight, amount eaten and drunk, passage of faeces and urine
- Handling and interaction with the animal should be minimized
  - To minimize stress
  - To avoid habituating the animal to humans
- The progress of the animal should be assessed daily with regard to continuation of treatment, fitness for release or requirement of euthanasia.

Legislation

Wildlife and Countryside Act 1981 (as amended 1988, 1991)

This makes it illegal to kill, injure, take, possess or sell certain UK native wild animals. An exception is made for those taking and possessing sick or injured animals, or euthanasing injured animals. The burden of proof falls on the person in possession of the animal, and so accurate and up-to-date records must be kept.

Section 8 of the Act states that birds should be kept in cages large enough for them to stretch their wings fully. A smaller cage may be used for transport or while undergoing veterinary treatment.

If diurnal birds of prey are taken under this Act, they must be ringed and registered if kept for more than 6 weeks; if for less than 6 weeks they may be held under an exemption for veterinary surgeons.

Non-indigenous species may not be released into the wild, unless they are listed in the Act as already established.

Dangerous Wild Animals Act 1976 and (Modification) Order 1984

A licence is required to keep certain species of venomous snakes, lizards and all crocodilians. This also includes all primates (except marmosets) and some poisonous spiders and scorpions. UK wildlife included are the wild cat and the adder. An exception is made if the animal is in a veterinary surgery for treatment.

Protection of Animals Acts 1911, 1988; Protection of Animals (Scotland) Acts 1912, 1988

This legislation makes it illegal to cause unnecessary suffering – which may include failure to provide food, water or veterinary treatment. Killing an animal is not an offence unless it is carried out inhumanely.

Abandonment of Animals Act 1960

This states that animals should not be abandoned in circumstances likely to cause them suffering. This is especially relevant when considering the release of a wildlife casualty.

Animal Health Act 1981; Transit of Animals Order 1973 (as amended 1988)

This states that animals (including invertebrates) must be transported without causing unnecessary suffering. Appropriate containers and vehicles must be used and adequate food, water, ventilation and temperature must be provided.

Veterinary Surgeons Act 1966

This Act restricts the veterinary treatment of mammals, birds and reptiles to veterinary surgeons and practitioners. Fish, amphibians and invertebrates may be treated by anyone, provided the Protection of Animals Acts are complied with. Owners may give minor treatment to their own animals. Anyone may give emergency first aid to an animal.

Medicines legislation: Medicines Act 1968; Medicines (Veterinary Drugs) (Prescription Only) Order 1985; Misuse of Drugs Act 1971; Misuse of Drugs Regulations 1985

Prescription-only drugs (POMs) must only be supplied by a veterinary surgeon to 'animals under his care'. These regulations apply to any animal for which the drugs are supplied – even the species that do not come under the Veterinary Surgeons Act.

Health and Safety at Work etc. Act 1974

Staff, volunteers or students working with non-domesticated species must be provided with additional safety procedures, depending upon risks involved. This includes training, working protocols and protective equipment.

Animals Act 1971

Those in possession of non-domesticated species (whether owned by them or not) that are likely to cause serious damage must ensure that damage to property and injuries to people are prevented.

Further reading

Beynon PH and Cooper JE (1991) *BSAVA Manual of Exotic Pets.* British Small Animal Veterinary Association, Cheltenham

Beynon PH, Forbes NA and Lawton MPC (1996) *BSAVA Manual of Psittacine Birds.* British Small Animal Veterinary Association, Cheltenham

Beynon PH, Lawton MPC and Cooper JE (1992) *BSAVA Manual of Reptiles.* British Small Animal Veterinary Association, Cheltenham

Butcher (1992) *BSAVA Manual of Ornamental Fish.* British Small Animal Veterinary Association, Cheltenham

Equine nursing

Tim Greet

This chapter is designed to give information on:

- The role of the veterinary nurse in equine practice
- The principles of handling and care of horses in the clinic
- Diagnostic techniques used in equine medicine and surgery
- Treatment techniques
- Vaccination schedules
- Parasite control schedules
- Equine anaesthesia
- Assessment and treatment of colic in the horse
- Equine theatre practice
- Equine intensive care
- Management of limb casts

Introduction

This chapter includes descriptions of techniques that cannot be legally performed by a nurse. At the time of writing, Schedule 3 of the Veterinary Surgeons Act specifically precludes veterinary nurses from treating equidae, although the veterinary nurse may carry out procedures within the clinic that do not constitute acts of treatment (for example, checking or replacement of bandages and diagnostic radiography). However, it is hoped that this legal barrier may soon be lifted. This is important, because horses and ponies form a considerable proportion of patients dealt with in veterinary practice. There is also an increasing number of specialist equine practices requiring specially trained nurses of high quality to provide support to veterinary surgeons. It is hoped that by reading this chapter a potential equine nurse will gain a detailed overview of the role of the nurse in modern equine practice.

The nature of the horse

The horse has evolved as a species that lives on large open plains. Accordingly, its sight and hearing are acute and by nature horses tend to be rather nervous. As herbivores, their teeth have developed to graze and chew a plant-based diet. The intestinal system is specialized to break down cellulose products in the hindgut and therefore the caecum and large colon are very well developed.

The soundness and athletic ability of horses and ponies are very important, because most of them are required to perform athletically to some degree and a few compete at the very highest level. This has a major influence on the way in which injury and disease are managed.

Horses and ponies can bite and kick and have the potential to cause serious injury to their handlers and to attending veterinary staff. Therefore great care must always be taken and horses must be approached and handled in a professional manner to avoid the risk of injury. Every equine nurse should endeavour to become familiar with horses and it is an advantage to have had some experience of riding them, as this tends to give much greater confidence when dealing with the veterinary aspects of equine patients.

Care of the equine patient

Horses are rewarding animals to work with but safe and correct handling is essential. Equine nurses should:

- Become confident at putting on headcollars and bridles
- Become competent in the use of a nasal twitch (a most valuable form of restraint for many patients) (Figure 9.1).

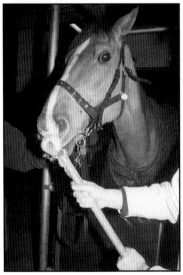

9.1
The application of a nasal twitch provides a very good means of restraint for many equine patients.

Where patients appear fractious it is essential that a veterinary surgeon should be consulted. Sedation may be appropriate in some animals before performing even the most basic procedures, as well as for carrying out more specialized treatments.

In some practices nurses may be expected to clean out stables and to groom equine patients. Grooming and care of equine patients is of great importance not only from the point of view of hygiene but also for equine welfare and good client relationships (a clinic's reputation is damaged if a horse is sent home looking uncared for). Nurses should be familiar with the application of rugs and limb bandages, as these will frequently be required for hospitalized patients, particularly during the winter months.

Routine clinical assessment

Nurses need to become familiar with horses' limbs, handling their legs and discerning heat in their feet. Equine patients are prone to limb swelling when they are hospitalized and early detection of the signs of laminitis, which is an occasional sequel to equine disease, may prove life-saving.

The following functions should be recorded on a daily basis on a hospital record chart.

- Rectal temperatures (normal range 37.2–37.8°C) should be monitored on at least a once-daily basis in patients under observation, or recovering postoperatively
- Resting pulse (normal 35–45 beats per minute) and respiratory rates (normal 8–16 breaths per minute) should be recorded
- The consistency of faeces produced by a horse should be monitored and the early signs of diarrhoea or constipation should be detected so that they may be remedied at the earliest opportunity
- The water intake and approximate urine production should be monitored (approximately 25 litres a day total fluid input and output for a 500 kg horse).

Diagnostic techniques

Veterinary nurses are frequently involved in the use of diagnostic imaging techniques in horses and they should have a working knowledge of the various procedures involved.

Radiography

Most radiographic examinations of horses are more satisfactorily and safely carried out with the horse sedated using a combination of an alpha-2 agonist (e.g. xylazine or detomidine) and an opioid (e.g. butorphanol).

Equine nurses must be particularly aware of the potential hazards of ionizing radiation. It is imperative that every care be taken with radiation protection, as exposure factors for horses are relatively large and patients are sometimes unpredictable.

- Owners are frequently asked to hold their horses during radiography. It is vital that the standard rules of radiation safety are always employed and clients should be instructed adequately
- The use of gowns and gloves by staff and owners, as appropriate, is mandatory
- Radiographic cassette holders should be used, to avoid exposure of hands
- Doses to staff and clients should be monitored continually.

Radiography of the foot
The standard projections of the foot are:

- Lateromedial projection with the foot in a weight-bearing position, usually on a wooden block
- Dorsopalmar upright projection of the pedal bone
- Upright dorsopalmar angled view with the beam centred at the coronary band to demonstrate the navicular bone (Figure 9.2)
- 'Skyline' projection of the navicular bone, obtained with the horse standing with its foot on the cassette and weight-bearing but in a more caudal position than normal. The X-ray tube is directed down through the bulbs of the heels. This demonstrates the flexor cortex of the navicular bone and its medullary cavity, which may be damaged in navicular disease (Figure 9.3).

In the latter two projections, the frog sulcus and clefts should be packed with modelling clay to avoid confusing air shadows on the radiographic image.

Radiography of the fetlock and carpus
Multiple views – usually a dorsopalmar, lateromedial and both 45 degree (oblique) projections – of the fetlock (Figure 9.4), cannon bone, 'splints' and carpus (Figure 9.5) are relatively easy to obtain. Sometimes flexed lateromedial views of both carpus and fetlock are helpful.

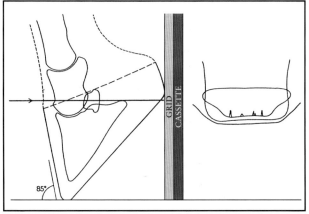

9.2 *An upright dorsopalmar view with the beam centred at the coronary band. This is a good view to demonstrate the navicular bone. Reproduced from Douglas et al. (1987)* Principles of Veterinary Radiography, *4th edn, with the kind permission of WB Saunders.*

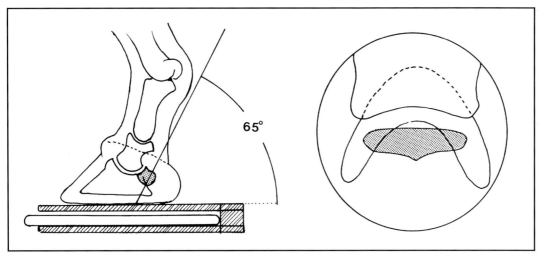

9.3

A skyline view of the navicular bone. This demonstrates the flexor cortex and the medullary cavity of the navicular bone; it is the most useful view of the bone. Reproduced from Douglas et al. (1987) Principles of Veterinary Radiography, 4th edn, with the kind permission of WB Saunders.

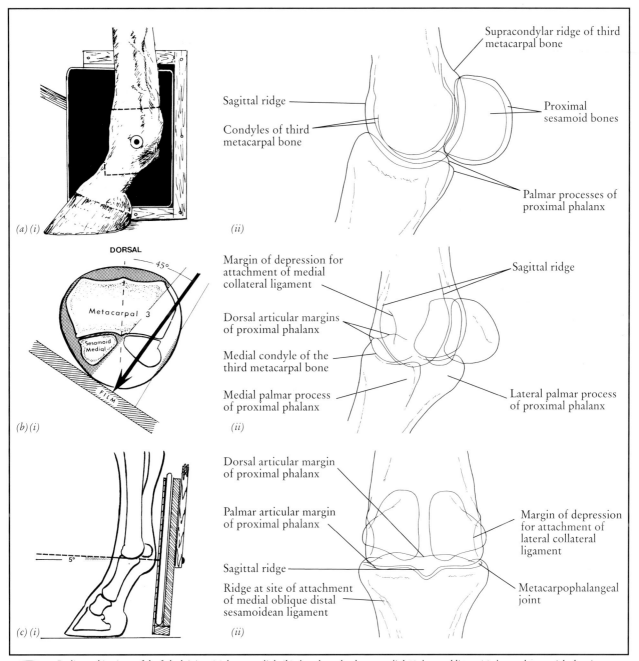

(a)(i)

DORSAL

45°

Metacarpal 3

Sesamoid Medial

FILM

(b)(i)

5°

(c)(i)

(ii)

Supracondylar ridge of third metacarpal bone

Sagittal ridge

Condyles of third metacarpal bone

Proximal sesamoid bones

Palmar processes of proximal phalanx

(ii)

Margin of depression for attachment of medial collateral ligament

Dorsal articular margins of proximal phalanx

Medial condyle of the third metacarpal bone

Medial palmar process of proximal phalanx

Sagittal ridge

Lateral palmar process of proximal phalanx

(ii)

Dorsal articular margin of proximal phalanx

Palmar articular margin of proximal phalanx

Sagittal ridge

Ridge at site of attachment of medial oblique distal sesamoidean ligament

Margin of depression for attachment of lateral collateral ligament

Metacarpophalangeal joint

9.4 Radiographic views of the fetlock joint: (a) lateromedial; (b) dorsolateral palmaromedial 45 degree oblique; (c) dorsopalmar weight-bearing. a(i), b(i), c(i) reproduced from Douglas et al. (1987) Principles of Veterinary Radiography, 4th edn, with the kind permission of WB Saunders. a(ii), b(ii), c(ii) reproduced from Butler et al. (1993) Clinical Radiology of the Horse, with the kind permission of Blackwell Science.

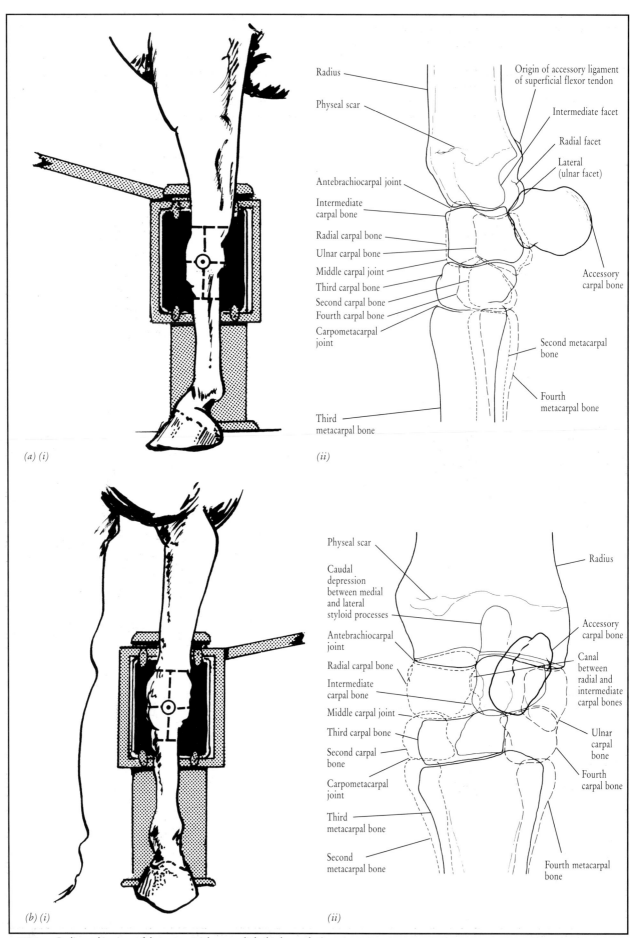

Radius

Physeal scar

Antebrachiocarpal joint

Intermediate carpal bone

Radial carpal bone

Ulnar carpal bone

Middle carpal joint

Third carpal bone

Second carpal bone

Fourth carpal bone

Carpometacarpal joint

Third metacarpal bone

Origin of accessory ligament of superficial flexor tendon

Intermediate facet

Radial facet

Lateral (ulnar facet)

Accessory carpal bone

Second metacarpal bone

Fourth metacarpal bone

(a) (i)

(ii)

Physeal scar

Caudal depression between medial and lateral styloid processes

Antebrachiocarpal joint

Radial carpal bone

Intermediate carpal bone

Middle carpal joint

Third carpal bone

Second carpal bone

Carpometacarpal joint

Third metacarpal bone

Second metacarpal bone

Radius

Accessory carpal bone

Canal between radial and intermediate carpal bones

Ulnar carpal bone

Fourth carpal bone

Fourth metacarpal bone

(b) (i)

(ii)

9.5 *Radiographic views of the carpus: (a) lateromedial; (b) dorsopalmar.*
a(i), b(i) reproduced from Douglas et al. (1987) Principles of Veterinary Radiography, *4th edn, with the kind permission of WB Saunders.*
a(ii), b(ii) reproduced from Butler et al. (1993) Clinical Radiology of the Horse, *with the kind permission of Blackwell Science.*

Radiography of the elbow and shoulder

Views of the elbow and shoulder are always obtained in a mediolateral direction, to facilitate positioning of the cassette.

Radiography of the hock, stifle and pelvis

The distal portion of the hindlimb is examined in much the same way as the forelimb. Four views of the hock – i.e. dorsoplantar, lateromedial and both 45 degree (oblique)

projections (Figure 9.6) – are standard for investigating this area.

The stifle is most frequently examined in a lateromedial projection. A caudocranial view (Figure 9.7) is also valuable but both views usually require a mobile or fixed X-ray generator to produce sufficient power to obtain a diagnostic view.

The pelvis is seldom examined radiographically and usually requires the horse to be anaesthetized.

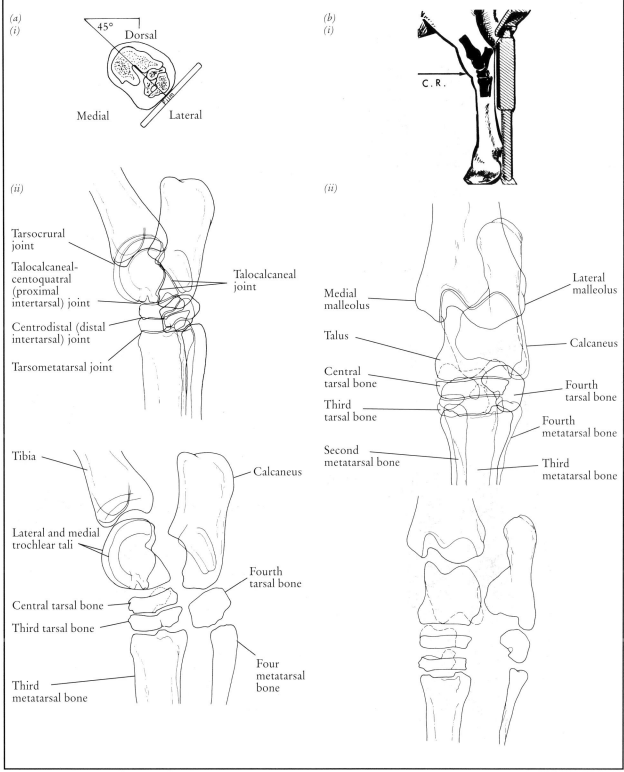

9.6 *Radiographic views of the hock: (a) dorsomedial plantarolateral oblique — this view is very useful for looking at lesions of OCD; (b) dorsoplantar.*
a(i), b(i) reproduced from Douglas et al. (1987) Principles of Veterinary Radiography, *4th edn, with the kind permission of WB Saunders.*
a(ii), b(ii) reproduced from Butler et al. (1993) Clinical Radiology of the Horse, *with the kind permission of Blackwell Science.*

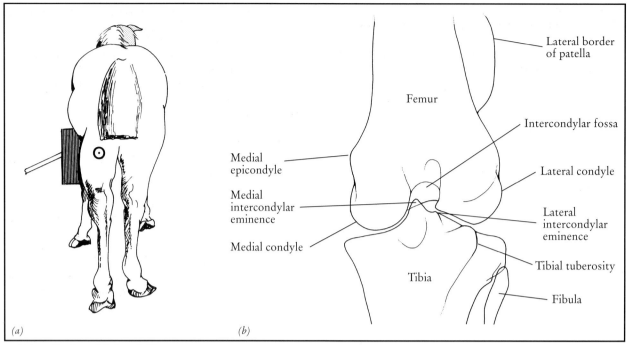

9.7 *Caudocranial view of stifle.*
(a) reproduced from Douglas et al. (1987) Principles of Veterinary Radiography, *4th edn, with the kind permission of WB Saunders.*
(b) reproduced from Butler et al. (1993) Clinical Radiology of the Horse, *with the kind permission of Blackwell Science.*

Radiography of the head

Even portable machines are capable of obtaining diagnostic images of the head, particularly for the paranasal sinuses and cheek teeth. Usually a lateral projection and oblique views illustrating the dental apices are required.

Lateral views of the neck and back are sometimes obtained but these views require relatively high-powered generators and are usually only performed in the clinic.

Endoscopy

Conventional flexible fibreoptic endoscopes can be used for investigation of problems associated with the upper airway, trachea, oesophagus, bladder and uterus; longer instruments (more than 2 metres long) can be used to examine the stomach.

Most commonly the instrument will be used to inspect the upper and lower respiratory tracts and this examination is usually performed with the horse either sedated or restrained by a nasal twitch. Sometimes it is useful to release the twitch once the endoscope has been inserted, as this may allow the horse to relax and allow easier assessment of laryngeal function.

When an endoscope is being used in the bladder it is important that the horse is adequately sedated, using an alpha-2 agonist/opioid combination or acetylpromazine.

Great care should be taken during oesophagoscopy and gastroscopy that the endoscope is not diverted into the oral cavity, with catastrophic and expensive consequences for the instrument.

Care of endoscopes

Veterinary nurses are frequently responsible for the care of flexible fibreoptic endoscopes. These are fragile, easily damaged and expensive instruments and it is advisable for nurses to attend a course on care of endoscopic equipment. Courses are run by the main manufacturers and they detail the principles of cleaning and maintenance. Awareness by the nurse of potential hazards to the endoscope along with regular cleaning and maintenance will help to avoid the need for costly repairs.

Diagnostic ultrasonography

The principles of ultrasonography are introduced in Chapter 5. Both linear and sector scanners are now widely used in equine practice. Initially they were used mainly for pregnancy diagnosis and the scanning of tendons and ligaments. There are very few areas of the horse that may not be imaged successfully using ultrasound, including most joints, the pelvis and the eye.

- The chest (particularly the heart) can be readily assessed
- Superficial areas of the abdomen may be examined transabdominally and deeper abdominal structures by use of the probe per rectum
- The bladder may be successfully imaged by ultrasound in the same way.

Generally speaking, any fluid-filled viscus is amenable to examination. However, air-filled cavities are impenetrable by ultrasound waves and so examination of the lungs is unrewarding unless the horse is suffering from a pleural effusion, pleurisy or peripheral abscessation.

Nurses should be familiar with the ultrasound machine, which should be cleaned and looked after carefully to ensure a longer working life.

Examination of lameness

Lameness is a common reason for veterinary examination of a horse and a variety of techniques are employed to assess the problem. Nurses are often involved in assisting with these procedures.

Trotting up

Firstly a horse is walked and trotted on a firm surface and then usually exercised on a lunge in order to identify the affected limb(s). Pressure on the sole of the foot using hoof testers may be reliable in identifying a source of pain such as a subsolar abscess. Palpation of the limb to identify sites of swelling and flexion of joints to identify pain or to exacerbate lameness following forced flexion are also standard procedures.

Nerve blocks

The use of perineural or intra-articular analgesia is also a fundamental part of lameness investigation. Most people are content to clean the skin carefully for perineural analgesia but when intrasynovial analgesia is performed it is mandatory to clip and prepare the site aseptically before the needle is inserted by a veterinary surgeon, who should be wearing sterile gloves. A sterile unopened bottle of local anaesthetic should always be used for intrasynovial analgesia.

Most joints can be injected. Regional nerve blocks can be carried out in the foreleg to just above the carpus and in the hindleg to just above the hock.

Some fractious patients may need to be restrained with a nasal twitch or by a low dose of sedative drug. The latter may make interpretation of nerve blocks more difficult.

Other diagnostic methods

Gamma scintigraphy

In recent years the use of gamma scintigraphy has become of great value, especially for assessing equine bone disease. In young racehorses in particular, detection of stress fractures which cannot be identified by other means has been revolutionized by this technology.

- The horse is hospitalized and injected intravenously with a radioactive bone label (methylene diphosphonate with ^{99m} technetium). This circulates round the body, localizing in areas of active bone turnover (so-called hot-spots)
- The horse is examined using a hand-held probe or a gamma camera, which detects the emitted gamma rays and counts them, producing a pattern of figures (probe) or an image (camera)
- Following the examination, the horse must be kept hospitalized for 36 hours
  - Any attendant must wear protective clothing and be monitored for radiation dose
  - Handling should be kept to a minimum in any case
  - All the urine and faeces must stay in the box for 72 hours before being mucked out normally.

See Chapter 5 for further details.

CT and MRI

In a few clinics, computerized tomography (CT) and magnetic resonance imaging (MRI) are available for use on horses. The techniques currently require the horse to be restrained under general anaesthesia but this technology is constantly improving and will certainly find much more widespread use in years to come.

Injection techniques

Most parenteral medications are administered by the intramuscular or intravenous route in horses.

Intramuscular injection

The best site for intramuscular injection is the semimembranosis/semitendinosis area at the caudal aspect of the thigh. This site involves slightly more risk to the injector compared with the use of the gluteal or pectoral muscles but can safely be used to administer a relatively large volume of drugs. Alternative sites include the gluteal region and the muscular portion of the neck just cranial to the scapula (pectoral muscles). All these sites are commonly employed and their use should be rotated in horses receiving multiple injections over a period of time.

Intramuscular injections can present particular problems in horses. For example, an intramuscular injection of procaine penicillin can result in acute excitement approximately 30 seconds to 2 minutes after the injection. This is thought to be due to the inadvertent intravenous injection of procaine. If the stable is rapidly evacuated of all personnel, and the top and bottom stable doors are closed, most horses will settle down without injury in 5 to 10 minutes.

Intravenous injections

Intravenous injections are almost always given into the jugular. As some horses develop reactions to intramuscular injection, the intravenous route is often preferred. However, it is imperative that a nurse checks with a veterinary surgeon about the suitability of a particular drug for intravenous injection, as many preparations are inappropriate for use by that route. Some drugs must be given by slow injection and others are extremely irritant if administered perivascularly. Great care must therefore be observed before administering any injection intravenously. The horse must be adequately restrained.

Blood collection

Samples of blood are most easily collected using proprietary evacuated blood collection tubes from the jugular vein. In hirsute equine patients, particularly in fat ponies with short necks, clipping the hair prior to venipuncture is advisable. Antiseptic preparation of the skin prior to introduction of the needle is also recommended.

Routine vaccination

A recommended programme is outlined in Figure 9.8.

- It is recommended that all horses are vaccinated against tetanus
- Vaccination against influenza in horses competing in all disciplines is mandatory
- Other diseases such as herpes virus infection are less effectively protected against by vaccination although commercial vaccines are available for both respiratory and abortion strains.

The schedule for influenza vaccination in Figure 9.8 is that required for horses entering competition grounds under Jockey Club rules. Although correct at the time of writing,

9.8 Recommended vaccination programme

Disease	Course	Timing
Tetanus	Primary course 1st dose 2nd dose Booster	 0 16–28 days 1–3-yearly
Influenza	Primary course 1st dose 2nd dose 3rd dose Booster	 0 21–92 days 150–215 days Not more than 1 year after 3rd dose of primary course and not less often than annually thereafter

these may change. Vaccination must not be given within 7 days of the event. Other bodies, such as the Pony Club and British Horse Society, apply the same regulations.

> ⚠️ Close adherence to the vaccination schedule and accurate certification are essential for competition horses, since they may otherwise be excluded from competition. Although the owner is responsible for this, practice personnel must be knowledgeable about the requirements.

Parasitism

Intestinal parasites are a universal problem in horses at grass. The use of effective anthelmintic drugs over the last 20 years has altered the typical equine worm burden. The development of resistance by some parasites to commonly used anthelmintics has made it necessary to alter anthelmintic strategy.

Parasitism may be responsible for weight loss, diarrhoea and the development of certain types of colic. The parasites that are of economic importance in horses include:

- Large strongyles whose larvae migrate through the cranial mesenteric artery, potentially leading to infarction of small areas of intestine. This manifestation is now uncommon
- Small strongyles that encyst and live in the mucosa of the large intestine (caecum and large colon). Mass emergence of larvae in spring can cause gross inflammation of the intestinal mucosa with consequent diarrhoea. This is the commonest cause of diarrhoea in adult horses and in extreme cases it can be fatal
- Tapeworms that attach to the mucosa of the caecum, particularly around the ileocaecal orifice. Tapeworms and small strongyles have been associated with caecocolic intussusception and tapeworms also with ileal impactions
- The lungworm of the donkey may cause severe bronchitis and bronchiolitis in horses. Donkeys with lungworm are often asymptomatic but represent an important source of infection for horses sharing grazing
- Larvae of the bot fly attach to the gastric mucosa, but have not been associated with any clinical problem.

Anthelmintic regimes are described in Figure 9.9.

 9.9 Anthelmintic regimes

Parasite	Regime
Tapeworms	Double dose pyrantel, spring and autumn
Bots	December treatment with an ivermectin or moxidectin
Large strongyles	Migrating larvae treated in autumn with benzimidazole-type or ivermectin or moxidectin
Small strongyles	Treat with 5-day course of benzimidazole-type in late autumn and again in early spring

Throughout grazing season, choose any of the anthelmintics and use at appropriate frequency as follows:

- 4–6 weeks pyrantel
- 8–10 weeks ivermectin
- 6–8 weeks fenbendazole
- 12 weeks moxidectin

Colic

Abdominal pain is a common presenting sign in equine patients. Typically horses may show a variety of signs, including:

- Looking uneasy
- Pawing the ground
- Rolling and sweating
- Getting up and down frequently
- Looking at the flanks.

Degree of pain

The degree of pain exhibited is important and extremely variable, depending on the initiating cause and the temperament of the patient. The implications for the patient are similarly wide-ranging. The initial aim of the veterinary surgeon is to provide appropriate analgesia to prevent unnecessary suffering.

Assessment and choice of treatment

More important than analgesia is the need to differentiate rapidly between conditions that will resolve with medical therapy and those that will need surgery. In the latter group, prompt referral for abdominal surgery may be life-saving. Alternatively, euthanasia may be appropriate under some circumstances (e.g. patient age, concurrent veterinary problems, economic factors).

The role of the equine nurse is to aid in:

- Observation of the patient
- Restraint of the patient to permit a thorough examination by a veterinary surgeon.

Vital signs

Associated with the degree of pain are the resting heart and respiratory rates, which should be assessed. Most horses with surgical intestinal lesions have high heart rates and high respiratory rates. Other signs of endotoxaemia may be apparent; for example, the mucous membranes may be brick-red or purple instead of pink.

Manual examination

Auscultation of the abdomen to assess the presence of intestinal motility may be useful and the veterinary surgeon will carry out a manual examination per rectum to assess distension of malposition of the intestine.

> ⚠️ These examinations may only be possible once the horse has been successfully restrained. Horses in pain are notoriously difficult to examine and so administration of sedation and/or analgesic medication may be a priority before a better assessment of the patient may be made.

Gastric distension

In horses with an upper intestinal obstruction, there is often gastric distension. Passage of a nasogastric tube will be performed by the veterinary surgeon to relieve this. Any horse that refluxes gastric contents down a nasogastric tube is probably suffering from a potentially surgical lesion.

Blood samples

Samples of blood may be assessed haematologically to evaluate the degree of dehydration. Blood biochemistry may be useful in evaluating the presence of any other organic disease.

Most horses with surgical lesions will have a metabolic acidosis but samples of arterial blood for blood gas analysis are usually only monitored in the anaesthetized patient.

Peritoneal fluid

The collection of a sample of peritoneal fluid, usually via a needle or cannula placed aseptically at the most dependent midline portion of the abdomen, may provide valuable information as to whether there has been strangulation of intestine or the presence of peritonitis. The gross appearance of bloodstained fluid is usually a sign of intestinal strangulation. Unfortunately, inadvertent injury to the spleen will also result in bloodstained peritoneal fluid but this is not usually homogeneous.

Ultrasonography

Additional aids to monitoring the horse with colic are the use of transabdominal and rectal ultrasound examinations. The transabdominal approach is particularly effective in foals or small ponies, in which a manual examination per rectum is impossible because of the patient's size.

Treatment

Horses with medical problems such as impaction of large intestine or tympanitic or spasmodic colic may be treated with a combination of spasmolytic (e.g. hyoscine/dipyrone) and analgesic drugs (e.g. phenylbutazone). In many cases this is combined with the administration of liquid paraffin and an electrolyte solution by nasogastric tube.

Patients suspected of requiring surgery should be referred promptly to a surgical unit or be destroyed without delay to prevent further suffering.

General anaesthesia

Many surgical procedures are most satisfactorily performed under general anaesthesia, although some operations are still commonly carried out under sedation and local analgesia. Particularly in the horse, the administration of a general anaesthetic represents a potential hazard to the patient's life. It is therefore critical that all members of the surgical team are sufficiently trained to facilitate the administration and monitoring of general anaesthesia in horses. They should be especially aware of current resuscitation techniques to cater for uncommon yet potentially catastrophic respiratory and cardiac arrests.

There is a surprisingly high mortality rate in elective equine surgical patients (approximately 1%) compared with small animals (approximately 0.1%). This emphasizes how vital are care and attention, no matter how routine the operation appears to be.

Preoperative assessment

Preanaesthetic evaluation of the patient should involve assessment of the patient's cardiovascular and respiratory systems in particular. A thorough clinical examination, including obtaining a rectal temperature, should always be performed. It is debatable whether blood samples should be analysed prior to anaesthesia. In the author's hospital this is done routinely for every patient undergoing general anaesthesia, to assess the presence of unsuspected disease processes that might compromise the patient during anaesthesia.

Insurance

It is important to know whether the horse is insured. If it is, the insurance company must be informed before the anaesthetic is administered. Some companies insist on a certificate of health prior to giving permission for general anaesthesia.

Insurance companies need not be informed in an emergency, but it is preferable to do so if the emergency arises during office hours.

Catheterization

Many equine patients undergoing general anaesthesia have a jugular vein catheterized to provide a convenient route for sedatives, anaesthetic agents and other medication and for intravenous fluids (Figure 9.10). Although anaesthetic drugs can be administered by needle, in most cases it is preferable to use a catheter to allow instant access to the circulatory system under all circumstances and to avoid the perivascular injection of irritant drugs such as thiopentone or phenylbutazone.

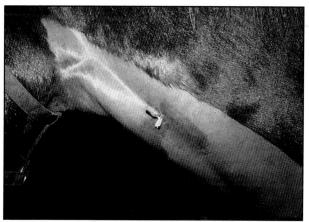

9.10 *Catheter placed aseptically prior to the administration of anaesthesia.*

- The best catheters are polyurethane, as they are least injurious to the vein, but polypropylene catheters are also used on a short-term basis
- The insertion of a jugular catheter (usually 14 or 16 gauge) for intravenous drug and anaesthetic administration should be done aseptically, as there is a risk of septic thrombophlebitis if care is not taken. This particularly applies if the catheter is to be used for postoperative fluid administration over a more prolonged period.

It is good practice to provide a continuous intravenous drip of Hartmann's solution (5 litres every 30 minutes) during surgery as this will reduce the incidence of postoperative myopathy.

Method of anaesthesia

A general anaesthetic may be administered in the field. The use of a to-and-fro anaesthetic circuit permits maintenance of anaesthesia using halothane/oxygen mixtures even under field conditions but injectable anaesthesia is more commonly used.

Horses will usually be anaesthetized in the clinic, where the conditions are more controlled.

- Most horses are initially sedated with acetylpromazine (with the notable exception of colic patients)
- Subsequently, heavy sedation with an alpha-2 agonist, such as romifidine or detomidine, is followed by injection of ketamine or thiopentone as a bolus for induction of the anaesthetic

- Some anaesthetists prefer to use the muscle relaxant glycerol guaiocolate (guaifenesin) prior to the injection of a bolus of inducing agent
- Once the horse has been anaesthetized, the mouth is opened with a gag and an endotracheal tube is passed into the trachea. The cuff is inflated and the patient is attached to an anaesthetic machine and circuit, which is either of a to-and-fro or circle type.

Prior to induction of anaesthesia, the nurse must always check that:

- The oxygen tank is adequately filled
- The soda lime cannister has not been exhausted
- Halothane levels are topped up
- The endotracheal tube has a functioning cuff.

Even in patients that are undergoing field anaesthesia, it is sensible to have an endotracheal tube available to provide an airway should a problem occur.

It is usual to restrain a horse with hobbles once anaesthesia has been achieved (Figure 9.11).

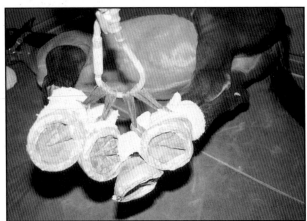

9.11 *Horse hobbled under general anaesthesia. Simple webbing hobbles, over padding, are held together with a carabine. This horse is ready for hoisting into the operating theatre.*

Total intravenous anaesthesia

There are other means of providing general anaesthetics which do not involve the administration of volatile gases. The most reliable of these is the so-called triple drip (Figure 9.12). This comprises an alpha-2 agonist, glycerolguaiocolate (guaifenesin) and ketamine. The combination is 'topped up to effect'. The drugs are administered in Hartmann's solution via an intravenous jugular catheter.

9.12 Constituents of 'triple drip' mixture

- 500 mg xylazine
- 1 g ketamine
- 5 g guiafenesin.

Combined in 1 litre Hartmann's solution, administered at about 2 ml/kg body weight/hour.

Positioning the patient

Horses are usually placed in lateral or dorsal recumbency, depending on the operation to be performed and the individual preference of the surgeon. In both positions muscle or nervous tissue may become compromised (myopathy or

neuropathy) because of pressure. This particularly applies during longer periods of anaesthesia or where the patient's blood pressure is low (e.g. in colic surgery).

- Adequate padding under the horse is mandatory to prevent myopathy or neuropathy
- Correct positioning of the limbs is essential (Figure 9.13)
- The use of continuous intravenous fluids in all horses under anaesthesia and positive inotropic drugs such as dobutamine in selected cases with low blood pressure will also help to reduce the incidence of these potentially life-threatening postoperative complications.

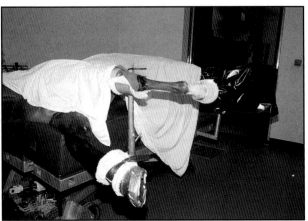

9.13 *Horse in lateral recumbency on heavily padded foam mat, with the underlying front leg extended. The hindlimb is supported in leg stands and the upper left forelimb is in a limb stand prepared for surgical procedure.*

Monitoring anaesthetic patients

Monitoring of anaesthesia (Figure 9.14) can be performed by assessing:

- Depth and rate of respiration
- Pulse rate and strength
- Eye position and response to surgical stimuli.

Auscultation of the heart is valuable but continual electrocardiographic monitoring is preferred. Assessment of blood pressure by digital evaluation of the facial or greater metatarsal arteries can be performed; however, in the clinic, direct monitoring of arterial blood pressure is preferred by the placement of an intra-arterial catheter connected to a monitoring device.

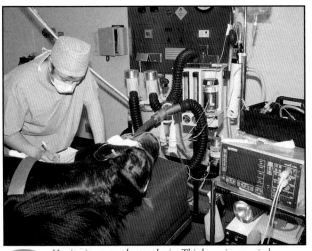

9.14 *Monitoring general anaesthesia. This horse is on a circle system. Blood pressure and ECG are constantly monitored.*

Soft tissue surgery

Instruments

The nurse's role in any surgical procedure may involve scrubbing up to assist the surgeons but in any case it should involve providing the appropriate instruments for the procedure. The instruments should be well maintained, sharp and, above all, sterile. After every surgical procedure it is important that:

- Instruments are inspected for mechanical faults and sharpness
- Each instrument is carefully cleaned before being resterilized.

Swabs

In equine surgery it is important in most circumstances to use large gauze swabs with radiographically detectable tags attached. Standard swabs used for small animal practice are inappropriate, as they are readily lost in surgical wounds. This particularly applies to their use in the equine abdomen. Swab counts are the responsibility of the nursing staff and should always be carried out.

Other equipment

Standard ancillary equipment, such as diathermy and suction pumps, is very useful for many equine operations and should be cleaned, sterilized and prepared prior to potential use in surgery. Nurses should have a thorough knowledge of wound healing, different suture materials and the types of drain available and their uses. Familiarity with surgical stapling devices will be necessary in those clinics where such instrumentation is used (typically for intestinal anastomosis).

Some common surgical procedures

Castration

Castrating colts is the commonest operation performed by veterinary surgeons in equine practice. There are two basic techniques:

- Castration under general anaesthesia
- Castration with the horse sedated in the standing position under local analgesia.

    Each method has its advantages and risks.

Castration under general anaesthesia

If the horse is to be operated on under a general anaesthesia, the testicles are removed via a scrotal incision. The testicular blood vessels are ligated before being cut and it is preferable that the vaginal tunic is closed to prevent catastrophic evisceration when the horse recovers from the anaesthetic. If the operation can be performed aseptically, closure of the skin wound is also beneficial – provided haemostasis is meticulous.

    The same technique is used for cryptorchid castration, except that the retained testicle is usually approached via an inguinal incision and retrieved from the abdomen by traction.

Castration of the standing horse

In the standing horse, local anaesthetic is injected subcutaneously into the testicle itself near its cranial pole. It is

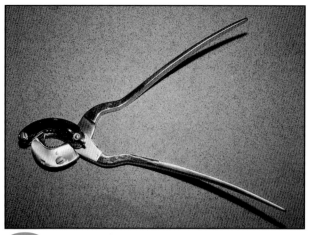

9.15 An emasculator.

very important that the horse is adequately restrained (i.e. with a bridle) to avoid injury to the surgeon. Most animals are sedated with acetylpromazine or a combination of an alpha-2 agonist and butorphanol. A bold incision is made into each testicle and the castration is performed using an emasculator (Figure 9.15).

Postoperative care

In most cases postoperative swelling is minimal and can be reduced further by the administration of non-steroidal anti-inflammatory drugs. A course of antibiotics for 3–5 days is also recommended. There is a small risk of intestinal herniation following open castration. If prolapse of intestine is suspected, the wound should be closed or packed and the horse referred immediately for emergency laparotomy under general anaesthesia. Fortunately this is a rare occurrence.

Skin wounds

Lower limb

Lacerations are commonly dealt with in equine practice. In the lower limb most of these wounds are best managed by careful cleansing and bandage support. Partial suturing is useful on some occasions.

    It is of vital importance that the anatomical structures related to the wound are assessed. In particular, penetration of synovial cavities may result in catastrophic infection and lameness if undetected or not treated with antibiotics and synovial lavage.

Body and thorax

Large flap wounds associated with the body and thorax are common in horses and in many cases these can be left open to heal by second intention or can be repaired (partially or completely) with the insertion of suitable drains. Penetration of the pleural or peritoneal cavity rarely occurs with these wounds but should be identified promptly, as the treatment strategy is significantly altered.

Face

Wounds associated with the face are also common and tend to heal well. Particular care should be taken with wounds associated with the lips, as these may result in significant disfigurement and possible interference with function if they are not managed appropriately. Surgical repair is indicated in most cases.

Exuberant granulation

Wounds of the limb below the carpus and hock are prone to developing exuberant granulation tissue ('proud flesh'). This may be managed by reducing mobility of the limb by using a cast or a Robert Jones bandage. Exuberant tissue may be removed by cauterization, using either chemical or diathermy methods and the application of corticosteroids. In some cases it may be possible to insert pinch grafts into a healthy bed of granulation tissue to reduce the time for re-epethialization.

Severe limb laceration

Severe lacerations of the distal limbs, particularly following entanglement in barbed-wire, are best managed by the application of a fibreglass cast (see later). Casts should be applied after the horse has been given a general anaesthetic and the wound has been scrupulously cleaned, debrided and partially repaired, if this is possible. Application of a fibreglass cast for 14 days will significantly improve the quality and speed of healing.

Respiratory tract surgery

Chronic paranasal sinusitis

Treatment of chronic paranasal sinusitis by copious lavage may be carried out with the horse standing, by inserting a catheter through the facial bones into the affected sinus. The catheter may be inserted through the facial bones after using an orthopaedic bone pin or a larger instrument, such as trephine, under local analgesia to create a hole into which a hose can be inserted or an indwelling balloon catheter placed.

Postoperative lavage (Figure 9.16) is effectively carried out using either a garden hose or a proprietary garden spray apparatus, which can be attached to a balloon catheter. The sinus should be lavaged with a 0.5% povidone/iodine solution.

In some cases it may be necessary to make a larger incision into the sinuses and this can be achieved by creation of a maxillary bone flap under general anaesthesia. This allows more careful inspection of the dental roots for periapical infections and the removal of a soft tissue mass such as a maxillary cyst or a progressive haematoma. In cases where the surgery creates major nasal haemorrhage, packing the maxillary sinus intraoperatively with a sterile bandage will prevent undue or potentially fatal haemorrhage. The packing may be removed at 2–3 days postoperatively.

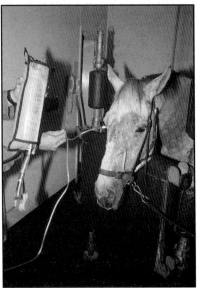

9.16
Flushing the maxillary sinus.

Laryngeal surgery

Laryngeal surgery such as cordoventriculectomy (Hobday's operation) can be carried out through a cricothyroid–laryngotomy incision. It is usually not necessary to insert a postoperative laryngostomy tube in these cases.

Laryngoplasty ('tieback') is a more complex procedure for treating left-sided laryngeal hemiplegia and requires to be performed under strictly aseptic conditions. An implant (usually a non-absorbable suture) is used to mimic the action of the abductor muscle of the larynx and this operation is usually combined with a cordoventriculectomy procedure.

Tracheotomy

Tracheostomy tubes may be inserted under local analgesia with the horse standing. This is a useful means of bypassing an obstruction of the upper airway.

The use of chronic permanent tracheostomy tubes has been recommended by some as a means of treating chronic conditions of the upper airway such as laryngeal hemiplegia or soft palate disease. Postoperatively the tubes must be removed on a daily basis to allow cleaning and to ensure that the tracheotomy site is inspected and cleaned. Occasionally emergency tracheotomy may be necessary because of acute upper airway dyspnoea.

Abdominal surgery

Abdominal surgery in horses is usually performed in referral centres rather than in veterinary practices.

Intestinal surgery can be performed through a ventral midline incision and this approach may also give access for removal of neoplastic ovaries and for caesarean section. Flank incisions for removal of ovaries are preferred by some surgeons but the wounds tend to heal less well than midline incisions and may be associated with incisional swelling. The removal of ovaries via the dorsal wall of the vagina (colpotomy) is now rarely used.

Castration of a cryptorchid testis is frequently performed via an inguinal approach and the testicle can usually be retrieved by traction. Some surgeons prefer a parapenile approach into the caudal abdomen, but this is more invasive and requires longer convalescence.

Intensive care

Adult horses

The provision of intensive care for equine patients is of vital importance in many postoperative situations and also in the support of horses with severe illness. A considerable proportion of a veterinary nurse's time will be spent in dealing with intensive care patients.

- It is crucial that the nurse should understand the principles of fluid therapy and electrolyte balance
- The more common complications which occur following colic surgery, such as paralytic ileus and diarrhoea, need careful management and the patient must be monitored closely
- The appropriate postoperative regimen for the management of major systemic infections, endotoxaemia and other complications such as laminitis, thrombophlebitis, pleurisy, peritonitis and incisional complications must also be understood.

As with other hospitalized patients, detailed records should be kept of rectal temperature, pulse, respiration, the degree of abdominal pain, the consistency of faeces and the condition of any surgical incisions. The general demeanour and appetite of each patient should be assessed carefully. Detection of the early signs of laminitis or other complications, such as an incisional hernia, may allow life-saving treatment.

A system should be devised for routine postoperative monitoring of intensive care patients. At the minimum, this should involve daily collection of a haematological sample. Periodic assessment of blood biochemical parameters may also be of value. In colic patients with endotoxaemia, clotting disorders may develop and secondary disease of liver or kidney may prejudice the outcome of the case. Equine nurses are referred to other more detailed works for reference values concerning haematology and blood biochemistry of horses.

It is integral to the management of critical care patients that a team of well trained observant and caring support staff are able to monitor the patient in an intensive or more extensive way, depending upon the severity of the patient's clinical condition.

Fluid therapy
Continuous intravenous fluid therapy using Hartmann's solution is a routine means of supporting critical care patients. The volume of fluid to be administered should be calculated upon the basis of maintenance levels plus fluid loss into the peritoneal cavity or into the intestinal lumen.

In postoperative colic patients, Hartmann's solution is usually supplemented with potassium chloride, but an electrolyte assessment should be made in each case and any deficiency corrected.

The use of hypertonic saline (7.2%) is very helpful as an emergency measure in restoring a depleted vascular compartment. It is most useful in a preoperative colic patient but may also be helpful postoperatively.

It is mandatory that hypertonic fluids are combined with administration of a large volume of isotonic fluid, otherwise intracellular fluids may become depleted, leading to organ failure.

Endotoxaemia
Hyperimmune plasma containing antibodies to a specific capsular type (J5) of the *Escherichia coli* bacterium has been shown to be very helpful in reducing the effects of endotoxaemia in horses with strangulating intestinal lesions.

- Usually broad-spectrum bactericidal antibiotic cover is given and the combination of penicillin and gentamicin is often used
- Non-steroidal anti-inflammatory drugs such as phenylbutazone or flunixin meglumine are often given three or four times daily at low dose levels to help reduce the effects of endotoxaemia
- Intestinal stimulants such as metaclopramide are administered with intravenous fluids to encourage normal intestinal motility to return
- If the large intestine is opened for any reason during surgery, metronidazole should be given; this is effective against anaerobic bacterial infections.

Foals
Foals present a special challenge for critical care. They are often premature or dysmature with low immunity levels. Plasma transfusions are frequently administered, along with broad-spectrum antibiotic cover. Convulsing foals may be treated with sedation.

Gastric ulceration
Any foal in the critical care unit is a prime candidate for gastric ulceration and possible rupture. It will therefore be given anti-gastric ulcer medication such as omeprazole or ranitidine. Non-steroidal anti-inflammatory medication must be used with great care in foals as this also contributes towards gastric ulceration.

Ruptured bladder
Foals may present with septicaemia or other infectious sequelae such as synovial sepsis, umbilical sepsis or even a ruptured bladder. Foals with ruptured bladders are hyperkalaemic and therefore it is essential that any intravenous fluid replacement should not contain potassium. Sodium chloride is the intravenous fluid of choice in such cases. Frequent assessment of the foal is required and in most cases continuous nursing care must be given if the foal's condition is poor.

Breathing problems
Premature foals may have difficulty in breathing and a face mask supplied with oxygen is useful. Frequent assessments of the chest by auscultation with a stethoscope and by radiography and ultrasonography are useful to monitor the development of secondary pneumonia.

Postoperative care
Foals represent a special challenge for the veterinary nurse and students are encouraged to refer to more specialized texts. The management of foals following major surgery is along similar lines to that of the critical care foal, and even for elective patients routine anti-gastric ulcer medication is administered.

Orthopaedic surgery

Orthopaedic surgery in the horse is being performed with increasing frequency. Although much of it is performed at referral centres, many practices carry out minor procedures under field conditions. In the hospital situation the nurse must become familiar with arthroscopic instrumentation and fracture repair techniques. This type of surgery is fairly specialized but nurses are vital elements in the orthopaedic team and familiarity with both the equipment and procedures is essential to successful completion of such operations. Nurses who are likely to be dealing with a significant orthopaedic caseload should refer to more specialized texts.

Arthroscopy
In the last 15 years arthroscopic examination has become a routine method for examining most equine joints (Figure 9.17). In addition to being a diagnostic procedure, arthroscopy is frequently used as a means of removing osteochondral fragments such as chip fractures or the lesions of osteochondrosis and in the treatment of septic arthritis and tenosynovitis.

The techniques are best carried out with the horse under general anaesthesia. In many circumstances it is useful to have the horse in dorsal recumbency although this will depend on the surgeon's preference.

- The telescope is inserted into the joint at an appropriate position to allow inspection of its surfaces or to allow the

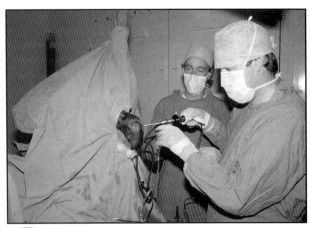

9.17 *Arthroscopic examination of a carpus.*

surgeon to triangulate with any lesion to be removed

• An instrument portal is then created to complete the triangulation, allowing removal of the chip fracture, curettage of a bone cyst or whatever the procedure to be undertaken
• The joint is distended using Hartmann's solution under pressure. The pressure is provided either manually or by a cuff using compressed air cylinders or with a specifically designed pump.

Instruments

A variety of specialized tools – such as rongeurs, small chisels, probes and curettes – is required to perform the procedures and the nurse should become familiar with the surgeon's routine in performing most operations.

In many situations the surgeon will perform arthroscopic procedures with the telescope attached to a chip camera and then to a television screen. This not only creates a focus of interest for the surgical team but also permits more satisfactory inspection and surgery within the joint. In addition, it permits a permanent videotape record to be made of the surgical procedure.

Most instruments, including some modern arthroscopes, can be sterilized in the autoclave. It is more common to use ethylene oxide or chemical agents such as glutaraldehyde. Although chip cameras can be sterilized with chemicals, these are corrosive and the longevity of the equipment can be preserved by sterilizing them with ethylene oxide or by using sterile shrouds.

Fragment removal

It may be necessary to monitor removal of fragments by radiography or image intensification intraoperativly, but many surgeons with experience do not use this facility in routine cases.

Closure

Following arthroscopic surgery, skin incisions are usually closed with either sutures or stainless steel staples. In most cases subcutaneous stitching is not required. Lower limb incisions are protected by bandages but upper limb incisions are usually left uncovered.

Fracture repair

Fractures are seldom repaired in equine practice except by those dealing with racehorses or in referral centres.

The use of ASIF (Association for the Study on Internal Fixation) techniques such as lag screw repair and the

application of dynamic compression plates is accepted as the standard method for managing fractures in horses. However, a number of horses can be managed conservatively or by the application of fibreglass casts.

Equipment

As fracture repair tends to be carried out relatively infrequently, it is of considerable value for nurses to attend courses on the use of ASIF equipment and its maintenance.

It is important that nurses working in clinics where fracture repair is carried out become familiar with the common techniques, such as inserting screws. They should also be familiar with the use of air drills, the sizes of drill bit and instruments such as countersinks and taps, which all form part of the standard equipment.

It is very helpful to the surgeon to have pre-packed screws labelled according to their size. If different diameter screws are used (e.g. 3.5 mm, 4.5 mm and 5.5 mm) they should be stored separately to avoid any risk of confusion.

Almost all fractures will be repaired under radiographic or image intensification control. Nursing staff need to be familiar with positioning radiographic cassettes and the tube head to obtain satisfactory views that allow intraoperative control of implant insertion (Figure 9.18).

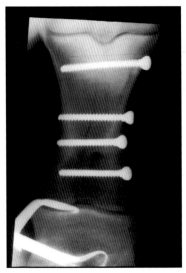

9.18 *Intraoperative radiographic view of proximal phalanx following the insertion of four 4.5 mm cortical screws.*

Orthopaedic equipment must be checked and cleaned routinely after every operation and implants that have been used should be replaced immediately to ensure that a complete kit is available. Instruments must be working satisfactorily and drill bits should be sharp. Great care should be taken to ensure that:

• Bits and taps are cleaned scrupulously and sterilized between operations
• Drills are lubricated to ensure that they work satisfactorily when the next patient is being treated.

Cast care

Following repair of the incision (which in some cases may only be a stab incision) most fractures of the distal limb are supported by application of a fibreglass cast. If this is required to remain in position for any length of time, an abrasion-resistant material should be used round the bottom of the foot to prevent the foot wearing though the cast, which would then have to be removed. Useful materials include synthetic hoof material.

Following surgery, nurses should also become familiar with monitoring a horse in a cast for signs of lameness or soreness and should be able to assist with the removal of casts using an oscillating saw. This may be done in the 12 hours following recovery from anaesthesia, or in some cases after several weeks. Most fibreglass casts are replaced, if this is necessary, under general anaesthesia. Radiographic monitoring of fracture healing is usually performed when the cast is removed or changed.

The same techniques are applicable to arthrodesis of low motion joints such as the proximal interphalangeal joint or the distal hock joints. Long bone fracture repair in adult horses is severely limited because of the physical size of the patient and therefore of the risk of catastrophic re-injury on recovery from anaesthesia. Economics also play a part, as such surgery is expensive. However, repair of the ulna is an exception and many horses with ulnar fractures can be managed successfully by the application of a dynamic compression plate to the caudal aspect of the bone.

Fractures in foals

Fractures in foals may be more amenable to surgical repair using plates but the rate of infection is quite high. This eventually results in implant loosening and failure of the repair.

Applying a fibreglass cast

Fibreglass casting material has revolutionized the external support of injured equine limbs. Most distal limb fractures will be supported in a cast at least for recovery from general anaesthesia. Many other injuries, such as tendon breakdowns and extensive wounds, may be supported in a cast for 10–14 days or even longer to ensure more satisfactory healing.

To apply a fibreglass cast:

- The hoof should be covered with a sterile or at least clean surgical glove and proprietary stockinette should be applied to the limb from above the level desired for the cast down to the hoof capsule
- This is then covered with two layers of conforming bandage and one layer of proprietary casting foam, which is wrapped an extra time at the proximal level of the cast
- Although some clinicians prefer to apply casts over a more heavily padded limb, this results in excessive movement and may potentially cause skin irritation or ulceration. Heavily padded casts do not give the support that can be expected from a cast applied as described here
- In the forelimb, most casts are applied from the hoof to the carpometacarpal joint. Occasionally a cast proximal to carpus may be applied – for example, for long bone fractures affecting the mid-third metatarsal region or a severe carpal injury
- In the hindlimb, casts are commonly applied to the tarsocrural joint but on occasion they may be applied to the level of the proximal tibia
- For a standard forelimb cast to the carpus, three rolls of casting material should be applied sequentially, having been prepared according to the manufacturer's instructions
  - The material can be applied circumferentially or using figure-of-eight technique, or occasionally using slabs of material
  - It is important that adequate support is given at the fetlock, which is the commonest site of fracture of casting material
- In a hindlimb (to the hock), four rolls of casting material

are generally used because this is subject to greater forces on recovery from anaesthesia
- Casting material will usually set and become able to bear weight within 20 minutes of application
- Before the last roll of casting material is applied, the top of the stockinette is rolled down and incorporated under the final layer of casting material, providing a neat non-irritant edge to the proximal margin of the cast
- Usually one layer of adhesive bandage is then applied from the top of the cast to the skin, to avoid debris such as shavings from gaining access to the skin beneath the cast and causing irritation or potential contamination of wounds
- The limb must be extended fully during cast application to ensure that the horse can bear weight correctly on the limb when standing.

Cast removal

Casts can be removed using an oscillating saw.

- A vertical cut can be made both medially and laterally in the casting material
- The material can then be levered apart and removed without much difficulty.

If a cast fractures, it is imperative that it be removed rather than repaired, as severe skin injuries may follow if the cast is not removed promptly.

Application of an Esmarch bandage and tourniquet

Although arthroscopy performed in dorsal recumbency has precluded the need for the use of a tourniquet in many situations, repair of distal limb fractures and orthopaedic procedures (except neurectomy) carried out with the horse in lateral recumbency are frequently facilitated by application of an Esmarch bandage and a tourniquet.

- The Esmarch bandage should be applied starting at the coronary band and wound round the leg, making sure that the bandage is not overlapped too much as this makes it difficult to remove (Figure 9.19)
- In the front limb, the tourniquet should be applied proximal to the carpus; in the hind limb the tourniquet should be applied proximal to the hock
- The most effective form of tourniquet is a pressure cuff (Figure 9.20), which can be inflated by a bicycle pump
- The Esmarch bandage is then removed, or at least unwound to the level of the pressure cuff

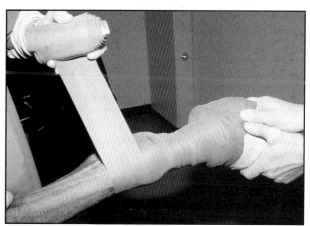

9.19 *Application of an Esmarch bandage.*

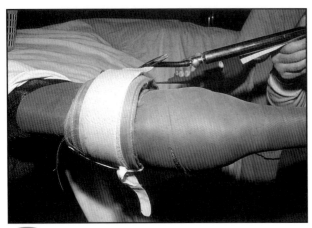

A pressure cuff used as a tourniquet.

- Applying a tourniquet to the middle portion of the cannon region should be avoided, as this may cause injury to the underlying flexor tendons
- It should be noted that application of a tourniquet proximal to the carpus or hock results in a flexed conformation of the distal limb, which should be taken into consideration when performing releasing surgeries such as a check ligament desmotomy. It is preferable not to use a tourniquet in such cases.

Other orthopaedic procedures

Patellar ligament desmotomy

Horses can suffer from intermittent (or even persistent) upward fixation of the patella. In some cases this requires surgical treatment which involves section of the medial patellar ligament (note that the horse has three patellar ligaments). In most patients this can effectively be achieved with the patient sedated and under local analgesia via a stab incision in the skin immediately axial to the ligament.

Neurectomy

Palmar digital neurectomy is occasionally performed in horses with incurable foot lameness and is carried out just proximal to the coronary band at the level of the pastern. In some cases both front legs may be treated similarly.

Neurectomy at other sites is much less common. Performing an ulnar neurectomy for a carpal problems or a tibial neurectomy for bone spavin may be performed on some occasions.

Flexural deformities

These deformities usually occur in young horses.

- In foals, the distal interphalangeal joint is usually involved and may be treated by section of the carpal head of the deep flexor tendon (inferior check ligament) and radical trimming of the affected heels
- Contracture of the fetlock tends to occur in yearlings and may be treated by surgical section of the carpal head of the deep digital flexor tendon and the radial head of the superficial flexor tendon
- There are usually few nursing problems with section of the carpal head of the deep digital flexor tendon, but a seroma may develop at the surgical site in some horses following section of the radial head of the superficial flexor tendon. To prevent sepsis and wound dehiscence, this incision will have to be monitored closely if seroma formation occurs.

Annular ligament desmotomy

One of the more common surgical procedures is the section of the fetlock palmar/plantar annular ligament for horses with annular ligament syndrome. The surgery is usually straightforward, with few complications postoperatively, although there is a risk of synovial fistulation in horses that are exercised too early following surgery.

Occasionally a similar procedure may be carried out on the palmar retinaculum of the carpus for horses with chronic carpal canal syndrome. In this case an elliptical portion of the retinaculum is removed.

Removal of splint bones

Removal of the distal portion of the third or fourth metacarpal/tarsal (splint) bone can be carried out in the horse where there has been a fracture. However, such injuries are often treated conservatively (i.e. by box rest for 3 months).

Management of angular limb deformities

These deformities are seen in young foals and are associated with angular limb deviations at the level of growth plates. They are classified as:

- Varus, where the deformity is concave on the medial aspect of the limb
- Valgus, where the concave deformity is on the lateral aspect of the limb.

The common sites are the distal radius, distal third of the metacarpus/metatarsus and distal tibia.

In many cases such mild deformities will correct when the foal is rested, but in severe deformities surgical treatment is indicated. Two basic procedures are involved:

- The more invasive is used for severe cases and involves temporarily bridging the physis (transphyseal bridge) on the convex side, using screws and wires or staples
- The alternative and less invasive method (carried out on the milder cases that are more commonly encountered in practice) is that of a hemicircumferential periosteal transection and elevation. This is performed on the concave side of the deformity just proximal to the affected physis.

Following the application of a transphyseal bridge the limb must be monitored very closely, with regular follow-up radiographic views. The implants must be removed before the limb is completely straight, otherwise overcorrection may occur – with catastrophic consequences.

Infected joints, tendon sheaths and bursae

Synovial sepsis represents a genuine emergency. Lavage of the synovial cavity involved should be carried out without delay.

Quite commonly, arthroscopic lavage may be used, as described previously, but in very acute situations it is often satisfactory to lavage the infected structure with a large-bore ingress/egress needle system using a large volume of Hartmann's solution containing penicillin and gentamicin.

The effectiveness of therapy can be monitored by repeated synoviocentesis and assessing the white cell and total protein counts within the joint. Assessment of the progress of these cases by the nursing staff can be very helpful to veterinary surgeons in evaluating the improvement following treatment.

Further reading

Brown JH and Powell-Smith V (1997) *Horse and Stable Management*. BSP Professional Books, Oxford

Butler JA, Colles CM, Dyson S, Kold SV and Paulos PW (1993) *Clinical Radiology of the Horse*. Blackwell Scientific, Oxford

Douglas SW, Herrtage ME and Williamson HD (1987) *Principles of Veterinary Radiography*, 4th edn. Baillière Tindall, London

Hall LW and Clarke KW (1991) *Vetrinary Anaesthesia*, 9th edn.

Baillière Tindall, London

McIlwraith CW (1990) *Diagnostic and Surgical Arthroscopy in the Horse*, 2nd edn. Lea and Febiger, Philadelphia

Nixon AJ (1996) *Equine Fracture Repair*. Saunders, Philadelphia

Rossdale PD and Ricketts SW (1980) *Equine Studfarm Medicine*. Baillière Tindall, London

Taylor FGR and Hillyer MH (1995) *Diagnostic Techniques in Equine Medicine*. WB Saunders, London

White NA (ed.) (1990) *The Equine Acute Abdomen*. Lea and Febiger, Philadelphia

Index